Y0-AER-412

Tranquillisers

TRANQUILLISERS: social, psychological, and clinical perspectives, ed. by Jonathan Gabe and Paul Williams. Tavistock/Methuen, 1986. 311p indexes 86-1843. 39.95 ISBN 0-422-79930-0. RM 333. CIP
An extremely valuable book that effectively deals with a topic of current concern. The editors have organized a collection of nicely conceived, well-written, previously published articles into five sections that proceed logically. Each section is preceded by an introduction, written by the editors, which provides a theoretical framework for the section and a description of the chapters within that theoretical perspective. The title of the book is somewhat misleading; although the focus is indeed on the use of tranquilizer drugs, the use and abuse of other psychotropic drugs are referred to throughout most of the chapters in a comparative format. As such, the value of the book is extended considerably beyond that implied by the title. Most of the articles included were initially written from a British perspective, using British data. However, without exception, the various authors include statistical information and literature from other countries, giving the volume an international perspective. All articles are well referenced; the few tables and figures are clearly presented and easily interpretable. This book will be of interest to upper-division and graduate students in the social and health sciences and would be a good acquisition for libraries wishing to maintain a well-rounded collection in the areas of substance abuse and addictions.—*T.D. DeLapp, University of Alaska, Anchorage*

Tranquillisers

Social, Psychological, and Clinical Perspectives

Edited by
Jonathan Gabe and Paul Williams

Forewords by Michael Shepherd
and Margot Jefferys

7S7B7O33O

RM
333
.T 74
1986

THE LIBRARY
SAINT JOSEPH'S COLLEGE
COLLEGEVILLE
RENSSELAER, IND. 47979

Tavistock Publications
London and New York

First published in 1986 by
Tavistock Publications Ltd
11 New Fetter Lane, London EC4P 4EE

Published in the USA by
Tavistock Publications
in association with Methuen, Inc.
29 West 35th Street, New York, NY 10001

© 1986 Jonathan Gabe and Paul Williams

Forewords © 1986 Michael Shepherd and Margot Jefferys

Typeset by Folio Photosetting, Bristol
Printed in Great Britain
at the University Press, Cambridge

All rights reserved. No part of this book may be reprinted or
reproduced or utilized in any form or by any electronic, mechanical or
other means, now known or hereafter invented, including photocopying
and recording, or in any information storage or retrieval system,
without permission in writing from the publishers.

British Library Cataloguing in Publication Data
Tranquillisers: social, psychological, and clinical
  perspectives.
  1. Tranquillizing drugs
  I. Gabe, Jonathan   II. Williams, Paul
  615'.7882   RM33

  ISBN 0-422-79930-0

Library of Congress Cataloging in Publication Data
Tranquillisers: social, psychological, and clinical
  perspectives.

  Includes bibliographies and index.
  1. Tranquilizing drugs. I. Gabe, Jonathan.
II. Williams, Paul, D.P.M. [DNLM: 1. Tranquilizing
Agents.   QV 77.9 T7725]
RM333.T74 1986 615'.7882   86-1843
ISBN 0-422-79930-0

Contents

List of contributors

Bernstein, Amy National Center for Health Services Research, Stop 3-50 Park Building, 5600 Fishers Lane, Rockville, MD 20857, USA.

Bond, Alison Research Assistant, University Department of Psychiatry, Warneford Hospital, Oxford, England.

Cafferata, Gail Lee National Center for Health Services Research, Stop 3-50 Park Building, 5600 Fishers Lane, Rockville, MD 20857, USA.

Catalan, Jose Clinical Lecturer in Psychiatry, University Department of Psychiatry, Warneford Hospital, Oxford, England.

Cooperstock, Ruth (deceased) Addiction Research Foundation, 33 Russell Street, Toronto, Ontario, Canada.

Edmonds, Gillian Research Assistant, University Department of Psychiatry, Warneford Hospital, Oxford, England.

Ennis, John Oxford Regional Health Authority, Headington, Oxford, England.

Ettorre, E.M. Research Sociologist, Addiction Research Unit, Institute of Psychiatry, Denmark Hill, London, England.

Fidell, Linda S. Department of Psychology, California State University, Northridge, California, USA.

Gabe, Jonathan Research Sociologist, General Practice Research Unit, Institute of Psychiatry, Denmark Hill, London, England.

Gath, Dennis Clinical Reader in Psychiatry, University Department of Psychiatry, Warneford Hospital, Oxford, England.

Helman, Cecil G. Clinical Lecturer in General Practice, Middlesex Hospital, London, and Honorary Research Fellow in Anthropology, University College, London, England.

Hemminki, Elina Department of Public Health Sciences, University of Tampere, Verkatehtaankatu 13, 33100 Tampere 10, Finland.

Hopkins, David R. General Practitioner, 50 Victoria Road, Worthing, BN11 1XE, England.

Kasper, Judith National Center for Health Services Research, Stop 3-50 Park Buildings, 5600 Fishers Lane, Rockville, MD 20857, USA.

Lader, M.H. Professor of Clinical Psychopharmacology, Institute of Psychiatry, Denmark Hill, London, England.

Lennard, Henry L. Center for Policy Research and Yeshiva University, New York, USA.

Lipshitz-Phillips, Susan Formerly Research Officer, Social Research Unit, Bedford College, Regents Park, London, England.

Martin, Pauline Research Assistant, University Department of Psychiatry, Warneford Hospital, Oxford, England.

Mucklow, John C. Consultant Physician, Department of Clinical Pharmacology, City General Hospital, Stoke-on-Trent, England.

Murray, Joanna Research Worker, General Practice Research Unit, Institute of Psychiatry, Denmark Hill, London, England.

Petursson, H. Geddeild, Borgarspitalinn, Reykjavik, Iceland.

Prather, Jane E. Professor of Sociology, California State University, Northridge, California, USA.

Raynes, Norma V. Hester Adrian Research Centre, University of Manchester, Manchester, M13 9PL, England.

Sethi, Kulwant B.S. General Practitioner, Highwood, Dunwood, Endon, Staffs., ST9 9AR, England.

Thorogood, Nicki Formerly Social Research Unit, Bedford College, Regents Park, London, England.

Williams, Paul Senior Lecturer, General Practice Research Unit, Institute of Psychiatry, Denmark Hill, London, England.

Foreword

Professor Michael Shepherd

The Oxford English Dictionary defines the adjective 'tranquil' as 'free from agitation or disturbance'. Its psychiatric associations, however, are less serene, for they hark back to the era of physical restraint and in particular to Benjamin Rush's 'tranquiliser', the notorious chair which he ~ommended in the following terms:

> 'The tranquiliser has several advantages over the strait waist coat or mad shirt. It opposes the impetus of the blood towards the brain, it lessens muscular action everywhere, it reduces the force of frequency of the pulse, it favours the application of cold water and ice to the head, and warm water to the feet . . . it enables the physician to feel the pulse and to bleed without any trouble, or altering the erect position of the patient's body; and lastly, it relieves him, by means of a close stool, half filled with water, over which he constantly sits, from the foetor and filth of his alvine evacuations.'

Rush's description can claim at least the merit of a clarity which has been missing from the more recent exploitation of the word. In the past thirty years the epithet 'tranquillising' has been widely applied to a number of pharmacologically diverse substances which induce sedation without impairment of consciousness. Devoid as it is of scientific meaning, the notion of 'tranquillisation' helped usher in the era of psychopharmacology as a favoured description of the effects of rauwolfia alkaloids and the phenothiazines on psychotic illnesses. It was not long, furthermore, before the 'major' tranquillisers were followed by a host of 'minor' tranquillisers, which quickly superseded the barbiturates in the management of states of anxiety, tension, and insomnia in the population at large. Among these compounds the benzodiazepines have become the most widely prescribed, principally because of their relative safety, and around them has been constructed another category of drugs, the 'anxiolytics'.

In recent years a sharp increase in the prescription of 'anxiolytics' has occurred in most industrialized countries. Explanations for this trend have varied. Some observers have stressed the sales techniques of the pharmaceutical industry and the gullibility of the medical profession in encouraging the consumption of relatively non-toxic, centrally acting drugs as a logical means of managing common, non-specific reactions to everyday problems in an 'age of anxiety' dominated by psychological and social stresses. Others, arguing that the lowering of class barriers has democratized the form, if not the content, of drug-taking behaviour, have invoked the vagaries of fashion; one of them has even concluded that psychotropic medication should be viewed in much the same light as 'the amount of claret and port consumed by the Victorian middle-classes'. The debate recalls John Ryle's comment on the causes and treatment of minor emotional disorders some forty years ago:

> 'Faults of upbringing, domestic stress, industrial fatigue, inadequate sleep and holidays, economic anxieties – factors eventually alterable by improved education, more ample accommodation for families, factory welfare and social insurance – have played their significant part. In the meantime we try to cope with their consequences with bottles of medicine and certificates and a multiplication of psychiatric clinics at an ever-increasing cost to the community.'

Here, then, is a social as well as a medical phenomenon. Its understanding calls for a medico-social perspective, which may be derived from this collection of papers. The editors have brought together material which deals with the wider significance of 'tranquillisation' from the standpoints of the providers, the consumers, and society as a whole. In so doing they have made it possible to identify and analyse the elements in a complex pattern which illustrates the continuing relevance of Thomas Carlyle's comment: 'Brothers, I am sorry I have got no Morrison's pill for curing the maladies of society.'

London
September 1985

Foreword

Professor Margot Jefferys

Anxiety, as a state of mind, evokes a variety of responses. It is taken to be of positive value when it implies solicitude or concern for others, or when it leads to cautious rather than foolhardy behaviour in situations of risk to life and limb. It is tolerated as an inevitable and hence legitimate state, too, if it is only temporary; for example, when waiting to compete in a sporting event, or for the outcome of an examination, or a diagnostic test. On the other hand, it meets with disapprobation if the level of arousal appears to be inappropriate to the real or perceived threat, especially if this becomes a habitual response to everyday problems.

Those who display chronic anxiety have always been likely to meet with social sanctions of a more or less severe kind. If the display is a mild one, it may merely evoke a verbal reassurance or the use of humour to reduce tension. There are also many folk remedies which can be combined with such measures. These include diversionary tactics and the performance of secular or religious rituals which have a symbolic significance. Also socially sanctioned in most societies is the ingestion of mood-changing substances. In western societies, alcohol and nicotine are two such substances whose selective use is generally permitted to adults. They can reduce dysfunctional levels of anxiety by engendering a mild euphoria. Of course, they are also often used prophylactically, and, as with other addictive drugs, this is the danger, because they become progressively less effective at every given dose level.

The 1960s was a period of therapeutic optimism, much of it justified: by relabelling many forms of obnoxious behaviour or unwelcome states of mind as pathological, it seemed as though it was possible to treat them effectively in a morally neutral, scientific way. Anxiety, when chronic, or inappropriate to the threat, was a prime candidate for what Zola termed the process of 'medicalisation'.[1] Moreover, in the same decade, as the editors of this volume of papers point out, the pharmaceutical industry produced and marketed new substances – the minor tranquillisers – which appeared to have none of the addictive properties nor unwanted side-effects of their predecessors in the pharmacopoeia of natural and artificial psychotropic drugs. It was not surprising that minor tranquillisers began to be prescribed on a massive scale by general practitioners in Britain and elsewhere.

We can now distance ourselves from the euphoria of the 1960s. Since then, tranquillisers have turned out to have some undesirable side-effects after all, and in some cases to be addictive. The pharmaceutical industry, its image tarnished by some catastrophic mistakes in drug developments, has been accused of peddling its products indiscriminately and of making vast profits from its tranquillisers. The profession responsible for regulating their use has been taken to task for either initiating or, at least, doing nothing to discourage an insatiable and ultimately futile demand for instant relief from even the mildest forms of mental or physical discomfort. Increasing self-consciousness and awareness among women, the main consumers of tranquillisers, about the social and psychological roots of their distress and help-seeking behaviour have also contributed to the climate of opinion which has now turned against tranquillisers and led to a reduction in their use, at least in western societies.

It is, of course, too early to predict what the future holds; but there are many aspects of current tranquilliser use which still require detailed analysis. This volume of papers, some already published elsewhere and some original, shows how much greater our understanding of the phenomenon of the last twenty years can be if we explore its social, psychological, and economic background and implications as well as its pharmacology. It is hoped that some of the editors' suggestions for research, which they make in the concluding chapter, will attract both research funders and workers from various disciplines, as well as those whose everyday work brings them into contact with the chronically anxious.

London
August 1985

Reference

1 Zola, I.K. (1972) Medicine as an institution of social control. *Sociological Review* 20: 487–504.

Preface

Traditionally the approach to psychotropic drug use in general, and tranquilliser use in particular, has been largely clinical. It is increasingly clear, however, that the biomedical perspective cannot provide an adequate framework for a comprehensive understanding of this phenomenon. What is required, we believe, is an approach which places tranquilliser use within a *social* context. This point of view is reflected in the selection of papers for this volume, although we have taken pains to avoid adopting any one particular theoretical perspective. Thus disciplines represented here include epidemiology, sociology, anthropology, and psychology, as well as clinical medical specialities such as psychiatry and general practice.

This is a collection of sixteen papers, twelve of which have been previously published elsewhere. It is structured as follows. In Part 1 we offer an epidemiological and sociological account of the history of tranquilliser use. This provides the necessary background for an understanding of the current situation. The remainder of the book is divided into four parts: each of these is prefixed by a short introduction, which highlights the contribution to understanding made by the papers within that part and relates them to the relevant body of literature. The sections reflect what are, we consider, the most important contemporary issues concerning tranquilliser use. This assessment is based on our own research experience and our knowledge and reading of the literature.

Part 2 focuses on long-term tranquilliser use from the epidemiological, clinical-pharmacological, and social-psychological points of view. Part 3 deals with factors which influence the use of tranquillisers from the point of view of the doctor, the patient, and the doctor–patient interaction. The papers in this section illustrate both macro- and micro-level approaches to the study of tranquilliser use.

Part 4 contains papers of particular interst to clinicians. They are concerned with alternatives to tranquilliser use, and illustrate a range of approaches from the exclusively clinical to the predominantly sociological.

In Part 5 we deal with the meaning of tranquilliser use. Meaning, in this context, refers to an interpretation which is constructed on a particular occasion by an individual interacting with others, and which may be subject to reformulation on subsequent occasions. Consideration of this aspect of tranquilliser use is important because it draws attention to the *processual* nature of drug use. The papers chosen in this section represent the first attempts in a hitherto undeveloped field to focus on such processes. In so doing they provide an initial basis for understanding *how* the association between prescribed drug use and the variables identified in the previous sections have come about.

The editors of any collection of previously published papers need to justify such an undertaking, and we believe that there are two reasons why this book is worthwhile. *First*, to our knowledge, there are no academic books currently available which focus on the aspects of tranquilliser use with which we are concerned. The few academic books (other than proceedings of conferences: Cooperstock 1974; Murray *et al*. 1981; Tognoni, Bellantuono, and Lader 1981) which have considered the use of prescribed psychotropic drugs have done so either from the perspective of social policy (Brunn 1983) or treated them as one issue among many to be included in a general analysis of drug prescribing (Mapes 1980; Melville and Johnson 1982). Thus our book will be filling a gap in the literature.

Second, this gap deserves to be filled because of the widespread interest in tranquilliser use in Britain and elsewhere. The broad spectrum of people interested in this issue has been borne in mind when selecting the papers for the book. In order to maximize international appeal we have chosen papers by authors from the United States, Canada, and Scandinavia as well as Britain. Our intention is that the papers chosen should appeal not only to researchers and lecturers with a medical or social science background but also to general practitioners, clinical psychologists, social workers, and other clinicians.

References

Brunn, K. (ed.) (1983) *Controlling Psychotropic Drugs: The Nordic Experience*. London: Croom Helm.

Cooperstock, R. (ed.) (1974) *Social Aspects of the Medical Use of Psychotropic Drugs*. Toronto: Addiction Research Foundation of Ontario.

Mapes, R. (ed.) (1980) *Prescribing Practice and Drug Usage*. London: Croom Helm.

Melville, A. and Johnson, C. (1982) *Cured to Death: The Effect of Prescription Drugs*. London: Secker & Warburg.

Murray, R.M., Ghodse, H., Harris, C., Williams, D., and Williams, P. (eds) (1981) *The Misuse of Psychotropic Drugs*. London: Gaskell Books.

Tognoni, G., Bellantuono, C., and Lader, M. (eds) (1981) *Epidemiological Impact of Psychotropic Drugs*. Amsterdam: Elsevier/North Holland Biomedical Press.

PART 1

Tranquilliser use: a historical perspective

1

Tranquilliser use: a historical perspective

Jonathan Gabe and Paul Williams

Introduction

Although this edited collection is concerned primarily with the use of tranquillisers, many of the studies referred to here have been concerned with 'psychotropic drugs' in general. This term is generally taken to include four categories of drug, classified according to their actions – tranquillisers, hypnotics, antidepressants, and stimulants. Tranquillisers are further subdivided into major tranquillisers, drugs used in the management of psychosis, and minor tranquillisers, used primarily in the management of anxiety. We shall not be concerned at all with major tranquillisers, and subsequently the term 'tranquilliser' will be taken to refer only to minor tranquillisers. In theory, drugs classed as minor tranquillisers, or anxiolytics, are indicated for the management of anxiety during the day while drugs classed as hypnotics are primarily intended for night sedation. In fact, the differences between these two categories of drug are less marked than the similarities – most anxiolytics will induce sleep when given in large doses at night, and most hypnotics will induce anxiety relief when given in smaller doses throughout the day (*British National Formulary* 1985).

At the present time the most frequently prescribed minor tranquillisers in Britain and other industrialized countries are the benzodiazepines: drugs with trade names like Valium, Librium, Mogadon, and Ativan. Although much has been written about these drugs and their predecessors from a biomedical standpoint, there have been relatively few attempts to place minor tranquilliser use within a *social* context. In doing so here, we hope to have created a basis for a comprehensive social understanding of the contemporary use of tranquillisers.

The early use of psychotropic drugs for medical purposes

Mood-altering drugs have been used for medicinal purposes throughout recorded history. Great physicians of classical antiquity like Dioscorides identified and listed the sedative and hypnotic properties of plants, their leaves and roots, thereby encouraging their therapeutic use (Belloni 1957). Knowledge of medical botany was developed further in the middle ages by Arab scholars who brought together the drug lore of many different countries (Parascandola 1977). In the sixteenth century the first attempts were made to isolate the 'quintessence' of botanical substances by chemical processes such as distillation and extraction (Parascandola 1977). These chemically prepared remedies were rejected by physicians at first but eventually came to be accepted and included in the pharmacopoeias of Europe in the seventeenth century. Thereafter minor complaints like sleeplessness were treated with chemically derived substances. By the nineteenth century drugs to calm or lift the spirits were in common use in Europe. Opium, for example, was frequently used 'to promote sleep and reduce nervous restlessness' (Berridge 1978: 441).

The beginning of the twentieth century witnessed the rapid development of 'mood-altering' chemicals as the pharmaceutical industry, governed by market economics, sought to maximize its profits (Rabin and Bush 1974). The bromides and chloral hydrate, which had replaced opium on the grounds that the latter was addictive (Berridge 1978), were themselves displaced in the 1930s by the barbiturates because the latter were considered 'safer'. By the 1950s the dependence-producing potential of barbiturates had also become clearly established, causing a great deal of concern (Hollister 1983). This encouraged the search for a suitable non-barbiturate, anti-anxiety, and hypnotic drug.

The first replacement was meprobamate (Miltown), a drug which was received enthusiastically by physicians and much used in the late 1950s as an anti-anxiety agent until it too was found to cause dependence (Hollister 1983). The second was the benzodiazepine group of drugs which quickly made meprobamate obsolete, once it became clear that they were safer and more effective in alleviating anxiety (Lader 1978). Chlordiazepoxide (Librium) was the first benzodiazepine to be introduced, in 1960, followed by diazepam (Valium), its even more successful stablemate, in 1963 (Cohen 1970). There are now eighteen generic benzodiazepine preparations available in Britain and their dominance in the field of anti-anxiety and hypnotic drugs indicates that we are unquestionably living in the 'benzodiazepine era' (Hollister 1983: 13).

The principal indication for the use of minor tranquillisers is the short-term management of anxiety. Short-term unwanted effects include drowsiness and impairment of psychomotor performance, but benzodiazepine drugs are extremely safe (certainly so when compared with their predecessors, the barbiturates) if taken in overdose. Long-term unwanted effects include tolerance and dependence, a problem which is dealt with elsewhere in this book. An important chemical basis for anxiety is thought to be hyperexcitability of certain neural pathways. Thus the most important mechanism associated with the anxiolytic properties of benzodiazepines is probably their action on the inhibitory neuro-transmission system involving gamma amino-butyric acid (GABA). Benzodiazepines bind to the GABA receptor, enhance the binding of GABA itself, and thus increase its inhibitory effect.

Further details of the medical aspects of tranquilliser and hypnotic use can be found in Crammer, Barraclough, and Heine (1982) and in the *British National Formulary* (1985), and more detailed accounts of their pharmacology can be found in Sullivan and Sullivan (1984).

The growth in tranquilliser and other psychotropic drug use

In this section we consider the changing pattern of psychotropic drug prescribing in Britain over the last twenty years, discuss the proportion of the population receiving and consuming these drugs, and suggest that current prescribing and use can be explained, at least in part, in terms of changes in drug-taking behaviour. Wherever possible we focus on tranquillisers. Much of the time, however, we have been forced to write in more general terms about 'psychotropic' drugs because of the failure of researchers to distinguish between different categories of drug (tran-quillisers, antidepressants, hypnotics, and stimulants).

The introduction of the tricyclic antidepressants in the late 1950s and the benzodiazepine tranquillisers in the early 1960s heralded the pheno-menon subsequently labelled by Trethowan (1975) as the 'relentless march of the psychotropic drug juggernaut'. Parish (1971) drew attention to this phenomenon as reflected in increases in the numbers of psychotropic drug prescriptions dispensed during the late 1960s in England and Wales. He observed:

> 'from 1965–70 inclusive, there was a 19 % increase in the prescribing of psychotropic drugs in England and Wales. In 1970, 43 % of all psychotropic drug prescriptions were for hypnotics, 36% for tran-quillisers, 7% for stimulants and appetite suppressants and 14% for antidepressants. Between 1965 and 1970, the prescribing of barbiturate hypnotics decreased by 24 % and stimulants and appetite suppressants by 36 %. There was an increase in the prescribing of non-barbiturate hypnotics of 145%, a 59% increase in tranquilliser prescribing and an 83% increase in antidepressant drug prescribing.' (Parish 1971: 2)

Parish based his analyses on DHSS prescription audits derived from a 1 in 200 sample of all prescriptions dispensed at retail pharmacies. Analyses of these data for subsequent years (Williams 1980a, 1980b; Marks 1983a) have demonstrated that prescriptions for tranquillisers and antidepressants continued to rise annually until the late 1970s. Much of the growth in tranquilliser prescribing has been due to the benzodiazepines, which have increased at the expense of the barbiturates. For example, in 1965 there were nearly 20 million prescriptions for barbiturates and less than 5 million for benzodiazepines dispensed at retail pharmacies in England and Wales; by 1975, the pattern had reversed (less than 5 million for barbiturates and over 20 million for benzodiazepines). Since the mid-1970s, there has been a levelling-off and then a decrease in the prescribing of tranquillisers, a pattern which has been found in most countries for which data are available (Marks 1983a).

As Williams (1979) has pointed out, such data should be interpreted with caution. For example, they overestimate consumption, because of non-compliance (Sackett and Haynes 1976); and overestimate the extent to which psychotropic drugs are prescribed 'to modify personal and interpersonal processes' (Trethowan 1975), since a significant proportion of psychotropic prescriptions are written as a response to physical ill-health (Solow 1975; Williams 1978). Conversely, DHSS prescribing data under-estimate psychotropic prescribing for the community as a whole, since they are derived only from retail pharmacies: prescribing in psychiatric outpatient clinics is thus largely excluded.

Most importantly, prescription data are based on prescriptions and not people. Thus the large annual increases in tranquilliser and antidepressant prescriptions that took place in the 1960s and 1970s could reflect an increase in the numbers of drug consumers, an increase in the average number of prescriptions per consumer, an increase in the amount of drugs prescribed but not consumed, or any combination of these factors. Differentiating between these patterns is important both for a sociological understanding of the 'psychotropic drug juggernaut' as well as for a public health policy approach to this and similar phenomena. To these ends, additional types of study are required.

Thus studies have also been conducted to investigate the proportion of the population receiving a prescription for a psychotropic drug over a given period. Many of these have been conducted by individual general practitioners in order to establish the prevalence of prescribing in their own practices (e.g. Harris *et al*. 1977; Wilks 1975; Varnam 1981). Given the wide variation in prescribing between general practitioners (Royal College of General Practitioners 1978) it is not possible to draw general conclusions about trends from these studies. However, there are two large-scale studies of general practitioner psychotropic prescribing in the United Kingdom from which such conclusions may be drawn (see *Table 1*).

Parish (1971) conducted a retrospective study of psychotropic drug prescribing by 48 Birmingham general practitioners during 1967–68.

Table 1 *Prevalence of psychotropic drug use in the United Kingdom*

	n, place, year of study	rate
1-year prevalence of prescribing		
Parish (1971)	13,259 Birmingham 1969	12.6%
Skegg, Doll, and Perry (1977)	36,280 Oxfordshire 1974	19.3%*
2-week prevalence of consumption		
Dunnell and Cartwright (1972)	1,412 England 1969	11.0%
Murray *et al.* (1981)	5,833 West London 1977	10.9%
Anderson (1980)	836 England 1977	12.0%

* Of those aged > 15 years.

Using information recorded during routine clinical practice, he found that 12.6 per cent of the population had received at least one prescription for a psychotropic drug (tranquilliser, hypnotic, antidepressant, or stimulant) during the study year. Skegg, Doll, and Perry (1977) used data obtained from the Prescription Pricing Authority to investigate psychotropic prescribing by 19 Oxfordshire general practitioners during 1974. When respondents aged less than 15 years are excluded (to make the results comparable with those of Parish), the one-year psychotropic prescribing prevalence rate was 19.3 per cent.

The validity of the conclusion that there was an increase in the prevalence of prescribing (as well as in the number of prescriptions dispensed) depends on whether the two studies can legitimately be compared. This was considered in detail by Williams (1983), who thought that they could.

In addition, there are also studies which provide evidence about the prevalence of consumption: that is, the proportion of the population who consume a drug on at least one occasion during a specified time period. Three large-scale studies in the United Kingdom have addressed this issue (*Table 1*). Their comparability has been assessed by Murray *et al.* (1981), who noted that each was based on a probability sample of the general population, that drug consumption data were collected in a comparable way in the three surveys, that each used a similar definition of 'psychotropic', and that each of the surveys was concerned with the previous two weeks.

It can be seen from *Table 1* that the three surveys all found the two-week prevalence of psychotropic drug consumption to be just over 10 per cent. Thus the conclusion is inescapable that the increases in prescriptions dispensed and in persons receiving prescriptions were *not* accompanied by an increase in persons consuming the drugs.

How are these findings to be explained? Williams (1983) has suggested that they reflect a pattern of drug use which stems from two factors: decreasing compliance and an increase in the duration of treatment. Compliance here is taken to mean that an individual does not consume the medicines prescribed for him/her. Indirect evidence from two sources suggests that compliance with psychotropic drug prescribing has decreased over recent years.

First, studies of primary non-compliance – that is, the extent to which prescriptions written are not dispensed – suggest, despite obstacles to comparison, that this behaviour is on the increase (see Williams 1983 for a detailed consideration of these studies). While such studies have been concerned with the prescribing of *all* drugs, rather than tranquillisers or even psychotropics, it is reasonable to assume, given the ample evidence that individuals with psychological problems are less likely than others to comply with medical advice (Sackett and Haynes 1976), that the same trend applies to the different categories of psychotropic drug.

The second source of indirect evidence for a trend of decreasing compliance is derived from Ann Cartwright's studies of general practice conducted in 1964 and 1977 (Cartwright 1967; Cartwright and Anderson 1981). In a recent paper, Cartwright (1983) compared the results of these studies and found that patients had become more critical of their doctors and their prescribing practices, and that patients and doctors both felt patients were more likely to question their doctor's judgement. Quoting case vignettes in support, she argued that such changes in attitude reflected changes in drug compliance.

There is also indirect evidence that the duration of drug treatment has changed. Anderson (1980) compared his data on 'how many prescriptions people had had for the same medicine' with those from the Dunnell and Cartwright (1972) survey. The results, while being 'similar', were not identical and, on average, there was an increase of 6 per cent in the number of prescriptions per consumer in the years between the surveys. While this relates to all prescribed drugs, a similar conclusion can be drawn from a comparison of the psychotropic prescribing studies of Parish (1971) and Skegg, Doll, and Perry (1977). The number of prescriptions per recipient almost doubled in the years between the two surveys, and when the changes in compliance are taken into account the relative increase is even greater (Williams 1983).

The implication of both these pieces of indirect evidence is that psychotropic consumers are each receiving more prescriptions latterly than formerly. This could be a consequence either of a decrease in the average quantity of drug per prescription, or of an inrease in the average duration of treatment. An analysis of factors relating to prescription cost (Williams 1982) suggests that the former is unlikely to be true, at least as far as tranquillisers are concerned, while studies of repeat prescribing support the latter interpretation (Drury 1982; Marks 1983b).

The weight of evidence, both direct and indirect, suggests that the 'psychotropic drug juggernaut' contains the two components of decreasing compliance (with its consequences both for resource utilization and for the doctor-patient relationship (Cartwright 1983)) and increasing long-term use. This latter has important implications in the light of recent findings on benzodiazepine dependence, an issue which is dealt with elsewhere in this volume.

The growth of concern about minor tranquillisers

In this section we map the growth of concern in Britain about benzodiazepines – currently the most frequently prescribed minor tranquilliser – and consider why the orchestrators of this concern have had a major impact on medical and public consciousness, particularly *after* the prescribing of these drugs had started to decline.

When benzodiazepines were introduced in the early 1960s, they were accepted enthusiastically by the medical profession as highly effective and safe anti-anxiety drugs which did not create physical or psychological dependence and which had few other unwanted side effects (Owen and Tyrer 1983). This impression was reinforced a few years later by favourable reports of clinical practice (Greenblatt and Shader 1974; Svenson and Hamilton 1966).

In the early 1970s, however, concern started to be expressed by social scientists and physicians (e.g. Dunlop 1970; Lennard *et al*. 1971; Jefferys 1973; *Lancet* 1973a, 1973b) about the extent of benzodiazepine prescribing. The social scientists talked of an 'overmedicated society' (Muller 1972) and suggested that benzodiazepines, by providing symptomatic relief, discouraged the search for a social solution to problems with social origins (Lennard *et al*. 1971). The physicians questioned whether the increase in tranquilliser prescribing reflected an increase in the number of people suffering from chronic anxiety, or a too-ready recourse to a prescription (*Lancet* 1973a) by doctors who saw tranquillisers as a suitable way of modifying personal and interpersonal processes (Trethowan 1975). If the latter was the case it was viewed as likely to fuel demand for tranquillisers among patients (Trethowan 1975). Also questioned were the therapeutic value (as opposed to the commercial value) of increasing the number of benzodiazepines available (Tyrer 1974), the cost to the British National Health Service of the mounting number of tranquilliser prescriptions dispensed (Trethowan 1975), and the possibility that tranquillisers were no more effective than placebos for those suffering from only minor mood changes (*Lancet* 1973b).

In the latter part of the 1970s the concern about tranquilliser prescribing levels abated, to be replaced at the start of the 1980s by a new concern: that of physical dependence on benzodiazepines. This possibility had, in fact, been acknowledged as far back as 1961 for those suddenly withdrawn from high dosages of benzodiazepines (Hollister, Motzenbecker, and Degon 1961). Thereafter, however, the number of cases and studies of dependence reported did not increase above a trickle and these generally referred to patients on high dosages (Tyrer 1980). Given the total number of benzodiazepines consumed, what impressed during this period, therefore, was the *rarity* of benzodiazepine dependence: a view endorsed by Marks (1978) who concluded, after a comprehensive review of published case histories of dependence, that benzodiazepines had a negligible dependence risk if used in therapeutic doses.

Two years after Marks had drawn this conclusion the picture started to change. The Committee on the Review of Medicines officially acknowledged for the first time a growing concern about physical dependence, even though it concluded that: 'on present available evidence the true addiction potential of benzodiazepines [is] low' (Committee on the Review of Medicines 1980: 910). Soon afterwards the evidence started to appear. Studies of relatively small numbers of people (usually about forty) agreeing to or requesting withdrawal from long-term benzodiazepine use at therapeutic dose have found that a significant number experienced symptoms of physical dependence (such as intolerance of noise and light, bad headaches, and dry mouth) on withdrawal (Petursson and Lader 1981; Tyrer, Rutherford, and Huggett 1981; Tyrer, Owen, and Dawling 1983), and that these symptoms can last a year or more (Ashton 1984). As a substantial number of people in the general population use benzodiazepines over a long period of time these findings suggest (bearing in mind that the sample was preselected rather than random) that as many as 45 per cent of such users are likely to be physically dependent (Tyrer, Owen, and Dawling 1983). From the standpoint of one of these researchers this represents an 'epidemic in the making' (Lader 1981).

Moreover, current concern has not been limited to academics and clinicians. Recent studies of tranquilliser users (see Helman 1981; Murray 1981; Gabe and Lipshitz-Phillips 1984, in this volume) and non-users (Gabe and Lipshitz-Phillips 1982, 1984) demonstrate a marked awareness of the side effects of tranquilliser use and, at best, an ambivalence about taking them. This kind of popular concern has not been reported before in Britain and suggests that tranquilliser use has become a public issue.

Why has this happened now, when the prescribing of tranquillisers is actually declining? One factor is the recent coverage of tranquilliser dependence in the mass media. Once discovered, this issue has featured regularly on television consumer programmes (Taking the Strain 1981; That's Life 1983, 1984a, 1984b, 1985), in the up-market and popular press (*Observer* 1980a, 1980b; *The Times* 1980; *Daily Mirror* 1980, 1981, 1982; *Mail on Sunday* 1982), and in women's magazines (*Woman's Own* 1984a, 1984b). Much of this coverage has been sensationalizing in tone, as the following newspaper and magazine headlines illustrate:

' "Hooked on the happy pill" (*Daily Mirror* 1980);
"Why the happy pills have had their day" (*Standard* 1981);
"Tranquillisers – the shocking truth" (*Woman's Own* 1984b).'

Furthermore, the impression has frequently been given that everyone on tranquillisers is likely to be dependent on them and will automatically have 'terrible' withdrawal symptoms if they try and stop. Indeed, one recent television programme began with the statement that 'kicking the tranquilliser habit can be harder than coming off heroin' (The London Programme 1984). As several commentators have recently remarked, this represents 'trial by media' (Lasagna 1980; Cohen 1983).

Second, concern has also recently been fuelled by mental health campaigning bodies like MIND and RELEASE. These organizations have, with the help of one or two sympathetic academics, produced pamphlets and booklets on tranquilliser dependence for the general public (RELEASE 1982; MIND 1984; Lacey and Woodward 1985), and have skilfully used and worked with the media in presenting their case.

Third, and finally, current concern also has to be set against the backcloth of wider cultural changes. Over the last fifteen years or so there seems to have been a shift in attitudes away from a belief in the right to happiness and an unwillingness to tolerate 'normal' discomfort and malaise towards a more puritanical view of life based on abstinence, stoicism, and self-reliance (Hall 1983). The latter view has encouraged an attitude to drugs which Klerman (1971) has described as 'pharmacological calvinism'. Simply stated, this means 'if it makes you feel good it is wrong' (Blackwell 1977). The development of this 'anti-drug culture' (Gabe and Lipshitz-Philips 1982) also coincides with increasing criticism of other forms of medical technology (Oakley 1980; Kennedy 1981) and the medical profession (Jefferys and Sachs 1983; Cartwright 1983), and an increasing enthusiasm for alternative medicines (Stanway 1982; Salmon 1985) and for self-help (Robinson 1978), at least among some social groups (Doyal 1983).

As one might expect, this concern about the danger of dependence is not shared to the same extent by all of those with an interest in tranquillisers. The pharmaceutical industry, for example, has been fighting back by financing researchers who might provide ammunition to challenge the risks of benzodiazepine dependence. Also, some academics and clinicians have independently questioned the evidence about the extent of dependence (Rickels 1981), the adequacy of existing studies (Kraüpl-Taylor 1984), and the availability of appropriate alternatives for chronic benzodiazepine users (Rickels *et al.* 1984). Even so, the future for benzodiazepines looks somewhat uncertain, given the level of current concern.

In Britain, this uncertainty is compounded by recent legislation concerning prescribing. As from 1 April, 1985, the prescription under the NHS of seven categories of drug – including the benzodiazepines – has been limited in range. That is, there now exists a 'whitelist' of drugs which can be prescribed under the NHS and a 'blacklist' of drugs which cannot (although such drugs can still be prescribed privately).

Prior to these regulations there were, as noted earlier, eighteen different benzodiazepines available in Great Britain. The government's initial proposal was to limit this to three although, in the event, generic preparations of seven benzodiazepine tranquilliser hypnotics were categorized as prescribable.

This legislation – and the way in which it was introduced – gives rise to a whole host of issues beyond the scope of this book (*British Medical Journal* 1984, 1985; Blane 1985). However, from the point of view of tranquilliser use, there is a preliminary suggestion that the regulations may have resulted in a sharp decline in prescriptions. Erlichman (1985) describes the results of a market research survey conducted in the few weeks following the legislation:

'Overall, the number of prescriptions written in the seven therapeutic classes covered by the limited list has fallen by 25%. Of greatest significance may be the real fall in the number of tranquillisers prescribed. Most branded tranquillisers like Valium and Librium have been banned ... generic replacements are not being prescribed at the same rate.'

It is, of course, too early for anything other than this very preliminary comment on the impact of the limited list legislation. It is, however, very important that its effects – especially those on long-term use – should be monitored closely.

The remainder of this book offers a selection of papers addressing what we regard as the most important contemporary issues concerning tranquilliser use. In the first part we present papers focusing on long-term tranquilliser use and the issue of benzodiazepine dependence, about which there is so much current concern. Subsequent parts deal with factors which influence the use of tranquillisers, the alternatives which are available, and the meaning which tranquillisers have for users and their doctors. The authors of most of these papers make an attempt to place tranquilliser use within a social context. This is particularly apparent in the papers in Part 5, whose authors draw heavily on ideas from sociology and anthropology.

References

Anderson, R.M. (1980) The use of repeatedly prescribed medicines. *Journal of the Royal College of General Practitioners* 30(219): 609–13.

Ashton, H. (1984) Benzodiazepine withdrawal: an unfinished story. *British Medical Journal* 288(6424): 1135–140.

Belloni, L. (1957) The Mandrake. In S. Garattini and V. Ghetti (eds) *Psychotropic Drugs*. Amsterdam: Elsevier Publishing Company.

Berridge, V. (1978) Victorian opium eating: responses to opiate use in nineteenth century England. *Victorian Studies* 21: 437–61.

Blackwell, B. (1977) Medical, social and ethical issues in minor tranquilizer use. Paper to the *World Congress in Mental Health*, Vancouver.

Blane, D. (1985) DHSS takes on the drug industry. *Medical Sociology News* 10(2): 11–14.

British Medical Journal Editorial (1984) Doctors, drugs and the DHSS. *British Medical Journal* 289(6456): 1397–398.

—— (1985) Doctors, drugs and government. *British Medical Journal* 290(6472): 880.

British National Formulary (1985) London: British Medical Association and the Pharmaceutical Society of Great Britain.

Cartwright, A. (1967) *Patients and their Doctors*. London: Routledge & Kegan Paul.

—— (1983) Prescribing and the doctor–patient relationship. In D. Pendleton and J. Hasler (eds) *Doctor–Patient Communication*. London: Academic Press.

Cartwright, A. and Anderson, R. (1981) *General Practice Revisited*. London: Tavistock Publications.

Cohen, I. (1970) The benzodiazepines. In F.J. Ayd and B. Blackwell (eds) *Discoveries in Biological Psychiatry*. Philadelphia: J.B. Lippincott.

Cohen, S. (1983) Current attitudes about the benzodiazepines: trial by media. *Journal of Psychoactive Drugs* 15(1–2): 109–13.

Committee on the Review of Medicines (1980) Systematic review of the benzodiazepines. *British Medical Journal* 280(6218): 910–12.

Crammer, J., Barraclough B., and Heine, B. (1982) *The Use of Drugs in Psychiatry*. London: Gaskell Books.

Daily Mirror (1980) Hooked on the happy pill, 18 March.

—— (1981) Are you a pill popper who just can't quit?, 7 May.

—— (1982) The dangers of the happiness pill, 11 March.

Doyal, L. (1983) Women's health and the sexual division of labour. *Critical Social Policy* 7 (Summer): 21–33.

Drury, V.M. (1982) Repeat prescribing – a review. *Journal of the Royal College of General Practitioners* 32(234): 42–5.

Dunlop, D. (1970) The use and abuse of psychotropic drugs. *Proceedings of the Royal Society of Medicine* 63(12): 1279–282.

Dunnell, K. and Cartwright, A. (1972) *Medicine Takers, Prescribers and Hoarders*. London: Routledge & Kegan Paul.

Erlichman, J. (1985) Sharp decline in prescriptions on the limited list. *Guardian*, 28 May.

Gabe, J. and Lipshitz-Phillips, S. (1982) Evil necessity? The meaning of benzodiazepine use for women patients from one general practice. *Sociology of Health and Illness* 4(2): 201–09.

—— (1984) Tranquillisers as social control. *The Sociological Review* 32(3): 524–46.

Greenblatt, D.J. and Shader, R.I. (1974) *Benzodiazepines in Clinical Practice*. New York: Raven Press.

Hall, S. (1983) The great moving right show. In S. Hall and M. Jacques (eds) *The Politics of Thatcherism*. London: Lawrence & Wishart.

Harris, G., Latham J., McGuinness, B., and Crisp, A. (1977) Relationship between psychoneurotic status and psychoactive drug prescription in general practice. *Journal of the Royal Colege of General Practitioners* 27(176): 173–77.

Helman, C. (1981) Tonic, fuel and food: social and symbolic aspects of the long term use of psychotropic drugs. *Social Science and Medicine* 15B(4): 521–33.

Hollister, L. (1983) The pre-benzodiazepine era. *Journal of Psychoactive Drugs* 15(1–2): 9–13.

Hollister, L.E., Motzenbecker, F.P., and Degon, R.O. (1961) Withdrawal reactions from chlordiazepoxide ('Librium'). *Psychopharmacologia* 2: 63–8.

Jefferys, M. (1973) Medicine takers. *Journal of the Royal College of General Practitioners* Supplement No. 2, 23: 9–11.

Jefferys, M., and Sachs, H. (1983) *Rethinking General Practice*. London: Tavistock Publications.

Kennedy, I. (1981) *The Unmasking of Modern Medicine*. London: George Allen & Unwin.

Klerman, G.L. (1971) Drugs and social values. *The International Journal of the Addictions* 5(2): 313–19.

Kraüpl-Taylor, F. (1984) Benzodiazepines on trial. *British Medical Journal* 288(6427): 1379.

Lacey, R. and Woodward, S. (1985) *That's Life Survey on Tranquillisers*. London: BBC Publications.

Lader, M. (1978) Benzodiazepines: the opium of the masses? *Neuroscience* 3(2): 159–65.

—— (1981) Epidemic in the making: benzodiazepine dependence. In G. Tognoni, C. Bellantuono, and M. Lader (eds) *Epidemiological Impact of Psychoactive Drugs*. Amsterdam: Elsevier/North Holland Biomedical Press.

Lancet Editorial (1973a) Unreasonable profit. *The Lancet* 1(7808): 867.

—— (1973b) Benzodiazepines: use, overuse, misuse, abuse? *The Lancet* 1(7812): 1101–102.

Lasagna, L. (1980) The Halcion story: trial by media. *The Lancet* 1(8172): 815–16.

Lennard, H.L., Epstein, L.J., Bernstein, A., and Ransom, D.C. (1971) *Mystification and Drug Misuse*. New York: Harper & Row.

The London Programme (1984) Tranquillizer addicts. *London Weekend Television*, 27 January.

Mail on Sunday (1982) The tranquillizer trap, 8 August.

Marks, J. (1978) *The Benzodiazepines: use, overuse, misuse and abuse*. Lancaster: MTP Press.

—— (1983a) The benzodiazepines: an international perspective.*Journal of Psychoactive Drugs* 15(1–2): 137–49.

—— (1983b) Benzodiazepines: for good or for evil? *Neuropsychobiology* 10: 115–26.

MIND (1984) *Tranquillizers: Hard Facts, Hard Choices*. London: National Association for Mental Health.

Muller, C. (1972) The overmedicated society: forces in the marketplace for medical care. *Science* 176(4034): 488–92.

Murray, J. (1981) Long-term psychotropic drug-taking and the process of withdrawal. *Psychological Medicine* 11(4): 853–58.

Murray, J., Dunn, G., Williams, P., and Tarnopolsky, A. (1981) Factors affecting the consumption of psychotropic drugs.*Psychological Medicine* 11(3): 551–60.

Oakley, A. (1980) *Women Confined*. Oxford: Martin Robertson.

Observer (1980a) The dangers of tranquillity, 24 February.

—— (1980b) Prescription risk, 2 March.

Owen, R.T. and Tyrer, P. (1983) Benzodiazepine dependence: a review of the evidence. *Drugs* 25(4): 385–98.

Parascandola, J.L. (1977) A brief history of drug use. In A.L. Wertheimer and P.J. Bush (eds) *Perspectives on Medicines in Society*. Hamilton: Drug Intelligence Publications.

Parish, P.A. (1971) The prescribing of psychotropic drugs in general practice.*Journal of the Royal College of General Practitioners* 21 (Suppl. 4): 1–77.

Petursson, H. and Lader, M. (1981) Benzodiazepine dependence. *British Journal of Addiction* 76(2): 133–45.

Rabin, D.L. and Bush, P.J. (1974) The use of medicines: historical trends and international comparisons. *International Journal of Health Services* 4(1): 61–87.

RELEASE (1982) *Trouble with Tranquillisers*. London: RELEASE.

Rickels, K. (1981) Are benzodiazepines overused and abused? *British Journal of Clinical Pharmacology* 11, Supplement 1: 71S–83S.

Rickels, K., Case, G.W., Winokur, A., and Svenson C. (1984) Long-term benzodiazepine therapy: benefits and risks. *Psychopharmacology Bulletin* 20(4): 608–15.

Robinson, D. (1978) Self-help groups. *British Journal of Hospital Medicine* September: 106–10.

Royal College of General Practitioners (1978) Practice activity analysis: psychotropic drugs. *Journal of the Royal College of General Practitioners* 28 (187): 122–24.

Sackett, D.L. and Haynes, R.B. (1976) *Compliance with Therapeutic Regimens*. Baltimore: John Hopkins University Press.

Salmon, J.W. (1985) Introduction. In J.W. Salmon (ed.) *Alternative Medicines: Popular and Policy Perspectives*. London: Tavistock Publications.

Skegg, D.C.G., Doll, R., and Perry, J. (1977) The use of medicines in general practice. *British Medical Journal* 1(6976): 1561–563.

Solow, C. (1975) Psychotropic drugs in somatic disorders. *International Journal of Psychiatry in Medicine* 6: 267–82.

Standard (1981) Why the happy pills have had their day, 16 October.

Stanway, A. (1982) *Alternative Medicine*. Harmondsworth: Penguin.

Sullivan, J.L. and Sullivan, P.D. (1984) *Biomedical Psychiatric Therapeutics*. Sevenoaks: Butterworth.

Svenson, S.F. and Hamilton, R.G. (1966) A critique of over-emphasis of side effects with the psychotropic drugs: an analysis of 18,000 chlordiazepoxide treated cases. *Current Therapeutic Research* 8: 455–64.

Taking the Strain (1981) *British Broadcasting Corporation*, 7 July.

That's Life (1983) *British Broadcasting Corporation*, 12 June.

—— (1984a) *British Broadcasting Corporation*, 13 May.

—— (1984b) *British Broadcasting Corporation*, 20 May.

—— (1985) *British Broadcasting Corporation*, 18 March.

The Times (1980) Doctors urged to cut use of tranquillizers, 28 March.

Trethowan, W.H. (1975) Pills for personal problems. *British Medical Journal* 3(5986): 749–51.

Tyrer, P. (1974) The benzodiazepine bonanza. *The Lancet* 2(7882):709–10.

—— (1980) Dependence on benzodiazepines. *British Journal of Psychiatry* 137: 576–77.

Tyrer, P., Owen R., and Dawling, S. (1983) Gradual withdrawal of diazepam after long-term therapy. *The Lancet* 1(8339): 1402–406.

Tyrer, P., Rutherford, D., and Huggett, T. (1981) Benzodiazepine withdrawal symptoms and Propranolol. *The Lancet* 1(8219): 520–22.

Varnam, M.A. (1981) Psychotropic prescribing. What am I doing? *Journal of the Royal College of General Practitioners* 31(229): 480–83.

Wilks, J.M. (1975) The use of psychotropic drugs in general practice. *Journal of the Royal College of General Practitioners* 25(159): 731–44.

Williams, P. (1978) Physical ill-health and psychotropic drug prescription – a review. *Psychological Medicine* 8(4): 683–93.

—— (1979) The extent of psychotropic drug prescription. In P. Williams and A.W. Clare (eds) *Psychotropic Disorders in General Practice*. London: Academic Press.

—— (1980a) Recent trends in the prescribing of psychotropic drugs. *Health Trends* 12(1): 6–7.

—— (1980b) The use of prescribed psychotropic medicines. *Public Health Reviews* 9(3): 215–47.

—— (1982) The cost of tranquillizers. *Social Science and Medicine* 16(22): 1955–958.

—— (1983) Patterns of psychotropic drug use. *Social Science and Medicine* 17(13): 845–51.

Woman's Own (1984a) The Valium vale of tears, 11 February.

—— (1984b) Tranquillisers: the shocking truth, 1 September.

© *1986 Jonathan Gabe and Paul Williams*

PART 2

Long-term tranquilliser use

2
Introduction

There is abundant evidence that most psychotropic drug use is short term, but that a significant minority of users are found to be still consuming their drugs many months, or even years, after the initial prescription. A number of studies provided estimates for the extent of such long-term use. For example. Parish (1971), in England, conducted a retrospective review of general practitioners' records regarding psychotropic drug prescription. He found that of those prescribed a psychotropic drug during the study year, 27 per cent received treatment for six months or more and 15 per cent for one year or more. Cooperstock (1978), in Ontario, found that 16 per cent of the women and 9 per cent of the men who 'received a prescription for a minor tranquiliser' during 1970–71 received ten or more prescriptions during that year. Mellinger, Balter, and Uhlenhuth (1984), in a cross-sectional study conducted in the United States, found that 20 per cent of respondents who admitted to consuming 'anti-anxiety agents' during the previous year had used them daily for '4 months or more'. An astonishingly high rate for long-term psychotropic drug use emerged from the national survey of England and Wales conducted by Anderson (1980): it can be calculated from data provided in his paper than nearly 60 per cent of psychotropic drug prescriptions had been initiated a year or more previously.

These data are all from cross-sectional studies. In the only longitudinal prospective study of psychotropic drug use that has been carried out in a British general practice setting, Williams, Murray, and Clare (1982) followed up a cohort of psychotropic drug recipients and found that 17 per cent of the tranquilliser and 28 per cent of the antidepressant users were still receiving prescriptions six months later.

The first paper in this section, which to some extent can be regarded as providing a context for the succeeding two, is concerned with factors which predispose people to become long-term psychotropic drug users. Using data from the longitudinal prospective study in general practice referred to above, Williams examines the influence on the duration of psychotropic drug treatment of demographic, social, and psychological characteristics of the patient, and the behaviour/attitudes of the general practitioner.

One especially important aspect of long-term use is the recent finding that treatment with benzodiazepines (the most commonly prescribed group of psychotropic drugs) can, at recommended therapeutic dose levels, give rise to problems of psychological *and* physical dependence.

In the second paper in this section, Petursson and Lader review the evidence for benzodiazepine dependence. While they consider briefly the relevant laboratory investigations, most of the work that they review is drawn from studies of patients who have ceased to consume (i.e. have withdrawn from) benzodiazepine medication. They focus on the symptomatology and temporal course of the benzodiazepine withdrawal syndrome. Since the publication of this paper, these authors have completed their clinical and physiological studies, which have been published in book form (Petursson and Lader 1984).

While the existence of a benzodiazepine dependence syndrome has become generally accepted, its extent and significance remain the subject of much dispute (see Part 1). The persisting confusion in evaluating research in this area is exemplified by the correspondence in the *British Medical Journal* which followed Ashton's recent (1984) descriptive study of benzodiazepine withdrawal phenomena. One correspondent (Snaith 1984) believed that the study 'highlighted the potential of benzodiazepines to cause harm', and indicated that the study supported his belief in the need for legislation to 'counteract the prescribing of benzodiazepines'. Another correspondent, in the same issue of the *British Medical Journal*, described the same study as 'far too seriously flawed to show anything' (Kraüpl-Taylor 1984).

Lader (1984) has noted that a major cause of the continuing confusion in this area is that much research on long-term psychotropic drug use has been conducted on selected, and hence biased, samples of patients. For this reason, he observed:

> 'it is not possible to distinguish retrospectively between patients becoming dependent on tranquillisers taken long-term and patients continuing long-term use because they have a withdrawal syndrome on attempted discontinuation. Patients coming to study tend to be self-selected or primary physician-selected because of severity, of withdrawal, chronicity of usage, and perhaps even the neurotic nature of their initial symptoms which led to the prescription of tranquillisers.'

The relevance of this observation is exemplified by the recent study of Rodrigo and Williams (1986). They administered a check list of (a) anxiety symptoms and (b) perceptual phenomena said to be specific to the benzodiazepine withdrawal syndrome to a sample of students just before an examination. They found that the so-called specific perceptual phenomena were commonly reported by the students, and that their occurrence correlated strongly with the measure of anxiety. An equivalent questionnaire, completed after the examination, showed decreases in both anxiety and perceptual symptoms.

As is discussed in Part 6, there is clearly a pressing need for studies on representative samples of long-term tranquilliser consumers. However, such studies will need to be informed by background information and hypotheses derived from studies of self-selected samples of consumers. There is also a need for studies concerned with broader aspects of the experience of long-term psychotropic drug use, i.e. studies which are not exclusively concerned with dependence. In particular, the views and perceptions of the long-term consumers themselves have been a relatively neglected focus of research. Murray takes up this issue in the third paper in this section. Using a self-selected sample, she investigates three aspects of the consumers' attitudes to and perception of their psychotropic drug use. *First*, she investigates what they believe the benefits of prolonged drug consumption to be, and *second*, the extent to which they wish to stop consuming the drugs and the factors they believe prevent them from doing so. *Third*, she compares current long-term psychotropic consumers with past users, i.e. those who have succeeded in discontinuing, in order to explore whether differences can be found in the behaviour or attitudes of the two groups.

Murray's work is in the tradition of empirical social epidemiology – that is, it is not grounded in any particular theoretical approach. There are, however, clear links between the issues investigated by her and those which are the concern of the more sociologically oriented studies in Part 4.

References

Anderson, R.M. (1980) The use of repeatedly prescribed medicines. *Journal of the Royal College of General Practitioners* 30(219): 609–13.

Ashton, H. (1984) Benzodiazepine withdrawal: an unfinished story. *British Medical Journal* 288(6424): 1135–140.

Cooperstock, R. (1978) Sex differences on psychotropic drug use. *Social Science and Medicine* 12B(3): 179–86.

Kraüpl-Taylor, F. (1984) Benzodiazepines on trial (Correspondence). *British Medical Journal* 288(6427): 1379.

Lader, M. (1984) Short-term versus long-term benzodiazepine therapy. *Current Medical Research and Opinion* 8 (Suppl. 4):120–26.

Mellinger, G.D., Balter, M.B., and Uhlenhuth, E.H. (1984) Anti-anxiety agents: duration of use and characteristics of users in the U.S.A. *Current Medical Research and Opinion* 8 (Suppl. 4): 21–36.

Parish, P.A. (1971) The prescribing of psychotropic drugs in general practice.*Journal of the Royal College of General Practitioners* 21 (Suppl. 4): 1–77.

Petursson, H. and Lader, M.H. (1984) *Dependence on Tranquillisers*, London: Institute of Psychiatry Maudsley Monograph No. 28, Oxford University Press.

Rodrigo, R. and Williams, P. (1986) Frequency of self-reported 'anxiolytic withdrawal' symptoms in a group of female students experiencing anxiety. *Psychological Medicine*, forthcoming.

Snaith, R.P. (1984) Benzodiazepines on trial (Correspondence). *British Medical Journal* 288(6427): 1379.

Williams, P., Murray, J., and Clare, A.W. (1982) A longitudinal study of psychotropic drug use. *Psychological Medicine* 12(1): 201–06.

3

Factors influencing the duration of treatment with psychotropic drugs in general practice: a survival analysis approach

Paul Williams

Synopsis   There have been few previous attempts to study factors which affect the duration of treatment with psychiatric drugs in general practice. In the present study 'duration of treatment' was regarded as analogous to 'survival time', and techniques of survival analysis were applied to data from a previously published study of psychotropic drug use in general practice (Williams *et al.* 1982). Methods of logistic modelling were used in an attempt to construct a comprehensive and parsimonious model to describe and predict the duration of psychotropic use. Such a model was found to include the effects of previous psychotropic treatment, social problems, duration of treatment and general practitioner behaviour. The implications of the findings, *vis à vis* the prevention of unnecessary long-term psychotropic drug use, are discussed.

Introduction

A variety of studies have documented the extent of psychotropic drug prescription and use in the community. In much of this work, a cross-sectional approach has been adopted: that is, the aim has been to establish the number and proportion of patients or respondents who received a prescription for, or who admitted to consuming, a psychotropic drug during a given period of time. Many of these studies have been reviewed by Williams (1979).

Another aspect of the extent of psychotropic treatment and use is its duration. There is evidence that much psychotropic drug use is short term

---

Reprinted, with permission, from *Psychological Medicine* 13: 623–33, 1983.

(Parish 1971; Williams *et al*. 1982), but a proportion of recipients are found to consume such drugs for many months, or even years (Parish 1971; Mellinger and Balter 1981).

There is indirect evidence (reviewed by Williams 1983) to suggest that patients treated with psychotropic drugs in the community (i.e. in general practice settings) are currently receiving treatment for longer periods of time than previously. For example, the number and proportion of drugs issued on an 'unseen repeat' basis have increased substantially over the past 10–15 years (Drury 1982): psychotropics are prescribed on this basis more commonly than any other kind of drug (Manasse 1974; Bain and Haynes 1975). Marks (1983) estimated that, while in the late 1960s about one-third of psychotropic recipients were getting their drugs on a 'long-term repeat' basis, this had risen to nearly two-thirds by the late 1970s. A similar conclusion, that there is an increase in the proportion of psychotropic consumers who receive drugs on a long-term basis (with a consequent increase in the average duration of treatment), can be drawn from comparing successive community surveys of psychotropic prescription and consumption (Williams 1983).

This trend is of particular importance in the light of recent concern about the problems associated with the long-term consumption of benzodiazepines (the most commonly prescribed type of psychotropic; Lader 1978). It is being increasingly realized that patients can become physically dependent on benzodiazepines (Petursson and Lader 1981): although the proportion of benzodiazepine consumers who become dependent is low (Marks 1978), it is thought to be rising. These and other concerns about the long-term effects of psychotropic drugs of various kinds indicate the need to study the duration of drug treatment and use, and the factors which influence it. Potentially influential factors can be considered under four headings.

1. Patient characteristics

Differences between patients are likely to constitute an important influence on the duration of treatment. For example, the duration of treatment may be related to the severity of the symptomatology, or to the presence or absence of associated social dysfunction, or to demographic factors such as age and sex (Parish 1971).

2. Treatment characteristics

It may be that the duration of treatment is related to the nature of the treatment itself. For example, there is evidence to suggest that tricyclic antidepressants should be continued for several months after clinical recovery (Mindham *et al*. 1973), whereas it is recommended that treatment with benzodiazepines should be short term (Committee on the Review of Medicines 1980).

3. Doctor characteristics

Doctors differ in their attitudes to psychiatric disorder in the extent to which they recognize it (Shepherd *et al*. 1966; Goldberg and Huxley 1980), and in the extent to which they prescribe psychotropics (Royal College of General Practitioners 1978). It is reasonable to suppose, as a hypothesis to be tested, that doctors will also differ in the extent to which their patients become long-term users of psychotropic drugs.

4. The passage of time

Consider two patients, identical except that one has received tranquillisers for one month and the other for six months. What are their respective chances of discontinuing drug treatment? It may be, for example, that the chances of discontinuing treatment decrease with time, because of a process which may loosely be termed 'dependence'. Conversely, it may be that the longer the duration of treatment the greater the clinical improvement and hence the greater the chances of stopping treatment.

The study of the duration of treatment with psychotropic drugs

Data on the duration of drug treatment can be regarded as *survival data*. The duration of treatment itself, i.e. the time elapsing between the initiation of treatment and some defined endpoint, can be regarded as 'survival time', and discontinuation of treatment regarded as analogous to 'failure' or 'death'. The duration of treatment can thus be investigated by methods of survival analysis (see Lee 1980; Kalbfleisch and Prentice 1980). Within medicine, these methods have been applied to topics as diverse as the study of mortality itself (e.g. Benjamin 1968), the analysis of controlled clinical trials (e.g. Peto *et al*. 1977), the duration of hospitalization (e.g. Eaton and Whitmore 1977), general practice consulting (Dunn and Skuse 1981), and the relationship between mental state and response time (Dunn and Master 1982).

In the present context, a survivorship curve or life table (a graph or table of the probability of an individual surviving (i.e. continuing treatment) at least until a given time, plotted or displayed against time) can be constructed for a cohort of patients receiving psychotropic drugs in general practice. Such curves can be constructed for defined subgroups of such patients, and comparisons can be made between them.

In this paper a variety of survival analyses are applied to data taken from a (previously published) 6-month longitudinal study of general practice patients who received psychotropic drugs either for the very first time or for the treatment of a new episode of illness (Williams *et al*. 1982). The aims of the analyses were:

(i)   to determine the utility of survival methods with this sort of data;
(ii)   to describe, using survivorship curves, the distribution of duration of treatment for various defined subgroup patients;
(iii)   to identify patient and treatment characteristics which influence the duration of treatment and the probability of discontinuing treatment;
(iv)   to assess the influence of the passage of time (as defined above) on the probability of discontinuing treatment;
(v)   to assess the extent of between-doctor variation in the duration of treatment and in the probability of discontinuing treatment;
(vi)   to utilize the results as a factual basis for a discussion of policies for further research into, and the possible reduction of, long-term psychotropic drug use.

Method

Data collection

This is described in detail by Williams *et al.* (1982), to which the reader is referred for a full account. In brief, 6 general practitioners were asked to record, over a period not exceeding 3 months, data about patients for whom they prescribed a psychotropic drug (antidepressant, hypnotic or tranquilliser, according to the DHSS (1976) classification), either for the first time ever or for a new episode of illness. Subsequent prescribing for these patients was monitored for a period of 6 months.

Variables used in the analysis

The dependent variable, duration of treatment, was calculated according to the method of Parish (1971). It was defined as the length of time elapsing between the initiation of treatment and the day on which medication would be used up if it were taken according to prescription (this is not, of course, necessarily the same as duration of use). The general practitioner was also treated as a variable in the analysis.

Patient characteristics
The patient characteristics studied were: (a) sex; (b) age; (c) severity of symptoms at the beginning of treatment (based on the GP's global assessment of severity, using a visual analogue scale, with the responses being standardized within doctor and expressed in standard deviation units); (d) social problems known to the doctor at the beginning of treatment (based on the GP's response to a checklist of 6 social problems and subsequently dichotomized as 'none or one' or 'two or more'); (e) the presence or absence of GP-diagnosed physical illness.

Treatment characteristics

The treatment characteristics studied were: (a) type of psychotropic prescribed at the beginning of treatment, categorized according to the DHSS Drug Master Index (1976) into 'antidepressants and antidepressant/ tranquilliser combinations' (referred to for simplicity as antidepressants) and 'tranquillisers and hypnotics' (referred to for simplicity as tranquillisers); (b) previous psychotropic drug use (according to the GP); (c) whether or not psychotropic drugs were requested by the patient.

Analysis

First, a survival curve was constructed for the entire patient cohort. Then, the relationship between the distribution of survival times (i.e. durations of treatment) and the patient and treatment characteristics were examined for each of the variables singly.

Each patient and treatment variable was treated as dichotomous, so that a pair of survival curves could be constructed for each. The significance of the difference between them was estimated by the log-rank test, according to the method described by Peto *et al.* (1977). Between-doctor differences in the distribution of treatment durations (a six-way comparison of survival distributions) were assessed by the method of Lee and Desu (1972).

Such a procedure, i.e. examining the effect of each explanatory variable singly, is quite adequate for simple descriptive purposes. It is, however, quite inadequate for explanation since variables may interact and exert joint effects on the duration of treatment, or the apparent effect of one variable may in fact be due to the effect of another related variable.

The joint effects of the predictor variables were studied by linear-logistic modelling (Cox 1970; Dunn 1981). Such a model is one in which the probability of an event, transformed to its logit, is modelled in terms of the joint effects of a number of explanatory, or predictor variables. Linear models for survival data have been described by Dunn and Skuse (1981) and by Dunn and Master (1982). In the analysis of survival the probability to be modelled is the hazard rate, defined as the probability of failure during a very small time interval per unit time, assuming that the individual has survived to the beginning of that interval (Lee 1980). In practice, and in the present context, it is estimated as the proportion of subects (patients) who fail (discontinue treatment) in a not necessarily very small time interval, per unit time, given that they had survived to (i.e. were receiving treatment at) the beginning of the interval.

A follow-up period can be divided into a series of successive time intervals, and a separate logistic model constructed for the hazard rate estimated from each interval (see Fienberg and Mason 1978). Alternatively, the set of models can be collapsed into one model, with the introduction of a variable to denote the interval from which the hazard rate was derived (time). This is the

Table 1   *The sample used in the analysis*

	no.
sex	
male	48
female	76
age (years)*	
< 45	60
⩾ 45	58
not known	6
severity of symptoms †	
< +1.5 S.D.	85
⩾ +1.5 S.D.	36
not known	3
social problems known to doctor	
0 or 1	97
2 or more	27
physical illness	
absent	70
present	54
drugs prescribed at inception	
antidepressants	43
tranquillisers	81
previous treatment	
no	54
yes	69
not known	1
drugs requested by patient	
no	67
yes	53
not known	4
doctors	
A	21
B	21
C	15
D	10
E	45
F	12

* Mean age = 46.6 ± 18.3 years.
† By definition, mean = 0, S.D. = 1.
  Median duration of treatment = 33 days.

technique described by Dunn and Skuse (1981) and Murray *et al*. (1982), and employed here: the model is essentially an analysis of covariance for a logistic transformation of the dependent variable.

In the present analysis, the follow-up period was divided into 3 successive 2-month intervals (i.e. T = 1, 2 or 3). First, a model involving patient and treatment variables and time was fitted. Standard hierarchical model building procedures were used to find the model of best fit (that model in which, according to this method of analysis, every term is necessary, and to which the addition of extra terms does not significantly improve the goodness of fit). Then, new cross-tabulations were prepared, involving only the variables in the model of best fit and the 'doctor' variable. The data from these were used to construct a model to assess the significance of between-doctor differences.

Results

153 patients were entered into the study. Their characteristics are described in detail by Williams *et al.* (1982). Of these, 124 (81 per cent) completed the 6-month follow-up (the drop-outs are discussed by Williams *et al.* (1982), and it is these who form the basis of the present study. *Table 1* summarizes them in terms of the variables used in the analysis.

Survival distributions

Figure 1 shows the survival curve for the entire cohort. It can be seen that about half of the respondents had discontinued treatment at or before 5 weeks, but that about one-fifth received treatment throughout the 6-month follow-up period. The hazard rate (per month) – the probability of discontinuing treatment during the following month, conditional on receiving treatment at the beginning of it – is also displayed in *Figure 1*, and can be seen to decrease as duration of treatment increases.

Figure 2 shows the relationships between the survival distribution of duration of treatment and the patient, treatment and doctor variables. It can be seen that symptom severity, type of psychotropic, and previous psychotropic use were each related to the duration of treatment (more severe, antidepressant prescription and previous history of psychotropic use each indicating longer duration of treatment). There was also significant heterogeneity between doctors with regard to the survival distributions.

Attention was then paid to the variables that appeared not to be significantly related to duration of treatment (sex, age, social problems, physical illness, and request for drugs). Assessments of each variable were then made for the two drug types separately (to investigate drug type $\times$ variable interactions). The only significant finding (*Figure 2j*) was of an association between increased age and duration of treatment for tranquilliser users only (log-rank $x^2 = 4.71$, df $= 1, P < 0.05$).

The effect of age, social problems, physical illness and request for drugs on duration of treatment was then assessed for each sex separately (to investigate sex $\times$ variable interactions). The only significant finding,

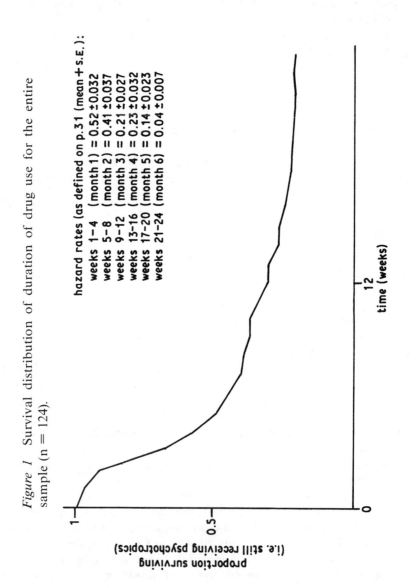

Figure 1 Survival distribution of duration of drug use for the entire sample (n = 124).

hazard rates (as defined on p.31 (mean + s.e.):

weeks 1–4   (month 1) = 0.52 ±0.032
weeks 5–8   (month 2) = 0.41 ±0.037
weeks 9–12   (month 3) = 0.21 ±0.027
weeks 13–16 (month 4) = 0.23 ±0.032
weeks 17–20 (month 5) = 0.14 ±0.023
weeks 21–24 (month 6) = 0.04 ±0.007

proportion surviving
(i.e. still receiving psychotropics)

time (weeks)

1

0.5

0

12

displayed in *Figure 2k*, was of an association between extent of social problems and duration of treatment for women only (log-rank $X^2 = 7.27$, df $= 1, P < 0.01$).

Linear-logistic modelling

Linear-logistic models were then fitted to the hazard rates, as described on p. 29. The variables included were sex, age, social problems, severity of illness, drug type, previous psychotropic use (as well as time). The model found to fit the data (deviance $= 103.5$, df $= 83$; deviance is a log-likelihood ratio criterion of goodness-of-fit, and is distributed as X^2) was:

$$\text{GRAND MEAN} + \text{PREV}(i) + \text{SEX}(j) + \text{SOC}(k) + \text{SEX}(j).\text{SOC}k) + t.\text{T}, (1)$$

where i takes the value 1 for no previous psychotropic use, and 2 for previous use; j takes the value 1 for men and 2 for women; k takes the value of 1 if 0 or 1 social problems and 2 if 2 or more social problems were identified by the GP; and t is a parameter whose value expresses the extent to which the hazard rate, independent of the effects of the other explanatory variables, changes with time ($T = 1, 2$ or 3). The estimated values of the parameters, their standard errors and significance levels are shown in *Table 2*.

Table 2 *Logistic modelling*

patient and treatment characteristics and time	parameter estimate	standard error	change in G^2	P (df = 1)
GRAND MEAN	1.573	0.478	—	—
SEX (2)	0.823	0.381	1.8	NS
SOC (2)	0.872	0.711	1.0	NS
PREV (2)	−1.033	0.358	10.0	< 0.01
T	−0.929	0.248	22.1	< 0.01
SEX (2) SOC (2)	−1.815	0.852	4.7	< 0.05

The variables are as defined in the text. Parameters of the models were constrained by GLIM to be zero whenever one of the class indicators in a model parameter took the value of 1.

As an example of the state of affairs predicted by this model, *Table 3* shows, for women only, the estimated probability of stopping psychotropic drug treatment within the subsequent 8 weeks, at the beginning and after 4 months of continuous treatment. It can be seen that a woman who had previously been treated with psychotropics, has social problems and has received psychotropic drug treatment for 4 months has little chance of early discontinuation of treatment (an example of the way in which these estimates can be obtained from the model is given in the Appendix).

Figure 2 Survival distributions of duration of psychotropic treatment

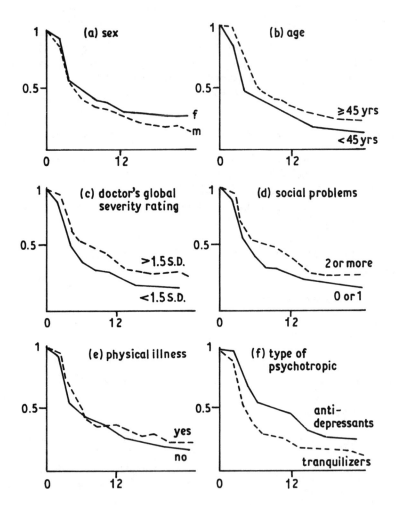

All vertical axes: probability of continuing treatment at least until time t. All horizontal axes: time (t) in weeks. (a) sex: log-rank $\chi^2 = 0.82$, df $= 1$, NS; (b) age: log-rank $\chi^2 = 1.98$, df $= 1$, NS; (c) doctor's global severity rating: log-rank $\chi^2 = 4.01$, df $= 1$, $P < 0.05$; (d) social problems: log-rank $\chi^2 = 1.54$, df $= 1$, NS; (e) physical illness: log-rank $\chi^2 = 0.41$, df $= 1$, NS; (f) type of psychotropic: log-rank $\chi^2 = 4.17$, df $= 1$, $P < 0.05$; (g) previous use: log-rank $\chi^2 = 10.23$, df $= 1$, $P < 0.01$; (h) request of drugs: log-rank $\chi^2 = 0.02$, df $= 1$, NS; (i) doctors: Lee & Desu's $\chi^2 = 13.19$, df $= 5$, $P < 0.025$; (j) age (tranquillizer recipients only): log-rank $\chi^2 = 4.71$, df $= 1$, $P < 0.05$; (k) social problems (women only): log-rank $\chi^2 = 7.27$, df $= 1$, $P < 0.01$.

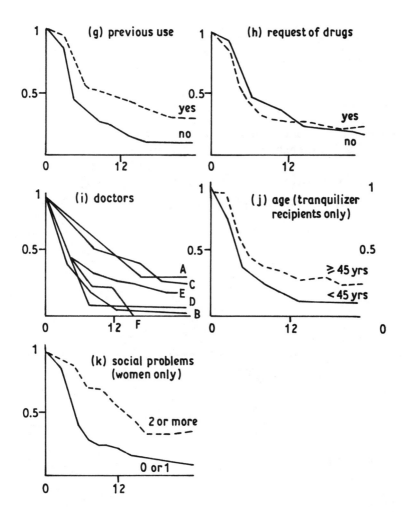

Table 3   *Probability of stopping psychotropic drug treatment within the next 8 weeks (women only) (estimated from the model)*

	social problems identified by GP	previous psychotropic use no	yes
(a) initiation of treatment	0 or 1	0.81	0.61
	2 +	0.91	0.38
(b) after 4 months of treatment	0 or 1	0.40	0.19
	2 +	0.62	0.09

A fresh set of cross-tabulations was prepared, as described on p. 31, and the significance of between-doctor variation assessed in the context of the previously described model. The model found to fit the data (deviance = 59.98, df =46) was model (1) above, with the addition of

$$+ \ DR(m) + DR(m)tT,$$

where m takes a value between 1 and 6, corresponding to doctors A–F. The parameter estimates, standard errors and significance levels are shown in *Table 4*. It can be seen that the main effect 'doctor' was significant at the 2 per cent level, and the doctor $\times$ time interaction at the 5 per cent level. Interactions betwen doctor and the other terms in the model were not significant (and hence are not shown in *Table 4*).

Table 4   *Logistic modelling*

patient and treatment characteristics, time, and doctor	parameter estimate	standard error	change in G^2	df	P
GRAND MEAN	0.226	0.942	—	—	—
SEX (2)	0.838	0.415	0.83	1	NS
SOC (2)	1.070	0.774	0.68	1	NS
PREV (2)	−0.859	0.391	6.03	1	< 0.02
T	−0.237	0.521	14.58	1	< 0.001
DR (2)	2.962	1.591			
DR (3)	2.015	1.130			
DR (4)	−8.077	39.620	14.49	5	< 0.02
DR (5)	−0.417	1.287			
DR (6)	9.818	33.760			
SEX (2) SOC (2)	−2.442	0.959	5.46	1	< 0.02
DR (2)t	−1.478	1.069			
DR (3)t	−1.329	0.708			
DR (4)t	9.410	39.600	10.62	4	< 0.05
DR (5)t	0.039	0.723			
DR (6)t	0	—			

The variables are as defined in the text. Parameters of the models were constrained by GLIM to be zero whenever one of the class indicators in a model parameter took the value of 1.

Discussion

On p. 28 were set out six aims of this study. They can conveniently be grouped into three categories for the purposes of discussion. The first (aim (i)) is concerned with the limitations of the data and the analysis; the second (aims (ii)–(v)) is to do with the substance of the findings; the third (aim (vi)) is concerned with their interpretation *vis à vis* the prevention of unnecessary long-term psychotropic drug use (it is not, of course, implied that all such long-term use is unnecessary).

The limitations of this data set have been discussed by Williams *et al.* (1982). They pointed out that the number of patients was, in epidemiological terms, relatively small. Also, they derive from a small and atypical (given their willingness to participate in research of this kind) sample of general practitioners. Furthermore, it was not possible to assess whether all the patients satisfying the entry criteria were in fact entered: for example, there were relatively few hypnotic users in the sample, although the distribution of prescribed drugs is not dissimilar to that found in cross-sectional studies (e.g. Skegg *et al.* 1977). It should also be borne in mind that the data concern the duration of treatment rather than the duration of drug use.

The relatively small sample size has implications for the interpretation of the logistic models. The deviance (G^2), by which the goodness of fit of the model is assessed, is regarded as following a χ^2 distribution. As the cell values of the contingency table from which the model is constructed decrease, so the distribution of G^2 deviates from that of χ^2. Caution is therefore required in the interpretation of the models (especially that in *Table 4*), particularly with regard to the interactions.

Within these limitations, this analysis has demonstrated that a survivorship approach is both appropriate to and feasible with data of this sort. Indeed, despite the constraints on the interpretation of the model described above, this approach is probably superior to alternative methods of analysis (for example, categorizing users into short and long-term, comparing mean durations with treatment – see Dunn and Master (1982) for a summary of the shortcomings inherent in such methods of analysis of survival data).

In the main, treatment with psychotropic drugs in general practice was a short-term affair, confirming the finding of Parish (1971). *Figure 1* shows that about half the patients had ceased treatment by the end of the first month. Subsequently, however, the rate at which treatment was stopped decreases sharply (as denoted by the decrease in the hazard rates displayed in *Table 1*), so that by the end of the follow-up period about one-fifth of the patients were found to have received drug treatment continuously.

A descriptive approach to factors which affect this distribution of duration of treatment was afforded by the comparison of survival curves.

With regard to patient characteristics, those rated by their doctor as more severely ill at the beginning of treatment were likely to receive treatment for longer than those rated as less severe. Similarly, women patients rated by their doctors as having two or more social problems were likely to receive treatment for longer than women with no or only one problem. The presence of physical illness was not related to the duration of treatment, but older recipients of tranquillisers were likely to receive treatment for longer than younger recipients (a finding that did not apply to recipients of antidepressant drugs).

Patients prescribed antidepressants received treatment for longer than those prescribed tranquillisers, and this may well reflect treatment policy. As mentioned earlier, the Committee on the Review of Medicines (1980) has recommended that treatment with benzodiazepines be kept short term wherever possible, while longer periods of treatment are recommended, for prophylactic purposes, with tricyclic antidepressants (Mindham *et al.* 1973). Previous users of psychotropic drugs were likely to be treated for longer than 'first timers', but there was no relationship between the patient requesting drug treatment and duration.

So far, the findings are in keeping with common sense and, in large part, with reasonably rational clinical behaviour. The marked differences between the doctors might perhaps be considered less rational, although not surprising. *Figure 2i* shows that the median duration of treatment ranged from just under 4 weeks (Doctor B) to just under 14 (Doctor A). This variation will be discussed in more detail later.

Such an analysis is quite acceptable for descriptive purposes. It allows us, for example, to answer questions of the form 'do patients with characteristic X tend to receive treatment for longer periods than those without it?' It is insufficient, however, for explanatory or analytical purposes, since no account is taken of relationships between variables and possible joint effects on the dependent variable (which, in the logistic models described above, is the probability of stopping treatment in a given time interval).

The only significant patient or treatment characteristics to emerge from the logistic modelling were previous treatment and, for women only, the extent of social problems. These two variables exerted independent (i.e. additive) effects on the probability of stopping drug treatment, effects exerted irrespective of the type of psychotropic prescribed or of symptom severity (variables which were not significant in the model). In addition to these, there was an independent effect of time: i.e. irrespective of the characteristics of the patient or the treatment, the probability of stopping treatment *decreases as the length of treatment increases*.

Ideally, the effect of between-doctor differences would have been included in the same model. Because of the already large numbers of variables and the relatively small sample size, it was decided to examine this by means of a separate model, as described on p. 31. The results of this model indicate that the effects of between-doctor differences on the probability of stopping psychotropic drug treatment are *independent of* those patient and treatment characteristics previously found to exert important influences. The model did reveal, however, that there was a significant interaction between doctor and time: that is, irrespective of the charcteristics of the patient or the treatment, the *rate* at which the probability of stopping treatment decreases with the duration of treatment differs between doctors. The implication of this finding is that, quite apart from the nature of the patient and his treatment, some doctors are less prepared than others to discontinue treatment with psychotropic drugs. The differences between doctors, then, are *not* merely due to differences between their patients.

These findings clearly require confirmation and replication on larger samples of patients. If similar findings emerge from larger studies, there are important implications for the prevention of unnecessarily long-term psychotropic drug use in general practice.

Consider first the role of the patient and treatment characteristics in influencing the duration of drug treatment. These two sets of characteristics are similar in that they are 'fixed' at the beginning of treatment. It follows, then, that to the extent that such factors are found to influence the duration of treatment, individuals at high risk of becoming long-term recipients of psychotropic drugs can be identified at the outset of treatment.

Consider now the effect of the passage of time. In this study the probability of stopping drug treatment (within a given interval) was found to decrease with time, independent of the characteristics of the patient or the treatment. It lends support to the concept of dependence on prescribed psychotropics and implies that the best time to prevent unnecessary long-term psychotropic drug use is early, rather than later, in the course of treatment. Compare, for example, the hazard rates (probabilities of discontinuing treatment) for the first and sixth months, as displayed in *Figure 1*, or the two sets of rates displayed in *Table 3*.

The between-doctor differences are also important from the preventive point of view. The findings suggest that some doctors may interact with their patients in such a way as to encourage, albeit not consciously, long-term use. If such a finding is confirmed, the identification of factors related to this, and their possible modification, is an important research priority.

This study, then, has identified important areas for further research into the problem of long-term psychotropic drug use in general practice. The identification of factors which increase the risk of long-term use, the effect of the passage of time and how it can be modified by techniques such as monitoring and surveillance, and the identification and possible modification of doctor characteristics have all been emphasized. There is a further issue, which is that it has been assumed that some long-term psychotropic drug use is at least unnecessary, at most harmful. There is still no universal agreement, let alone clear criteria, to enable a doctor to distinguish between 'necessary' and 'unnecessary' psychotropic drug treatment. This problem clearly merits the close attention of all those concerned with the use (and misuse) of psychotropic drugs.

Acknowledgements

Grateful thanks are due to the general practitioners who took part in the study. Thanks are also due to Dr N. Raynes and Ms V. Cairns, who commented helpfully at various stages in the data collection phase of the study, and to Professor A. Clare and Ms J. Murray who participated in the data collection.

Grateful thanks are also due to Dr G. Dunn for helpful discussions and for commenting on the manuscript. The study was carried out as part of a research programme funded by the Department of Health and Social Security, under the direction of Professor M. Shepherd, to whom thanks are due for advice, comment and support throughout the study.

Appendix

Calculation of probability estimates from the model parameters

The model whose parameter estimates are displayed in *Table 2* is equation (1) on p. 33, i.e.

$$\ln\left(\frac{p}{1-p}\right) = \text{GRAND MEAN}+\text{PREV}(i)+\text{SEX}(j)+\text{SOC}(k)+ \text{SEX }(j).\text{SOC }(k)+t.\text{T}.$$

Example 1
Consider a woman ($j = 2$), with no previous psychotropic treatment ($i = 1$), with no social problems ($k = 1$) at the beginning of treatment ($T = 1$):

$$\ln\left(\frac{p}{1-p}\right) = \underset{\substack{\text{GRAND}\\\text{MEAN}}}{1.573} + \underset{\text{PREV}(1)}{0} + \underset{\text{SEX}(2)}{0.823}$$
$$+ \underset{\text{SOC}(1)}{0} + \underset{\text{SEX}(2).\text{SOC}(1)}{0} + \underset{t.\text{T}}{(-0.929\times1)}$$
$$= 1.467.$$

So $\qquad p = \dfrac{\exp(1.467)}{1+\exp(1.467)} = 0.81,$

the value displayed in the upper left-hand cell of *Table 3a*.

Example 2
Consider a woman ($j = 2$) with a history of previous psychotropic treatment ($i = 1$), with 2 social problems ($k = 2$) who has been on treatment for 4 months (T = 3):

$$\text{In} \left(\frac{p}{1-p}\right) = \underset{\substack{\text{GRAND} \\ \text{MEAN}}}{1.573} + \underset{\text{PREV(2)}}{(-1.033)} + \underset{\text{SEX(2)}}{0.823}$$

$$+ \underset{\text{SOC(2)}}{0.872} + \underset{\text{SEX(2).SOC(2)}}{(-1.815)} + \underset{t.\text{T}}{(-0.929\times3)}$$

$$= -2.367.$$

So $\qquad p = \dfrac{\exp(-2.367)}{1+\exp(-2.367)} = 0.09,$

the value displayed in the lower right-hand cell of *Table 3b*.

References

Bain, D.J. and Haynes, A.J. (1975) A year's study of drug prescribing in general practice using computer-assisted records. *Journal of the Royal College of General Practitioners* 24: 203–07.

Benjamin, B. (1968) *Health and Vital Statistics*. London: Allen & Unwin.

Committee on the Review of Medicines (1980) Systematic review of the benzodiazepines. *British Medical Journal* 280 (6218): 910–12.

Cox, D.R. (1970) *Analysis of Binary Data*. London: Chapman & Hall.

Department of Health and Social Security (1976) Drug Master Index. Unpublished.

Drury, V.W.M. (1982) Repeat prescribing – a review. *Journal of the Royal College of General Practitioners* 32 (234): 42–5

Dunn, G. (1981) The role of linear models in psychiatric epidemiology. *Psychological Medicine* 11: 179–84.

Dunn, G. and Master, D. (1982) Latency models: the statistical analysis of response times. *Psychological Medicine* 12: 659–66.

Dunn, G. and Skuse, D. (1981) The natural history of depression in general practice: stochastic models. *Psychological Medicine* 11: 755–64.

Eaton, W.W. and Whitmore, G.A. (1977) Length of stay as a stochastic process: a general approach and application to hospitalisation for schizophrenia. *Journal of Mathematical Sociology* 5: 273–92.

Fienberg, S.E. and Mason, W. (1978) Identification and estimation of age, period and cohort models in the analysis of discrete archival data. In K.

Schüssler (ed.) *Sociological Methodology*: 1–67. San Francisco: Jossey-Bass.

Goldberg, D. and Huxley, P. (1980) *Mental Illness in the Community*. London: Tavistock.

Kalbfleisch, J.D. and Prentice, R.L. (1980) *The Statistical Analysis of Failure Time Data*. New York: Wiley.

Lader, M.H. (1978) Benzodiazepines: the opium of the masses? *Neuroscience* 3 (2): 159–65.

Lee, E.T. (1980) *Statistical Methods for Survival Data Analysis*. Belmont, California: Lifetime Publications.

Lee, E.T. and Desu M.M. (1972) A computer program for comparing *K* samples with right-censored data. *Computer Programs in Biomedicine* 2: 315–21.

Manasse, A.P. (1974) Repeat prescriptions in general practice. *Journal of the Royal College of General Practitioners* 24: 203–07.

Marks, J. (1978) *The Benzodiazepines*. Lancaster: MTP Press.

—— (1983) Benzodiazepines – for good or for evil? *Neuropsychobiology* 10: 115–26.

Mellinger, G.D. and Balter M.B. (1982) Prevalence and patterns of use of psychotherapeutic drugs. In G. Tognoni, C. Bellantuono, and M. Lader (eds) *The Epidemiological Impact of Psychotropic Drugs*: 117–36. Amsterdam; Elsevier.

Mindham, R.H.S., Howland C., and Shepherd, M. (1973) An evaluation of continuation therapy with tricyclic antidepressants in depressive illness. *Psychological Medicine* 3: 5–17.

Murray, J., Dunn, G., and Tarnopolsky, A. (1982) Self-assessment of health: an exploration of the effect of physical and psychological symptoms. *Psychological Medicine* 12: 371–78.

Parish, P.A. (1971) The prescribing of psychotropic drugs in general practice. *Journal of the Royal College of General Practitioners* 21: Suppl. 4: 1–77.

Peto, R., Pike, M.C., Armitage P., Breslow, N.E., Cox, D.R., Howard, S.V., Mantel, N., McPherson, K., Peto, J., and Smith, P.G. (1977) Design and analysis of randomised clinical trials requiring prolonged observation of each patient: 11. Analysis and examples. *British Journal of Cancer* 35: 1–39.

Petursson, H., and Lader, M.H. (1981) Benzodiazepine dependence. *British Journal of Addiction* 76 (2): 133–45.

Royal College of General Practitioners (Birmingham Research Group) (1978) Practice activity analysis: 4. Psychotropic drugs. *Journal of the Royal College of General Practitioners* 28 (187): 122–24.

Shepherd, M., Cooper, B., Brown, A.C., and Kalton, G. (1966) *Psychiatric Illness in General Practice*. London: Oxford University Press.

Skegg, D.C.G., Doll, R., and Perry, J. (1977) Use of medicines in general practice. *British Medical Journal* 1 (6976): 1561–563.

Williams, P. (1979) The extent of psychotropic drug prescription. In P. Williams and A.W. Clare (eds) *Psychosocial Disorders in General Practice*, 151–60. London: Academic Press.

—— (1983) Patterns of psychotropic drug use. *Social Science and Medicine* 17(13): 845–51.

Williams, P., Murray J., and Clare, A.W. (1982) A longitudinal study of psychotropic drug prescription. *Psychological Medicine* 12 (1): 201–06.

4

Benzodiazepine dependence

H. Petursson and M.H. Lader

Summary Benzodiazepines, the most widely used of all drugs, are powerful anxiolytics, anticonvulsants, and muscle relaxants. Dependence is difficult to induce in animals but has been induced by high doses in man. Case reports of benzodiazepine dependence are rare compared with the usage of these drugs, but do not provide a proper epidemiological framework for the estimation of risk. Patients taking these drugs for four months or more may develop a physical withdrawl syndrome, characterized by anxiety, dysphoria, malaise, depersonalization, and by perceptual changes such as hyperacusis and unsteadiness. In our experience drawn from over 20 patients, withdrawal from therapeutic doses of benzodiazepine may be attended by a fully-developed physical withdrawal syndrome.

Benzodiazepine dependence

The benzodiazepines comprise a group of drugs which are the most widely used of all prescribed drugs. The first was introduced in 1960 when the clinical effectiveness of chlordiazepoxide was established. This drug was soon followed by its even more successful congener, diazepam. Several thousand other benzodiazepines have been synthesized and tested for potential clinical use. At present about 25 different types have been marketed throughout the world and others are at an advanced state of development.

The benzodiazepines have largely replaced the barbiturates because of the following advantages: they are more effective in alleviating anxiety and stress responses; they have fewer and less severe side-effects; they are much safer in overdosage; they induce liver enzymes much less and so do not interact with other drugs: and finally, they are believed to be less liable to

---

Reprinted, with permission, from the *British Journal of Addiction* 76: 133–45. 1981.

induce dependence. However, one is immediately reminded of the typical life-cycle of most sedative/hypnotics and tranquillisers. Introduced as major innovations or hailed as vast improvements, their effectiveness may prove limited or side effects seem appreciable, and finally the drug's abuse potential is belatedly recognized. This has happened with the bromides, paraldehyde, chloral, barbiturates and meprobamate. Escalation of dosage has been noted, tell-tale signs of drug-seeking behaviour have been detected, and charasteristic withdrawal syndrome has been described.

This paper reviews the evidence concerning the dependence-inducing properties of the benzodiazepines, focusing in particular on the therapeutic situation. The discussion is biased towards the biological phenomena, i.e. tolerance, dependence and withdrawal, whereas little is known about the potential roles of phychosocial factors in a benzodiazepine dependence syndrome. The definitions used of dependence-related terms are those currently accepted by the WHO [1].

Extent of usage

The importance of this topic directly reflects the extent of usage of the benzodiazepines. Several surveys have suggested that about one in ten adult males and one in five adult females take tranquillisers or hypnotics, mainly benzodiazepines, at some time during the course of each year. Of these people between a half and two-thirds take tranquillisers for at least a month at a time. Perhaps 2 per cent of the adult population, say 600,000 people, are taking tranquillisers every day or night of the year [2, 3]. Over 4 per cent of all prescriptions are for diazepam alone [4]. Finally, the commonest drugs on repeat prescriptions are the benzodiazepines. Such widespread and chronic use is to be expected with common, recurrent or continuing conditions such as anxiety states, tension, insomnia and vague psychosomatic complaints [5, 6]. Nevertheless, the cynic, recalling the history of the barbiturates and meprobamate and their predecessors, might posit the involvement of some process of dependence. This possibility will be reviewed under the usual headings of animal evidence, tolerance, withdrawal symptoms, etc.

Pharmacological aspects

Benzodiazepines are rapidly absorbed after oral administration and most are extensively bound to plasma proteins. They are highly lipid soluble and are readily distributed in body tissues. There are two main kinetic properties which define their clinical profile. Firstly, the formation of pharmacologically active metabolites, and secondly, the length of elimination half-lives which vary, with consequent variation in length of action.

The metabolism of the various benzodiazepines is interconnected. Some undergo N-dealkylation in the liver to N-desmethyldiazepam (nordiazepam) or its halogenated homologues. These metabolites are then hydroxylated to oxazepam or its halogenated homologues. Finally, the drugs are excreted after conjugation with glucuronic acid. The 7-nitro, 1,4-benzodiazepines have a different metabolic pathway with no pharmacologically active metabolites. N-desmethyldiazepam accumulates during chronic treatment and probably accounts for a considerable proportion of the side-effects of benzodiazepines.

The benzodiazepines act primarily on subcortical structures, such as the amygdala and hippocampus of the limbic system. Recently specific benzodiazepine receptors have been identified in the brain and the existence of an endogenous benzodiazepine-substance has been postulated. Biochemical data indicate that the benzodiazepines indirectly potentiate and prolong the synaptic actions of GABA, an inhibitory neurotransmitter. The potent anticonvulsant effect of benzodiazepines is possibly due to their effect on GABA-ergic mechanisms. Furthermore, the benzodiazepines lower the turnover of both brain NA and 5-HT, perhaps through a primary action on GABA mechanisms. The initial sedative effects of the benzodiazepines tend to produce tolerance, and are probably the result of an effect on NA mechanisms. The rebound phase, seen when animals are withdrawn from long-term benzodiazepine administration, consists of enhanced release and decreased uptake of NA, DA and 5-HT [7]. Preliminary studies suggest that changes in benzodiazepine receptors cannot explain the development of tolerance and dependence following chronic treatment [8,9].

Behavioural effects
The main behavioural effects of benzodiazepines in animals are characterised by an increase in behavioural responses that are normally depressed by response contingent punishment or conditioned fear.

Clinically, the benzodiazepines have an anxiolytic action in doses which do not produce sedation, although higher doses cause drowsiness and lethargy. They are also effective as hypnotics without the 'knock-out' action of the barbiturates, although they may subsequently cause subjective 'hangover' symptoms. There is a deterioration in psychomotor performance with increasing plasma benzodiazepine concentrations. Amnesia has been reported following the intravenous administration of lorazepam [10]. Acute and chronic doses reduce R.E.M. sleep, followed by a rebound phase during withdrawal. Other clinical indications include: (a) muscle spasm, especially that secondary to musculo-skeletal lesions; (b) status epilepticus; (c) intravenous administration of diazepam or lorazepam is widely used preoperatively and as a soporific during dental and endoscopic procedures. Diazepam can substitute for alcohol during withdrawal and, unfortunately, during the self-induction of intoxication. Effects on mood, sex, aggression, and sociability are complex and are probably influenced by expectation. In general benzodiazepines decrease rather than increase hostility and aggression, but there is also evidence that paradoxical release of aggression can occur. The latter is probably modulated by sex, route of administration and the social setting [11].

Drug addicts who take large doses of diazepam, either alone or in conjunction with narcotics, experience a pleasant, relaxed sensation which they describe as a 'high' [12]. Large doses produce drowsiness, sleep, incoordination, muscle weakness, ataxia and dysarthria. Our patients have described a 'rush' effect in response to 10 mg intravenous diazepam, with euphoria, flight of ideas, pressure of speech, enhanced self-confidence, pleasant relaxation and calmness, followed by increasing drowsiness.

Dependence-inducing properties

Animal models can be used to demonstrate whether a drug is potentially liable to induce dependence. As the extrapolation to man is fairly valid such studies are a valuable introduction to the study of dependence potential. One simple model is to induce rats to drink fluids containing drugs. This can be achieved with barbiturates and morphine but not with benzodiazepines [13, 14].

A more sophisticated model consists of implanting an indwelling catheter into a vein. When the animal presses a lever or carries out some other operation, a bolus of drug-containing solution is injected into the bloodstream. Rats will bar-press at a very high rate in order to maintain an input of a powerful dependence-inducing agent such as heroin and other opiates, amphetamines and cocaine. Alcohol and barbiturates are associated with moderate rates of operant behaviour whereas no bar-pressing is produced by antipsychotic drugs. The benzodiazepines show low activity in this model. In one experiment, rhesus monkeys were given chlordiazepoxide intravenously in doses of 1mg/kg every 3 hours. Then two animals were given a choice of bar-pressing to continue on the benzodiazepine or of switching to barbiturate: the animals changed to barbiturate [15]. Another study using a similar method found evidence for dependence, but very high doses of benzodiazepines were used [16].

Animal models of withdrawl have also been studied and a definite withdrawal syndrome can be recognized on discontinuation of benzo-diazepines. They can also be cross-substituted in animals previously rendered dependent on other drugs [17].

It seems, therefore, that benzodiazepines do have a potential to induce dependence but this is more clearly seen as physical dependence with a withdrawal syndrome than as drug-seeking or maintaining behaviour.

Studies in humans

Several hundred papers are extant reporting cases of dependence on the benzodiazepines. Marks [18] comprehensively reviewed this literature and found that only 118 of these publications contained fully verified cases of physical dependence with a definite withdrawal syndrome or carefully documented cases of psychological dependence. The cases collected by Marks fell into two categories:

1. Those occurring in a therapeutic situation.
2. Those arising within the context of the 'drug scene' with evidence of multiple drug abuse or alcoholism.

We have largely adhered to this classification, but within the clinical situation we have also distinguished between withdrawals from high- and low-doses of benzodiazepines because of the clinical importance of the latter group. Experimental investigations are reported first, followed by less systematic studies and case reports. A third group, habituation, consists of cases in which only psychological dependence is documented.

Polydrug abuse

Marks collected 151 cases worldwide of benzodiazepine dependence within the framework of multiple drug abuse or alcoholism, plus 250 less definite cases [18]. As he points out it is difficult to assign individual cases to the 'abuse' or the 'therapeutic' group, the main criterion being whether the supplies of benzodiazepines come via a prescription or from illicit sources. It is also not clear how many individuals become dependent within the clinical situation, and then turn to the 'black market' for supplies and this classification probably underestimates the extent of clinical dependence. More importantly, however, it is difficult to assess the nature and degree of possible benzodiazepine dependence in people who are concurrently dependent on other drugs and/or alcohol. A detailed review of this part of the literature is therefore beyond the scope of this paper. In the vast majority of cases excessive doses of benzodiazepines have been used [19, 20, 21, 22, 23, 24, 25, 26, 27]. The duration of use has varied from a few months to a few years. A few individuals have stayed within the therapeutically recommended doses for several years [27, 28]. In some instances neither dose nor duration has been stated [29, 30, 31, 32, 33, 34, 35, 36, 37].

Clinical dependence

Cases of benzodiazepine dependence reported to have occurred solely within the therapeutic situation, and in which other forms of drug dependence do not seem to have played a major contributory role, constitute a minority of the several hundred cases reported in the literature. Each case has been assigned to one of three groups, withdrawal from high-

and low-doses, and cases in which the dependence appears to have been largely psychological.

High dose   Attempts have been made in the past to induce dependence in humans. In the most vigorously pursued study [38], psychiatric patients in hospital were treated with chlordiazepoxide, 100 to 600 mg daily for 1 to 7 months, most patients for over 3 months. Dizziness, weakness, sleepiness and tiredness were common side-effects usually following too rapid a dosage increase. At high doses of 300 mg or more, three patients became agitated necessitating a reduction in dose. Eleven patients were abruptly switched to placebo after being on 300 to 600 mg/daily, 6 patients receiving the highest dose. Ten of the 11 patients reported new symptoms or developed new signs following placebo substitution. Psychoses were aggravated in 5 patients, insomnia and agitation supervened in 5, and 4 lost their appetite. Two patients had major epileptiform convulsions on the seventh and eighth day following discontinuation. Symptoms following benzodiazepine withdrawal were more belated and less severe than those following withdrawal of barbiturates or meprobamate but were of the same type. A study by Burke and Anderson [39] failed to confirm these findings in 25 chronic alcoholics. However, in this study lower doses were used and the drug was only administered for two weeks.

Patients within the high dose category have usually taken 2–5 times the normal therapeutic doses of the various benzodiazepines. Several reports indicate that on such doses physical dependence can develop within 2–3 weeks [12, 40], and certainly within four months [41]. In the majority of cases, however, the drugs have been taken for much longer, usually a few years [35, 42, 43, 44, 45, 46, 47, 48, 49, 50]. Finally, two reports have described apparent withdrawal symptoms in neonates following maternal exposure to benzodiazepines [51, 52].

Low dose   There are few systematic studies of benzodiazepine withdrawal following ingestion of therapeutic doses. Covi *et al.* [53, 54] investigated the effect of abrupt discontinuation of chlordiazepoxide treatment, 45 mg daily for twenty weeks. They found a mild abstinence syndrome, consisting mainly of subjective feelings of anxiety and tension as well as minor symptoms, such as trembling, poor appetite and faintness or dizziness. A recent study by Tyrer [55] investigated benzodiazepine dependence on patients seen in general practice and psychiatric out-patients clinics. Eighty-six patients satisfied the inclusion criteria, namely that they had taken either diazepam or lorazepam regularly for four months or longer, were not on any other psychotropic drugs, and were not considered to need the drug on clinical grounds. Only forty agreed to be withdrawn, of whom eighteen dropped out and returned to taking their benzodiazepine again. Of the 40 patients a substantial minority, as much as 45 per cent, suffered a withdrawal syndrome when their medication was abruptly stopped. After two weeks follow-up three groups of patients were identified. Firstly, those whose condition remained unchanged, or were improved, after withdrawal (32.5 per cent). Secondly, those whose former anxiety symptoms gradually increased, and thirdly, patients with a withdrawal symptoms gradually increased, and, thirdly, patients with a withdrawal pain, extreme dysphoria, persistent headache or sensory changes.

Maletzky and Klotter [56] reviewed 27 articles in which diazepam was claimed to be free of addicting properties, and concluded that none had used adequate methods. Systematic withdrawal was not carried out, and in some no data regarding tolerance were collected. One reason why signs of benzodiazepine dependence may be missed or misdiagnosed is the fact that unlike withdrawal from opiates or alcohol, anxiety is the cardinal symptom of the benzodiazepine withdrawal syndrome. Furthermore, the temporal relationships of the respective syndromes are quite different because of pharmacokinetic differences.

Several papers are extant reporting cases of physical withdrawal reactions from short-term (weeks-months) [12, 57, 58, 59, 60], and long-term (years) [59, 61, 62, 63, 64, 65, 66, 67, 68], low-dosage benzodiazepine treatment. It is of significance that in most instances these abstinence phenomena are qualitatively and quantitatively identical to those on withdrawal from high-doses of benzodiazepines.

Habituation   A number of papers do not document any direct evidence of a physiological withdrawal syndrome, perceptual distubrances, fits or psychosis. In these cases the dependence appears to be mainly psycho-logical [61, 69, 70, 71, 72, 73, 74, 75, 76]. The withdrawal syndrome consists essentially of anxiety and/or depression and sometimes signs of drug-seeking behaviour are reported.

Tolerance

Although relatively few studies have looked directly at the process of tolerance to benzodiazepines, some degree of tissue (receptor-site) tolerance or adaptation probably occurs in most people exposed to these drugs. Subjective drug effects may depend more upon the rate at which blood concentrations are achieved following a single dose of benzo-diazepine than upon the concentration measured at the time that the subjective effect is assessed [77]. Similar findings are reported regarding the extent of psychomotor impairment, the effect being far greater on the upswing of the plasma concentration curve [78, 79].

Tolerance to the sedative effects can be demonstrated in animals as the depression of exploratory and general motor activity induced by benzodiazepines wears off after a few days [80]. Most patients reporting initial drowsiness find it wanes over a few days [81, 82, 83, 84]. Normal subjects given a single dose of a long acting benzodiazepine such as clorazepate report progressively fewer subjective effects of drowsiness over the next few hours despite plasma concentrations of the drug hardly diminishing [85]. It is possible that tolerance to the anxiolytic effects of the benzodiazepines may develop less readily although this has not been reliably documented within the clinical situation.

In a study by Lader *et al.* [86] using normal subjects, clorazepate was administered as a single dose (7.5 or 15 mg) every morning for 15 days and compared with placebo. Electroencephalographic effects such as increase in fast-wave activity and decrease in auditory evoked responses were much less apparent following the 15th dose than the first. Perceptual impairment was also less although subjective reports tended to increase with repetition of the dose. Plasma concentrations were elevated following the dose at least as much on the 15th day as on the first showing that the tolerance was not pharmacokinetic.

Further support for a non-pharmacokinetic tolerance comes from case studies of acute overdosage [87]. Finally, there is cross-tolerance between the benzodiazepines and barbiturates and alcohol [88, 89]. Patients with histories of drug abuse of the alcohol/sedative type tend to use benzo-diazepines if the opportunity arises but still prefer barbiturates or alcohol.

Animal studies indicate that excessive doses of benzodiazepines can produce enzyme induction [88]. This effect probably does not occur in clinical use. Investigations of whether benzodiazepines stimulate the metabolism of other drugs have been negative [88, 90]. It is unclear whether the benzodiazepines stimulate [91, 92] or inhibit [93] their own metabolism. The effect of nicotine on the biotransformation and elimination of the benzodiazepines is equally controversial [94, 95].

Most patients maintain themselves on a fairly constant dose of benzodiazepine while others steadily escalate their dosage [96]. Clinical observations suggest that increase in dose is associated with increased problems and stresses. When these resolve, the dosage is reduced in most patients [97]. Some patients, however, seem to become rapidly tolerant to the anxiolytic effects and do not reduce their dosage when the stress is relieved. Thus, a relevant question may concern the factors which govern variations in the rate of acquiring tolerance.

The practical implications of these various studies and observations mainly concern patients with previous histories of drug abuse or alcoholism. Such patients are more likely than others to become tolerant to benzodiazepines and to escalate the dose. Other methods of management and alternative medications should be considered.

Withdrawal syndrome

The fully-developed benzodiazepine withdrawal syndrome has been described as a severe sleep disturbance, irritability, increased tension and anxiety, panic attacks, hand tremor, profuse sweating, difficulty in concentration, dry retching and nausea, weight loss, palpitations, and muscular pains and stiffness. Instances are also reported of more serious developments such as epileptic fits [19, 24, 38, 59, 60, 63, 98], psychotic reactions [19, 38, 49, 50, 57, 59, 62, 64, 66, 98] and even death [40].

During the last year we have withdrawn, under doubleblind, placebo-controlled conditions, 24 patients (13 males, 11 females) from low-dosage, long-term benzodiazepine treatment. Their psychiatric diagnosis was anxiety neurosis, depression, or personality disorder, and none was alcoholic or took other drugs. They had all received benzodiazepines in therapeutic doses for at least one year (range: 1-16 years). All have experienced some form of withdrawal reaction, but more importantly, the changes on withdrawal of normal doses have in most cases been indistinguishable from those on withdrawal of high doses in other patients [99], either in quality or quantity. The withdrawal reaction has ranged from anxiety and dysphoria to severe affective and perceptual changes. Anxiety ratings rise as the drugs are discontinued but usually subside to pre-withdrawal levels over the next two to four weeks. This in itself suggests that the symptoms represent a true withdrawal syndrome and not a revival of the original anxiety symptoms. Furthermore, some of the symptoms are untypical of anxiety. The dysphoria is an amalgam of anxiety, depression, nausea, malaise and depersonalization. Perceptual changes are common; patients complain of intolerance to loud noises, bright lights and touch, numbness, paresthesia, unsteadiness, and a feeling of motion. Some patients have complained of strange smells and a metallic taste; some chronic, heavy smokers have even given up their cigarettes temporarily.

EEG changes comprised marked reduction in fast-wave activity as the drugs were withdrawn. At the same time auditory evoked responses to clicks increased from very small pre-withdrawal values to normal values. Galvanic skin responses (GSR, an indirect measure of sweat gland responses to stimuli) gradually rose to a peak level during the withdrawal syndrome and then returned to pre-withdrawal levels. After withdrawal improvement in psychomotor performance was noted as demonstrated by the digit symbol substitution test.

Plasma concentrations of the benzodiazepines and any pharmacologically active metabolites were measured by a radioreceptor technique. The drugs on some occasions could still be detected in plasma up to ten days after they had been discontinued, reflecting the relatively long elimination half-lives of most benzodiazepines. The syndrome was maximal 4-6 days after cessation of medication and subsided after 8-10 days.

Epidemiology

The peak of reporting of cases of possible benzodiazepine dependence was in 1969–73, that is, about ten years after the introduction of the first benzodiazepine. Numbers since then have been few despite increasing use of the drugs. This presumably reflects lack of concern among the medical profession rather than lack of cases. Marks estimated that the usage of benzodiazepines in the United Kingdom was about 150 million patient-months since their introduction in 1960 to mid-1977 [18]. About 28 cases of dependence were recorded in the U.K. over this period making the risk one case per 5 million patient-months for all forms of dependence. For dependence arising solely in the therapeutic context, the risk was put at one case per 50 million patient-months.

Two reviews of the pre-1965 studies of chlordiazepoxide [100], and diazepam [56], did not detect any cases of dependence. Survey data have also suggested little general concern. In the Boston Collaborative Drug Surveillance Program, trained nurses monitored data on medical patients in nine hospitals in North America, New Zealand and Israel. Of 25,000 interviewed, 4,500 patients were taking benzodiazepines but no signs of dependence were detected [94, 101]. Two other large-scale surveys of patients have only reported 2–3 cases of benzodiazepine dependence [102, 103].

In contrast to these findings more recent reports appear to show that a substantial proportion of patients taking benzodiazepines will develop some form of dependence [55, 56].

Finally, benzodiazepines are commonly used by drug abusers. Thus, for example, Woody *et al.* [104], found up to 40 per cent of their narcotic addicts used diazepam. A survey of 113 drug abuse patients found that 30 per cent used street-purchased diazepam [12]. The 'street' use of diazepam has been described with 10 mg tablets of diazepam selling for 50¢. Doses of 100 to 500 mg per day produced a 'pleasurable state of intoxication' [105].

Conclusion

As with their predecessors, benzodiazepines are fully capable of inducing both physical and psychological dependence. Human experimental studies confirm those in animals that definite dependence can be induced by giving high doses for a prolonged period but that dependence on therapeutic doses is more apparent as a syndrome complex on withdrawal rather than as marked drug-seeking behaviour. Even so, the withdrawal syndrome is often underplayed as a recrudescence of the original anxiety for which the benzodiazepine was prescribed [106].

In view of the extremely wide usage of these drugs, documented cases of dependence are rare, although more recent studies indicate that the incidence of dependence may be substantially higher. Despite this apparent lack of published evidence, the extent of chronic usage of the benzodiazepines – although reflecting the chronic nature of their indications – may mean that a proportion of users become dependent, even at normal therapeutic dosage. In view of the psychological impairment associated with chronic sedative ingestion [107] and the socioeconomic implications, a careful examination of the problem in an epidemiological framework is a matter of urgency.

References

1 WHO Expert Committee on Drug Dependence (1974) Twentieth Report. *WHO Technical Report Series*. no.551.

2 Balter, M.B., Levine, J., and Manheimer, D.I. (1974) Cross-national study of the extent of anti-anxiety/sedative drug use. *New England Journal of Medicine* 290: 769–74.

3 Lader, M. (1978) Benzodiazepines – the opium of the masses? *Neuroscience* 3: 159–65.

4 Skegg, D.C.G., Doll, R., and Perry, J. (1977) Use of medicines in general practice. *British Medical Journal* 2:1561–563.

5 Shepherd, M., Cooper, B., Brown, A.C., and Kalton, G.W. (1966) *Psychiatric Illness in General Practice*. London: Oxford University Press.

6 Taylor, Lord and Chave, S. (1964) *Mental Health and Environment*. London: Longmans.

7 Rastogi, R.B., Lapierre, Y.D., and Singhal, R.L. (1978) Synaptosomal uptake of norepinephrine and 5-hydroxytryptamine and synthesis of catecholamines during benzodiazepine treatment. *Canadian Journal of Physiology and Pharmacology* 56: 777–84.

8 Braestrup, C. and Nielsen, M. (1980) Benzodiazepine receptors. *Arzneimittel Forschung. Drug Research* 30(1): 852–57.

9 Möhler, H., Okada, T., and Enna, S.J. (1978) Benzodiazepine and neurotransmitter receptor binding in rat brain after chronic administration of diazepam or phenorbarbital. *Brain Research* 156: 391–95.

10 Heisterkamp, D.V. and Cohen P.J. (1975) Effect of intravenous premedication with lorazepam, pentobarbitone or diazepam on recall. *British Journal of Anaesthesia* 47: 79.

11 Valzelli, L. (1967) In S. Garattini and P.A. Shore (eds) *Advances in Pharmacology*. New York: Academic Press, 79–108.

12 Woody, G.E., O'Brien, C.P., and Greenstein, R. (1975) Misuse and abuse of diazepam: An increasingly common medical problem. *The International Journal of the Addictions* 10(5): 843–48.

13 Stolerman, I.P., Kumar, R., and Steinberg, H. (1971) Development of morphine dependence in rats: Lack of effect of previous ingestion of other drugs. *Psychopharmacologia* 20: 321–36.

14 Harris, R.T., Glaghorn, J.L., and Schoolar, J.C. (1968) Self administration of minor tranquillisers as a function of conditioning. *Psychopharmacologia* 13: 81–8.

15 Findley, J.D., Robinson, W.W., and Peregrino, L. (1972) Addiction to secobarbital and chlordiazepoxide in the Rhesus monkey by means of a self-infusion preference procedure. *Psychopharmacologia* 26: 93–114.
16 Yanagita, T. and Takahashi, S. (1973) Dependence liability of several sedative-hypnotic agents evaluated in monkeys. *Journal of Pharmacology and Experimental Therapeutics* 185: 307–16.
17 Deneau, G.A. and Weiss, S. (1968) A substitution technique for determining barbiturate-like physiological dependence capacity in the dog. Pharmakopsychiatrie, *Neuro-Psychopharmakologie* 1: 270–75.
18 Marks, J. (1978) *The Benzodiazepines. Use, Overuse, Misuse, Abuse.* Lancaster: MTP Press.
19 Barten, H.H. (1965) Toxic psychosis with transient dymnestic syndrome following withdrawal from valium. *American Journal of Psychiatry* 121: 1210–211.
20 Bakewell, W.E. and Wikler, A. (1966) Incidence in a university hospital psychiatric ward. *Journal of the American Medical Association* 196(8): 710–13.
21 Bartholomew, A.A. and Reynolds, W.S. (1967) Four cases of progressive drug abuse. *The Medical Journal of Australia* 54: 653–57.
22 Clare, A.W. (1971) Diazepam, alcohol, and barbiturate abuse. *British Medical Journal* 4: 340.
23 Petzold, E. (1972) Valiumsucht. *Internist Praxis* 12: 355.
24 Nerenz, K. (1974) Ein Fall von Valium-Entzugsdelir mit Grand-mal-aufällen. *Nervenarzt* 45: 384–86.
25 Selig, J.W.(1966) A possible oxazepam abstinence syndrome. *Journal of the American Medical Association* 198(8): 279–80.
26 Lingjaerde, O. (1971) Bruk og misbruk av benzodiazepiner. *Nordisk Medicin* 16:(37):1065–092.
27 Rechenberger, H.G. (1972) Valiumsucht. *Internist Praxis* 12: 354.
28 Feuerlein, W. and Busch, H. (1972) Valiumsucht. *Internist Praxis* 12: 353.
29 Eichner, H.L. and Aebi, E. (1970) Septic retinitis due to injection of a homemade alcoholic beverage. *Journal of the American Medical Association* 213(10): 1644–646.
30 Malcolm, M.T. (1972) Temporal lobe epilepsy due to drug withdrawal. *British Journal of Addiction* 67: 309–12.
31 Maletzky, B.M. (1974) Assisted covert sensitization for drug abuse. *The International Journal of the Addicitions* 9(3): 411–29.
32 Hallberg, R.J., Lessler, K., and Kane, F.J. (1964) Korsakoff-like psychosis associated with benzodiazepine overdosage. *American Journal of Psychiatry* 121: 188–89.
33 Holmberg, G. (1969) Missbrukas diazepam? *Lakartidningen* 66: 77–81.
34 Noble, P.J. (1970) Drug-taking in delinquent boys. *British Medical Journal* 1: 102–05.
35 Kryspin-Exner, K. (1966) Missbrauch von Benzodiazepin-derivaten bei Alkoholkranken. *British Journal of Addiction* 61: 283–90.
36 Lefevre, C.G. (1971) A factual study of drug dependence and drug abuse during 1965–1969 in New South Wales: a summary. *The Medical Journal of Australia* 58: 395–97 and 715.

37   Hoover, J.P. (1972) College drug scene. *New York State Journal of Medicine* 72: 1866–872.
38   Hollister, L.E., Motzenbecker, F.P., and Degan, R.O. (1961) Withdrawal reactions from chlordiazepoxide ('Librium'). *Psychopharmacologia* 2: 63–8.
39   Burke, G.W. and Anderson, C.W.G. (1962) Response to librium in individuals with a propensity for addiction: a pilot study. *Journal of Louisana State Medical Society* 114: 58–60.
40   Relkin, R. (1966) Death following withdrawal of diazepam. *New York State Journal of Medicine* 66: 1770–772.
41   Hayashki, T., Higashki, T., and Kadota, K. (1974) 3 Cases of chronic chlordiazepoxide intoxication and their withdrawal symptoms. *Clinical Psychiatry* 16: 77–83.
42   Aivazian, G.H. (1964) Clinical evaluation of diazepam. *Diseases of the Nervous System* 25: 491–96.
43   Slater, J. (1966) Suspected dependence on chlordiazepoxide hydrochloride (Librium). *Canadian Medical Association Journal* 95: 416.
44   Gordon, E.B. (1967) Addiction to diazepam (Valium). *The British Medical Journal* 1: 112.
45   Mader, Von, R. (1972) Primäre Valiumabhängigkeit bei einem Jugendlichen. *Wiener Medizinische Wochenschrift* 122: 699–700.
46   Venzlaff, V. (1972) Valiumsucht. *Internist Praxis* 12: 349.
47   Badura, H.O. (1972) Valiumsucht. *Internist Praxis* 12: 352.
48   Misra, P.C. (1975) Nitrazepam (Mogadon) dependence. *British Journal of Psychiatry* 126: 81–2.
49   Preskorn, H. and Denner, J. (1977) Benzodiazepines and withdrawal psychosis. Report of three cases. *Journal of the American Medical Association* 237: 36–8.
50   Allgulander, C. and Borg, S. (1978) Case Report: A delirious abstinence syndrome associated with clorazepate (Tranxilen). *British Journal of Addiction* 73: 175–77.
51   Athinarayanan, P., Pierog, S.H., Nigam, S.K., and Glass, L. (1976) Chlordiazepoxide withdrawal in the neonate. *American Journal of Obstetrics and Gynecology* 124: 212–13.
52   Rementeria, J.L. and Bhatt, K. (1977) Withdrawal symptoms in neonates from intrauterine exposure to diazepam. *Journal of Pediatrics* 90: 123–26.
53   Covi, L., Park, L.C., Lipman, R.S., Uhlenhuth, E.H., and Rickels, K. (1969) Factors affecting withdrawal response to certain minor tranquillisers. In J.O. Cole and J.R. Wittenborn (eds) *Drug Abuse: Social and Psychopharmacological Aspects*. Springfield, Illinois: Thomas. 93–108.
54   Covi, L., Lipman, R.S., Pattison, J.H., Derogatis, L.R., and Uhlenhuth, E.H. (1973) Length of treatment with anxiolytic sedatives and response to their sudden withdrawal. *Acta Psychiatrica Scandinavica* 49: 51–64.
55   Tyrer, P.J. (1980) Benzodiazepine dependence and propranolol. *Pharmaceutical Journal* 225: 158–60.
56   Maletzky, B.M. and Klotter, J. (1976) Addiction to diazepam. *The International Journal of the Addictions* II(1): 95–115.
57   Fruensgaard, K. and Vaag, U.H. (1975) Abstinenspsykose efter nitrazepam. *Ugeskrift for Laeger* 137: 633–34.

58 Haskell, D. (1975) Withdrawal of diazepam. *Journal of the American Medical Association* 233: 135.

59 Fruensgaard, K. (1976) Withdrawal psychosis: a study of 30 consecutive cases. *Acta Psychiatrica Scandinavica* 53: 105–18.

60 Rifkin, A., Quitkin, F., and Klein D.F. (1976) Withdrawal reaction to diazepam. *Journal of the American Medical Association* 236(19): 2172–173.

61 Peters, U.H. and Boeters, U. (1970) Valium-Sucht. Eine Analyse anhand von 8 Fällen. Pharmakopsychiatrie. *Neuropsychopharmakologie* 3: 339–48.

62 Darcy, L. (1972) Delirium tremens following withdrawal of nitrazepam. *The Medical Journal of Australia* 2: 450.

63 Vyas, I. and Carney, M.W.P. (1975) Diazepam withdrawal fits. *British Medical Journal* 4: 44.

64 Dysken, M.W. and Carlyle, H.C. (1977) Diazepam withdrawal psychosis: a case report. *American Journal of Psychiatry* 134(5): 573.

65 Bant, W. (1975) Diazepam withdrawal symptoms. *British Medical Journal* 4: 285.

66 Floyd, J.B. and Murphy, M. (1976) Hallucinations following withdrawal of valium. *Journal of the Kentucky Medical Association* 74: 549–50.

67 Pevnick, J.S., Jasinski, D.R., and Haertyen, C.A. (1978) Abrupt withdrawal from therapeutically administered diazepam. *Archives of General Psychiatry* 35: 995–98.

68 Winokur, A., Rickels, K., Greenblatt, D.J., Snyder, P.J., and Schatz, N.J. (1980) Withdrawal reaction from long-term low-dosage administration of diazepam. *Archives of General Psychiatry* 37: 101–05.

69 Guile, L.A. (1963) Rapid habituation to chlordiazepoxide (Librium). *The Medical Journal of Australia* 50: 56–7.

70 Hanna, S.M. (1972) A case of oxazepam (Serenid D) dependence. *British Journal of Psychiatry* 120: 443–45.

71 Quitkin, F.M., Rifkin, A., Kaplan, J., and Klein, D.F. (1972) Phobic anxiety syndrome complicated by drug dependence and addiction. *Archives of General Psychiatry* 27: 159–62.

72 Smith, A.J. (1972) Self-poisoning with drugs: A worsening situation. *British Medical Journal* 4: 157–59.

73 Morgan, H.G., Bouluois, J., and Burns-Cox, C. (1973) Addiction to prednisone. *British Medical Journal* 2: 93–4.

74 Wätzig, H. and Michaels, R. (1973) TAVOR: Kein problem-loses Benzodiazepine – Derivat. *Nervenarzt* 44: 499–500.

75 Bowes, H.A. (1965) The role of diazepam (Valium) in emotional illness. *Psychosomatics* 6: 336–40.

76 Kellett, J.M. (1974) The benzodiazepine bonanza. *Lancet* ii: 964.

77 Greenblatt, D.J. and Shader, R.I. (1978) Dependence, tolerance and addiction to benzodiazepines: clinical and pharmacokinetic considerations. *Drug Metabolism Reviews* 8(1): 13–28.

78 MacLeod, S.M., Giles, H.G., Patyalek, G., Thiessen, J.J., and Sellers, E.M. (1977) Diazepam actions and plasma concentrations following ethanol ingestion. *European Journal of Clinical Pharmacology* II: 345–49.

79 Bliding, A. (1974) Effects of different rates of absorption of two benzodiazepines on subjective and objective parameters. *European Journal of Clinical Pharmacology* 7: 201–11.

80   Vellucci, S.V. and File, S.E. (1979) Chlordiazepoxide loses its anxiolytic action with long-term treatment. *Psychopharmacologia* 62: 61–5.

81   Hillstad, L., Hansen, T., and Melsom, H. (1974) Diazepam metabolism in normal man. II. Serum concentrations and clinical effect after oral administration and cumulation. *Clinical Pharmacology and Therapeutics* 16: 485–89.

82   Kaplan, S.A., Jack, M.L., Alexander, K., and Weinfeld, R.E. (1973) Pharmacokinetic profile of diazepam in man following single intravenous and oral and chronic oral administration. *Journal of Pharmacological Science* 62: 1789–796.

83   Gamble, G.A.S., Dundee, G.W., and Gray, R.C. (1976) Plasma diazepam concentrations following prolonged administration. *British Journal of Anaesthesia* 48: 1087–090.

84   Eatman, F.B., Colburn, W.A., Boxenbaum, H.G., Postmanter, H.H., Weinfeld, R.E., Ronfeld, R., Weissman, L., Moore, J.D., Gibaldi, M., and Kaplan, S.A. (1977) Pharmacokinetics of diazepam following multiple-dose oral administration to healthy human subjects. *Journal of Pharmacokinetics and Biopharmacology* 5: 481–94.

85   Greenblatt, D.J., Shader, R.I., Harmatz, J.S., and Georgotas, A. (1979) Self-rated sedation and plasma concentrations of desmethyldiazepam following single doses of clorazepate. *Psychopharmacology* 66: 289–90.

86   Lader, M.H., Curry S., and Baker, W.J. (1980) Physiological and psychological effects of clorazepate in man. *British Journal of Clinical Pharmacology* 9: 83–90.

87   Greenblatt, D.J., Woo, E., Allen, M.D., Orsulak, P.J., and Shader, R.I. (1978) Rapid recovery from massive diazepam overdose. *Journal of the American Medical Association* 240(17): 1872–874.

88   Greenblatt, D.J. and Shader, R.I. (1974) *Benzodiazepines in Clinical Practice*. New York: Raven Press.

89   Greenblatt, D.J. and Shader, R.I. (1975) Treatment of the alcohol withdrawal syndrome. In R.I. Shader (ed.) *Manual of Psychiatric Therapeutics*. Boston: Little Brown. 211–35.

90   Vesell, E.S., Passamanti, G.T., Vian, J.P., Epps, J.E., and Di Carlo, F.J. (1972) Effects of chronic prazepam administration on drug metabolism in man and rat. *Pharmacology* 7:197–206.

91   Kanto, J., Iisalo, E., Lektinen, V., and Salminew, J. (1974) The concentrations of diazepam and its metabolites in the plasma after an acute and chronic administration. *Psychopharmacologia* 36: 123–31.

92   Sellman, R., Kanto, J., Raijola, E., and Pekkarinen, A. (1975) Induction effect of diazepam on its own metabolism. *Acta Pharmacologia and Toxicologia* 37: 345–51.

93   Klotz, U., Antonin, K.H., and Bieck, P.R. (1976) Comparison of the pharmacokinetics of diazepam after single and subchronic doses. *European Journal of Clinical Pharmacology* 10: 121–26.

94   Boston Collaborative Drug Surveillance Program (1973) Clinical depression of the central nervous system due to diazepam and chlordiazepoxide in relation to cigarette smoking and age. *New England Journal of Medicine* 288: 277–80.

95 Klotz, U., Avant, G.R., Hyumpa, A., Schenker, S., and Witkinson, G.R. (1975) The effects of age and liver disease on the disposition and elimination of diazepam in adult man. *Journal of Clinical Investigations* 55: 347–59.

96 Winstead, D.K., Anderson, A., Eilers, M.K., Blackwell, B., and Zaremba, A.L. (1974) Diazepam on demand. Drug-seeking behaviour in psychiatric inpatients. *Archives of General Psychiatry* 30: 349–51.

97 Allgulander, C. (1978) Dependence on sedative and hypnotic drugs. A comparative clinical and social study. *Acta Psychiatrica Scandinavica*, Supplement 270.

98 De Bard, M.L. (1979) Diazepam withdrawal syndrome: a case with psychosis, seizure and coma. *American Journal of Psychiatry* 136: 104–05.

99 Hallstrom, C. and Lader, M.H. (1981) Benzodiazepam withdrawal phenomena. *International Pharmacopsychiatry* 16: 235–44.

100 Svenson, S.E. and Hamilton, R.G. (1966) A critique of overemphasis on side-effects with the psychotropic drugs: an analysis of 18,000 chlordiazepoxide-treated cases. *Current Therapeutics Research* 8: 455–64.

101 Miller, R.R. (1973) Drug surveillance utilizing epidemiologic methods. *American Journal of Hospital Pharmacy* 30: 584–92.

102 Miller, R.R. (1974) Hospital admissions due to adverse drug reactions. *Archives of Internal Medicine* 134: 219–23.

103 Grant, I.N. (1969) Drug habituation in an urban general practice. *Practitioner* 202: 428–30.

104 Woody, G.E., Minty, J., O'Hare, K., O'Brien, C.P., Greenstein, R.A., and Hargrave, E. (1975). In Problems in Drug Dependence, 37th Annual Meeting, Washington, May, 1975. Washington, D.C: *National Academy of Science*, 1144.

105 Patch, V.D. (1974) The dangers of diazepam, a street drug. *New England Journal of Medicine* 290: 807.

106 Rickels, K., Downing, R.W., and Winokur, A. (1978) Antianxiety drugs: clinical use in psychiatry. In L.L. Iversen, S.D. Iversen, and S.H. Snyder (eds) *Handbook of Psychopharmacology*. New York: Plenum, 395–430.

107 McNair, D.M. (1973) Antianxiety drugs and human performance. *Archives of General Psychiatry* 29: 609–17.

5

Long-term psychotropic drug-taking and the process of withdrawal

Joanna Murray

Synopsis Perceived efficacy and reliance on psychotropic drugs is explored in a sample of mainly long-term consumers. A comparison of past and present users elucidates some of the factors involved in prolonged usage and the experiences of those who withdraw from the medication.

Introduction

Studies of dependence on psychotropic drugs have tended to address the clinical aspects of drug abstinence syndromes (Marks 1978; Lader 1980), while sociomedical studies have provided demographic profiles of consumers. It is known that twice as many women consume these drugs as men and that consumption increases with age (Balter *et al.* 1974; Skegg *et al.* 1977; Murray *et al.* 1981). While the majority of patients have ceased to take the medication at one month, Parish (1971) showed that approximately 15 per cent continued for over a year. Both Parish (1971) and Woodcock (1970) found that those aged over 40 constituted approximately 80 per cent of the long-term consumers, and that women were more than twice as likely as men to enter this group.

A recent longitudinal study (Williams *et al.* 1982) compared some characteristics of long-term and short-term users in an attempt to identify factors which might predict the duration of treatment at onset. Those who continued with the drugs for over 6 months were extensively interviewed and given a psychiatric assessment, but their number was too small to permit a broad exploration of the behaviour and attitudes of the long-term users. The dearth of information on the health, attitudes and drug-usage

Reprinted, with permission, from *Psychological Medicine* 11: 853–58. 1981.

patterns of this group led to the present study. This paper will focus on only some of the topics explored:

(1)   What benefits do consumers believe they derive from prolonged drug-taking?

(2)   Do they wish to withdraw from the drugs and, if so, what do they claim prevents their doing so?

(3)   Comparing present with past 'chronic' users, can differential factors be identified in the behaviour or attitudes of the two groups?

Method

A postal survey offered a rapid and inexpensive method of testing questions for a future large-scale study of psychotropic drug-takers. A display panel was placed in a popular women's magazine (*Woman's Own*) in August 1979, briefly outlining the survey and asking those willing to participate to write in. As a result, 300 questionnaires were despatched to respondents of whom approximately one-third were past users. It was, therefore, necessary to produce two versions of the questionnaire, one for past and one for present users.

Both questionnaires contained the 30-item Symptom Rating Test (SRT) (Kellner and Sheffield 1973), a modified version of the Belloc Physical Status Inventory (Belloc *et al.* 1971), questions on the use of medical services, attitudes to the drugs, and social networks. Present users additionally answered questions on current and perceived future use of the drugs, desire to give up and attempts made, and side-effects. Past users were asked about the process of withdrawal.

Results

Of the 300 questionaires despatched, 261 (87 per cent) were completed, 183 by present users and 78 by past users. Only 38 (15 per cent) respondents were aged between 16 and 30, with the largest group (120, 46 per cent) being 30–44 years. None was aged over 65. Since only 20 respondents (7.6 per cent) were male, no attempt has been made to consider the results separately for men and women.

Symptoms and illness
There was evidence of widespread physical impairment as measured by the Belloc scale: only 6 people scored as having no disability or physical symptoms. Present users tended more towards the upper 3 (of 7) levels of disability than past users.

Scores on the SRT were dichotomized into high (13 or over) and low (12 or less), these being the cut-off scores yielding the best 'case'/'non-case' classification on the basis of Cochrane's (1980) data. There was a higher prevalence of psychiatric symptoms among present users (152, 83 per cent), although 42 (55 per cent) past users scored as probable 'cases'. A strong association was found between physical and psychological morbidity, particularly among present drug-takers.

Drugs taken currently
103 (56 per cent) present users were taking one psychotropic drug, the majority of these being minor tranquillisers (89, 86 per cent). A further 42 (34 per cent) were taking 2 psychotropic drugs and the remaining 18 (10 per cent) respondents were taking 3 or more. Antidepressants were rarely taken alone (6 out of 49 cases). Hypnotics were taken by only 29 respondents (16 per cent).

The duration of drug-taking was similar for past and present users, the majority having been consumers for over 5 years. The sample thus consisted primarily of chronic tranquilliser users.

Reasons for prescribing and perceived benefits
Respondents stated in their own words why they believed their doctors had prescribed the drugs (*Table 1*). The two samples were remarkably similar, apart from the higher reporting of depression among past users.

Approximately three-quarters of both samples considered that the drugs had helped them. However, 13 (7 per cent) present users and 14 (18 per cent) past users were adamant that the drugs had not helped. *Table 2* shows the uniformity between past and present users in the order of importance of 6 benefits assigned to the drugs (the benefits were pre-selected).

Table 1   *Perceived reasons for psychotropic drug prescription*

	present users (n = 183)		past users (n = 78)	
	no.	(%)	no.	(%)
for anxiety, tension, nerves	70	(38)	31	(40)
for depression	24	(13)	23	(29)
to calm me down	21	(11)	8	(10)
to help me sleep	16	(9)	5	(6)
following a nervous breakdown	20	(11)	4	(5)
for agoraphobia	5	(3)	3	(4)
for a physical illness	31	(17)	8	(10)
marital problems	7	(4)	7	(9)
family problems/bereavement	20	(11)	9	(11)
they help me (unspecified)	11	(6)	—	—
I cannot manage without them	13	(7)	—	—
GP too busy to offer other help	20	(11)	6	(7)
prescribed by psychiatrist/hospital	15	(8)	1	(1)
other reasons	16	(9)	17	(22)

Table 2   *Ways in which the drugs helped*

	present users (n = 183)		past users (n = 78)	
	no.	(%)	no.	(%)
calm(ed) me down	115	(64)	46	(59)
make (made) me less worried or tense	105	(58)	43	(55)
help(ed) me sleep	98	(54)	35	(45)
make (made) me less irritable	52	(29)	18	(23)
make (made) me more confident	43	(24)	15	(19)
make (made) me feel happier	28	(16)	14	(18)
no help	13	(7)	14	(18)

Table 3   *Tasks in which respondents felt a need for psychotropic drugs*

	present users (n = 183)		past users (n = 78)	
	no.	(%)	no.	(%)
travelling	81	(44)	19	(24)
going shopping	78	(43)	22	(28)
mixing with people	75	(41)	29	(37)
running their homes	65	(36)	20	(26)
doing their work	61	(33)	31	(40)
family problems	61	(33)	32	(41)
meeting strangers	50	(28)	17	(22)
their marriages	40	(22)	21	(27)
money problems	20	(11)	11	(14)
housing problems	13	(7)	2	(3)
additional spontaneous responses				
tension; anxiety	50	(27)	7	(9)
physical symptoms	27	(15)	5	(6)
agoraphobia	16	(9)	3	(4)
depression	15	(8)	6	(8)
sleep problems	16	(9)	1	(1)
a specific event	17	(9)	15	(19)

A second list presented respondents with 10 practical tasks and personal problems. They were asked to indicate whether they (had) needed to take psychotropic drugs to cope with each area. *Table 3* shows that the highest rates of need indicated by present users were in response to activities outside the home (travelling, going shopping) and mixing with people. Past users were more likely to nominate family problems and carrying out their work.

Side-effects
The reporting of perceived side-effects was more common among past

Table 4 *Side-effects reported*

	present users (n = 183)		past users (n = 78)	
	no.	(%)	no.	(%)
none reported	78	(42)	18	(23)
drowsiness/lack of energy	41	(22)	25	(32)
impairment of memory/concentration	23	(13)	24	(31)
withdrawal/unsociability	9	(5)	18	(23)
depression	12	(7)	12	(15)
anxiety/panic attacks	2	(1)	10	(13)
irritability	4	(2)	8	(10)
emotional flatness	9	(5)	7	(9)
depersonalization	5	(3)	6	(8)
loss of inhibitions	6	(3)	6	(8)
altered libido	12	(7)	5	(6)
weight change, in-coordination, sweating, urinary problems, headache, giddiness, blurred vision, aggression, palpitations, gastrointestinal disorders, dry mouth, nightmares, and loss of interest	each reported by up to 6% in the 2 samples			

users; 60 (77 per cent) believed that the drugs had had a 'bad effect on (their) health, personality or behaviour', compared with 105 (58 per cent) present users. They were asked to describe these effects in their own words and the most commonly reported effects have been categorized in *Table 4*.

Attitudes to the drugs
The views of respondents on 5 statements about psychotropic drug taking and prescribing were elicited by means of a 4-point scale (agree strongly, agree, disagree, disagree strongly). The first 2 statements, designed to indicate their degree of reliance on the drugs, discriminated most between present and past users, although not to the extent that might have been predicted (*Table 5*). There was little difference between the 2 groups in the extent to which they regarded the taking of such drugs as a 'sign of weakness', although slightly more past users strongly agreed that 'a good heart-to-heart talk about your problems' did more good than taking tablets. Approximately 70 per cent overall agreed that doctors are too ready to prescribe pills for 'personal problems'.

Reliance on the drugs
The majority of present users (105, 58 per cent) said they would find it very difficult to manage without the drugs, while an additional 59 (33 per cent) claimed they would not be able to manage at all. This self-assessed reliance

Table 5 Extent of agreement with 5 attitude statements

	users	agree strongly no.	(%)	agree no.	(%)	disagree no.	(%)	disagree strongly no.	(%)	not answered no.	(%)
(1) 'I don't like taking these tablets but I could not manage without them'	present	81	(44)	78	(43)	19	(10)	2	(1)	3	(2)
	past	14	(18)	36	(48)	14	(18)	11	(14)	3	(4)
(2) 'I find I can cope with things much better when I take these tablets'	present	60	(33)	104	(57)	14	(8)	1	(1)	4	(2)
	past	9	(11)	39	(50)	14	(18)	9	(11)	7	(9)
(3) 'Taking tablets for your nerves is a sign of weakness'	present	15	(8)	35	(19)	80	(44)	50	(27)	3	(2)
	past	8	(10)	12	(15)	36	(46)	18	(23)	4	(5)
(4) 'A good heart-to-heart talk about your problems does you more good than taking tablets'	present	27	(15)	52	(28)	80	(44)	18	(10)	6	(3)
	past	18	(23)	23	(29)	31	(40)	3	(4)	3	(4)
(5) 'Doctors are too ready to give out pills to people with personal problems'	present	50	(27)	74	(40)	43	(23)	12	(7)	4	(2)
	past	29	(37)	27	(35)	20	(26)	1	(1)	1	(1)

Present users, $n = 183$; past users, $n = 78$.

varied little with physical disability or illness, as measured by the Belloc scale, or with psychiatric symptomatology (SRT score).

If psychotropic drugs were not available, 163 (89 per cent) present users said that they would take some other action to try to cope with their problems. Most asserted that they would take some other substance: herbal remedies (11 per cent), alcohol (12 per cent), painkillers or other non-prescription drugs (14 per cent), alternative prescribed drugs (11 per cent).

Only 17 (9 per cent) present users could foresee their medication ending within the next few months; indeed, 74 (40 per cent) believed they would always need to take the drugs. Reponses showed only small variations in the previous duration of treatment. Most present users (160, 88 per cent) claimed they would like to stop, this desire being most strongly expressed by those with over 5 years' consumption. The principal reason for not stopping involved fears of the return of symptoms.

Those who had made attempts to give up the drugs (148, 82 per cent) had generally managed without them for only a few weeks. The shorter the drug-free period, the greater the likelihood of claiming they had felt worse without the tablets.

There was widespread belief in the general practitioner's acquiescence in continued drug-taking: more than three-quarters (149) of the present users claimed that their doctors either wished them to continue or did not mind. Only one in five said their general pracitioners had ever tried to 'get (them) off the tablets'.

The process of withdrawal
Just under half of the past users had stopped taking the drugs more than a year ago; only 16 (20 per cent) had stopped within the previous 3 months. Only a quarter recalled having felt better without the drugs, although a further 26 (34 per cent) conceded that they had felt 'better in some ways but worse in others'. Those who had felt worse were asked to describe their experiences. The most commonly reported symptoms were anxiety, panic attacks and tremor, although a wide variety of somatic and functional complaints were mentioned. Half had gradually reduced the dosage and half had abruptly stopped the medication. Those who had been taking the drugs daily were more likely to report having felt worse after stopping than less frequent consumers, yet the duration of drug-taking appeared to have little influence on the assessment of withdrawal effects.

Just over one-third of past users believed they would need to take psychotropic drugs again in the future, although those who had achieved at least one year without them were more adamant than the rest that they were unlikely to start again. The most common reasons given for anticipated future use were the likelihood of life events and stress leading to a return of symptoms. Indeed, 33, (42 per cent) past users believed that the problem or complaint which had led to their taking the drugs had not been resolved.

Discussion

There were fewer elderly respondents than would have been anticipated from prevalence studies (e.g. Parish 1971; Woodcock 1970; Murray *et al.* 1981); this is probably a reflection of the readership of the magazine. The relatively low proportion of current hypnotic takers is also likely to stem from the younger age profile of the present sample compared with that of long-term psychotropic drug-takers in the community (Anderson 1980).

Both past and present users exhibited substantial physical and psychological symptoms, although the latter group was more impaired. The co-existence of physical, psychiatric and psychosocial disorders among psychotropic drug takers is well documented (Shepherd *et al.* 1960; Munro 1969; Williams 1978; Solow 1975).

They claimed frequency of drug-taking appears high, although Sackett and Haynes (1976) have demonstrated frequent discrepancies between patient reports and biochemical measures of consumption. The present users' reports of unpleasant symptoms during drug-free periods suggest that regular daily consumption is more commonly linked to these symptoms when the drug is withdrawn, although the duration of drug-taking appeared to have little influence. Their descriptions of effects experienced after withdrawal are consistent with those described by Marks (1978) as indicative of physical dependence on benzodiazepines, although he does emphasize the difficulties in distinguishing between abstinence syndrome and a return of the original symptoms.

The high proportion who were satisfied that the drugs had helped them accords with the findings of Parry *et al.* (1973) that 77 per cent of psychotropic users claimed that the drugs had helped 'a great deal' or 'quite a bit'. A high level of psychological dependency seemed to have developed among present users. They tended to see their drug-taking extending indefinitely into the future: psychotropics had become a means of sustaining daily life, rather than representing a determinate course of treatment. Although professing a desire to stop, many claimed they were unable to do so without a return of symptoms. Experiences during brief drug-free periods confirm to the patient that the symptoms are still present. It is suggested that a vicious cycle has developed, with possible withdrawal symptoms implicated in the rapid retreat to drug-taking.

Marks (1978) emphasizes the need for gradual withdrawal over a period of 1–2 weeks. Among the past users in our sample who gradually withdrew, there was a higher proportion reporting that they felt better without the drugs. The role of the general practitioner is crucial in this process; educating the patient about possible short-term symptoms and providing support during this period might enhance the long-term drug-taker's chance of withdrawal. Only a minority of present takers claimed their general practitioners would like them to give up, and only a third of past users said they had received any assistance in the process from their general practitioner. These findings should be treated with caution; the desirability of complying with medical advice might lead chronic users to interpret repeat prescribing as evidence of their doctor's approval of continued use.

The majority of respondents had been taking psychotropic drugs for over 5 years and many present users expressed anxiety about prolonged use. There was marked ambivalence towards the drugs; a desire to give up coupled with pessimism about their ability to do so, and with the belief that the drugs were helping them to function in daily life.

A longitudinal study of psychotropic drug recipients is currently being planned; this will allow a systematic exploration of the processes leading to chronic drug-taking.

Acknowledgements

This project was undertaken as part of a research programme, funded by the Department of Health and Social Security, under the direction of Professor M. Shepherd.

I would like to record my thanks to Dr Paul Williams for help in designing the questionnaires and categorizing symptoms and drugs, and to Professor Shepherd, Dr Williams, and Dr Anthony Clare for their helpful comments on drafts. Miss Gillian Andrews provided invaluable help in coding the questionnaires. I am indebted to the respondents for completing the questionnaires in such detail.

References

Anderson, R.M. (1980) The use of repeatedly prescribed medicines. *Journal of the Royal College of General Practitioners* 30: 609–13.

Balter, M.B., Levine J., and Manheimer, D. (1974) Cross-national study of the extent of anti-anxiety/sedative drug use. *New England Journal of Medicine* 290: 769–74.

Belloc, N.B., Breslow, L., and Hochstim, J.R. (1971) Measurement of physical health in a general population survey. *American Journal of Epidemiology* 93: 328–36.

Cochrane, R. (1980) A comparative evaluation of the Symptom Rating Test and the Langner 22-item Index for use in epidemiological surveys. *Psychological Medicine* 10: 115–24.

Kellner, R. and Sheffield, B.F. (1973) A self-rating scale of distress. *Psychological Medicine* 3: 88–100.

Lader, M. (1980) *Dependence on Prescribed Psychotropic Drugs*. Welwyn Garden City: SKF Publications.

Marks, J. (1978) *The Benzodiazepines. Use, Over-Use, Mis-Use, Abuse.* Lancaster: MTP Press.

Munro, A. (1969) Psychiatric illness in gynaecological out-patients. *British Journal of Psychiatry* 115: 807–09.

Murray, J., Dunn, G., Williams, P., and Tarnopolsky, A. (1981) Factors affecting the consumption of psychotropic drugs. *Psychological Medicine* 11: 551–60.

Parish, P.A. (1971) The prescribing of psychotropic drugs in general practice. *Journal of the Royal College of General Practitioners* 21, supp. 14: 1–77.

Parry, H.J., Balter, M.B., Mellinger, G.D., Cisin, I.H., and Manheimer, D.I. (1973) National patterns of psychotherapeutic drug use. *Archives of General Psychiatry* 28: 769–83.

Sackett, D.L. and Haynes, B. (1976) *Compliance with Therapeutic Regimens.* Baltimore: John Hopkins University Press.

Shepherd, M., Davies, B., and Culpan, R. (1960) Psychiatric illness in a general hospital. *Acta Psychiatrica et Neurologica Scandinavica* 35: 518–25.

Skegg, D., Doll, R., and Perry, J. (1977) Use of medicines in general practice. *British Medical Journal* i: 917–19.

Solow, C. (1975) Psychotropic drugs in somatic disorder. *International Journal of Psychiatry in Medicine* 6: 267–82.

Williams, P. (1978) Physical ill-health and psychotropic drug prescription: a review. *Psychological Medicine* 8: 683–93.

Williams, P., Murray, J., and Clare, A. (1982) A longitudinal study of psychotropic drug prescription. *Psychological Medicine* 12(1): 201–06.

Woodcock, J. (1970) Long-term consumers of psychotropic drugs. In M. Balint, J. Hunt, D. Joyce, M. Marinker, and J. Woodcock (eds) *Treatment or Diagnosis*, 147–76. London: Tavistock Publications.

## PART 3

Influences on tranquilliser use

6
Introduction

A substantial amount of research effort has been devoted to the investigation of a wide range of factors which have been thought to influence tranquilliser prescribing, and it is this topic that is addressed in this section. These factors can be considered in four non-mutually exclusive categories (*Figure 1*), 'the socio-cultutal milieu', 'the patient', 'the doctor', and 'the doctor-patient interaction'. As *Figure 1* shows, these categories can be thought of as arranged in a hierarchy of three levels of 'distance' from the act of prescribing itself. Thus the socio-cultural milieu can be thought of as exerting an influence on prescribing via the doctor and the patient at the second level, and via the doctor-patient interaction at the third level; doctor and patient influences on prescribing can themselves be thought of as operating via the doctor-patient interaction. It is worth noting that, as indicated by the direction of the arrows in *Figure 1*, influence is not all one-way: experience of specific doctor-patient encounters will inform and modify the views and attitudes of individual patients and doctors, which collectively shape and determine the prevailing social consensus.

Two types of influence can be considered under the heading 'the socio-cultural milieu'. First are the prevailing attitudes to and the beliefs about tranquilliser use itself: changes in these attitudes were discussed in Part 1. As was made clear, the general trend in recent years has been towards a more questioning and more critical view of tranquilliser use (as indeed it has with regard to doctors and health care in general (Jefferys and Sachs 1983, Cartwright 1983)). This has been associated with a deceleration and more recently a reversal in the trend of increasing tranquilliser prescribing that characterized the late 1960s and early 1970s. While there is no definite evidence that the association is causal, such a conclusion would be hard to escape.

It is not only prevailing attitudes about drugs themselves that may influence tranquilliser prescribing: generally prevailing views on other issues, which themselves are related to tranquilliser use, may be important. For example, the sex difference in tranquilliser recipients (women > men)

Figure 1 Influences on tranquilliser prescribing

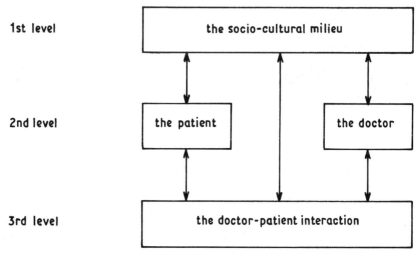

is one of the most consistent findings in the literature, and one of the many explanations that has been advanced is in terms of the stereotyped attitudes of many (male) physicians towards women (see, for example, Cooperstock 1971; Gabe and Lipshitz-Phillips 1984). The position of women in society has changed in recent years (Oakley 1981; Stacey and Price 1981; Whitelegg *et al.* 1982), and there is certainly evidence to suggest that such change has resulted in an attenuation of the sex difference in depression (Kessler and Macrae 1981, and a similar finding can be adduced from Hagnell *et al.*'s (1982) data). Such changes may well form part of the matrix of factors responsible for the changes in tranquilliser prescribing.

The 'socio-cultural milieu' may be presumed to exert an influence on tranquilliser prescribing via the *doctor* and the *patient* at the second level.

Since the prescription of a tranquilliser always (in the United Kingdom) requires the sanction of a doctor, it is clear that s/he will exert an important influence on the extent of tranquilliser prescribing. In the first paper in this part, Hemminki reviews the literature on factors which affect a doctor's propensity to prescribe. These include education, personal characteristics, the influence of colleagues, and, importantly, the influence of the pharmaceutical industry, exerted primarily by means of advertising.

Drug advertisements for psychoactive and other prescribed drugs have been the subject of much research effort. The second paper in this section, by Prather and Fidell, was one of the earliest studies on this topic. Their study, which demonstrates the influence of sex role stereotypes on the content of drug advertisements, exemplifies one way in which generalized societal attitudes (conceptualized at the first level in *Figure 1*) may exert an influence on the doctor (conceptualized at the second level in *Figure 1*) and hence on the prescription of tranquillisers. Other recent papers on drug advertising include those by Mant and Darroch (1975), Stimson (1975), Smith and Griffin (1977), and Chapman (1979).

Influences on tranquilliser prescribing which are associated with or derived from the patient also require comment. First, there are those aspects directly related to the patient's perceived and reported health. It is a truism that ill-health is an important factor in drug prescribing: indeed, in the United Kingdom, there is evidence that some 90 per cent of patients who are treated with tranquillisers by their general practitioner have levels of psychological ill-health that would be regarded as significant by a psychiatrist (Williams, Murray, and Clare 1982; Catalan *et al.*, this volume). Furthermore, there is strong evidence (reviewed by Williams 1978) that tranquillisers (and antidepressants) are widely prescribed in response to physical, as opposed to psychological, ill-health.

It would be naïve to assume, however, that health is the only factor requiring consideration, since there is increasing evidence that a variety of social influences is important. Foremost among these are the growing level of 'social stress' (Waldron 1977); the impact of being without a full-time paid job (Cooperstock 1976); living alone and being deprived of social stimulation (Webb and Collette 1975); and the experience of an unhappy marriage (Murray, Williams, and Clare 1982; Linn and Davis 1971).

The third paper in this section, by Cafferata and her colleagues, describes the investigation of some of these features. By means of secondary analysis (Hyman 1972) of national (USA) health survey data, they demonstrate that for women, family role responsibilities, structures, and stressful events significantly affect the chance of receiving a psychotropic drug. Such findings applied even when health status was taken into account.

The *doctor-patient* interaction is conceptualized on the third level in *Figure 1*. While this has been the subject of a great deal of research – much of it ably reviewed in Pendelton and Hasler (1983) – relatively little attention has been directed to the relationship between the doctor-patient interaction and the prescription of tranquillisers. There is, however, some indirect evidence. For example, Goldberg and Huxley (1980) demonstrated that certain aspects of a general practitioner's 'interviewing style' were important determinants of the accurate identification of patients with psychological ill-health. The final study in this section, by Raynes, is one of the few attempts to investigate directly the relationship between psychotropic drug prescribing and what happens during the consultation.

References

Cartwright, A. (1983) Prescribing and the doctor–patient relationship. In

D. Pendleton and J. Hasler (eds) *Doctor–Patient Communication*. London: Academic Press.

Chapman, S. (1979) Advertising and psychotropic drugs: the place of myth in ideological reproduction. *Social Science and Medicine* 13A(6): 751–64.

Cooperstock, R. (1971) Sex differences in the use of mood modifying drugs: an explanatory model. *Journal of Health and Social Behaviour* 12(3): 238–44.

—— (1976) Psychotropic drug use amongst women. *Canadian Medical Association* 115: 760–63.

Gabe, J. and Lipshitz-Phillips, S. (1984) Tranquillisers as social control? *The Sociological Review* 32(3): 524–46.

Goldberg, D. and Huxley, P. (1980) *Mental Illness in the Community: The Pathway to Psychiatric Care*. London: Tavistock Publications.

Hagnell, O., Lanke, J., Rorsman, B., and Ojesjo, L. (1982) Are we entering an age of melancholy? *Psychological Medicine* 12(2): 279–90.

Hyman, H.H. (1972) *Secondary Analysis of Sample Surveys*. New York: John Wiley & Sons.

Jefferys, M. and Sachs, H. (1983) *Rethinking General Practice*. London: Tavistock Publications.

Kessler, R.C. and Macrae, J. (1981) Trends: The relationship between sex and psychological distress 1957–1976. *American Sociological Review* 45(4): 443–52.

Linn, L.S. and Davis, M.S. (1971) The use of psychotherapeutic drugs by middle-aged women. *Journal of Health and Social Behaviour* 12(4): 331–40.

Mant, A. and Darroch, D.B. (1975) Media images and medical images. *Social Science and Medicine* 9(11/12): 613–18.

Murray, J., Williams, P., and Clare, A. (1982) Health and social characteristics of long-term psychotropic drug takers. *Social Science and Medicine* 16(18): 1595–598.

Oakley, A. (1981) *Subject Women*. Oxford: Martin Robertson.

Pendelton, D. and Hasler, J. (eds) (1983) *Doctor–Patient Communication*. London: Academic Press.

Smith, M.C. and Griffin, L. (1977) Rationality of appeals used in the promotion of psychotropic drugs. A comparison of male and female models. *Social Science and Medicine* 11(6/7): 409–14.

Stacey, M. and Price, M. (1981) *Women, Power, and Politics*. London: Tavistock Publications.

Stimson, G. (1975) The message of psychotropic ads. *Journal of Communication* 25(3): 153–60.

Waldron, I. (1977) Increased prescribing of Valium, Librium and other drugs – an example of the influence of economic and social factors on the practice of medicine. *International Journal of Health Services* 7(1): 37–61,

Webb, S.D. and Collette, J. (1975) Urban ecological correlates of stress alleviative drug use. *American Behavioral Scientist* 18(6): 750–70.

Whitelegg, E., Arnot, M., Bartels, E., Beechey, V., Birke, L., Himmelweit, S., Leonard, D., Ruehl, S., and Speakman, M.A. (eds) (1982) *The Changing Experience of Women*. Oxford: Basil Blackwell.

Williams, P. (1978) Physical ill-health and psychotropic drug prescription – a review. *Psychological Medicine* 8(4): 683–93.

Williams, P., Murray, J., and Clare, A. (1982) A longitudinal study of psychotropic drug prescription. *Psychological Medicine* 12(1): 201–06.

7

Review of literature on the factors affecting drug prescribing

Elina Hemminki

Abstract   A review of the literature on the factors affecting drug prescribing in Western countries is given. Factors discussed are education, advertising, colleagues, control and regulation measures, demands from society and patients and doctor's characteristics. On the basis of the available literature the role of the drug industry seems especially important. Suggestions for futher studies are given.

Drug consumption is continually increasing in Western countries [1]. Most of the drugs are issued on prescription [1]. Whatever the fundamental causes for increasing drug consumption are, it is largely regulated by the physicians, because they control the prescriptions. If doctors are in such a key-position it is worth studying the factors which affect their prescribing habits. In the following a review on the literature on the factors affecting drug prescription is given.

Great variation in the prescribing practices of doctors has been found [2–5]. For instance, Maronde *et al.*, studying excessive prescribing, found that of a prescribing population of 870 physicians, 30 accounted for about 50 per cent of them [4]. Balter *et al.* discovered that the *top* 25 per cent of prescribers might account for as much as 50 per cent of the psychotropic drug prescriptions written [2].

If only medical factors influenced prescribing, the variation in prescribing practice might be explained by differing patient populations but many other factors (education, advertising, colleagues, working-circumstances, personality etc.) have been found to affect prescribing. A model of the factors affecting prescribing has been given in an earlier paper [6]. The different factors interlace to such an extent that their

Reprinted, with permission, from *Social Science and Medicine* 9: 111–15, 1975.

individual effects are difficult to evaluate. However, in order to influence drug prescribing habits it is important to know the mutual preponderance of the different factors. Very little is known of this aspect. The study made by Wilson *et al.* in England at the beginning of the 1960s indicated that the doctors obtained 32 per cent of their therapeutic information from their medical training, 28 per cent from drug firms, and 40 per cent from other sources (consultant advice, textbooks, periodicals etc.) [7]. The recently qualified doctor depended less on the information derived from the pharmaceutical industry. Jenssen *et al.* [8] reported that the doctors selected their drugs for standard therapy most commonly from the commercial drug catalogues, short review articles and advice from other colleagues. In a study made by Dunnell *et al.*, a quarter of the general practitioners considered information from drug firms and a quarter considered medical journals as the most helpful source of information about new drugs [9]. According to Linn *et al.* [10] the sources of information physicians prefer to use in learning about new drugs were significantly related to certain attitudes and beliefs about drugs in general. The real effects of the different sources cannot, however, be evaluated by direct questioning. In addition, the components of medical training, consultant advice, text books and periodicals should be considered.

Education

Education should provide basic therapeutic skills and maintain them. But its success varies between countries and universities. Some people have worried about the imbalance between accessibility to potent drugs and professional training in the use of those drugs [11]. The popularity of drugs is often short; the average market life of a drug – from its time of introduction to its withdrawal from the market – is only 5 years in Sweden and in the USA [12, 13]. Many drugs in current use did not exist when today's practising doctors were students. In many countries, including Finland, compulsory postgraduate education is lacking and is up to the individual doctor. Consequently in these countries education cannot have any decisive effect on prescribing.

In few studies has the effect of education been investigated. But in England, Lee *et al.* found no significant differences in prescribing patterns among doctors graduating from different medical schools [3]. On the other hand Joyce found that higher educational qualifications were associated with less prescribing of drugs of all kinds [14]. Becker *et al.* found that physicians with patterns of higher appropriateness ratings and lower chloramphenicol use were found to be younger and to have fewer years of professional experience but with more postgraduate training [15]. These studies suggest that education positively influences the quality of prescribing.

Advertising

The contribution of advertising to prescribing is debatable. Some representatives of the drug industry have said the effect of advertising to be slight or that it helps in keeping doctors up to date [16, 17]. Yet the pharmaceutical industry trusts in sales promotion to the extent of investing in it from 12–40 per cent of sales (depending on the country and the method of calculation) [18–22]. Marketing expenditure is not the same for all product categories. It tends to increase from highly potent and medically effective remedies to palliative substances [22]. A major proportion of the sales promotion funds is directed to professional advertising. Financially the most important form is the drug representatives [19–21]. In Finland there were 309 drug representatives (one per 10 doctors) in 1968 [23, 24].

Much of the rivalry between drug firms is more apparent than real. The real enemies to the profits of drug firms are those institutions which attempt to decrease and control drug consumption. This became evident at the time of the thalidomide disaster. Other drug firms felt discomfort, since the case 'might throw suspicion' on the whole international pharmaceutical industry [25]. The common interest of drug firms and retailers is also seen in the founding of cooperational organizations at the national as well as the international level [26]. The purpose of advertising is to affect doctors' prescribing habits, to make them prescribe as many profitable preparations as possible [27]. To reach this goal advertising has escalated from pure communication to manipulation of the conscious and unconscious opinions which create new needs and habits of consumption. According to the constructors of advertisements:

> 'medical men are subject to the same kind of stress, the same emotional influences as affect the laymen. Physicians have, as part of their self-image a determined feeling that they are rational and logical, particularly in their choice of pharmaceuticals. The advertiser must appeal to this rational self-image, and at the same time make a deeper appeal to the emotional factors which really influence sales.' [28]

Advertising techniques are used which force doctors to prescribe drugs on the basis of attributes other than their therapeutic activities, and, from a medical point of view, the quality of drug advertisements is often questionable [29–31]. The effect of advertising is potentiated by other means as well: at least two kinds of social reward exist for over-prescribing: client approval and dissonance from rereading advertisements for drugs already prescribed [32].

Advertising ignores the fact that there are other forms of patient management than drug therapy [33]. But to increase drug consumption it is not enough to treat all illnesses with drugs, new illnesses must be created [32]. The sales and market research departments of drug firms employ medical advisers and use market research companies to carry out field work on doctors' prescribing and attitudes [34]. Market research by those companies is highly sophisticated. A seminar on the marketing of pharmaceutical products gives some indication of the level of study. For example, there were papers on: segmentation of doctors' types, the development of a technique for measuring the reactions of general practitioners to marketing prices and journal advertising, a simulation model of the doctors' prescribing, the differing promotional requirements for consultants, hospital doctors and general practitioners [34]. Garai, a former Senior Writer in a drug firm, stated:

> 'As an advertising man, I can assure you that advertising which does not work does not continue to run. If experience did not show beyond doubt that the great majority of doctors are splendidly responsive to current ethical advertising, new techniques would be devised in short order. And if indeed, candor, accuracy, scientific completeness and a permanent ban on cartoons came to be essential for the successful promotion of ethical drugs, advertising would have no choice but to comply.' [19]

The questionable nature of the contents and techniques of advertising is disquieting because of the positive and trustful attitudes of doctors [10, 35–38]. Generally, the representatives are appreciated most, although in one study, among medical students, journal advertising was rated above the representatives as a source of drug information [39]. Sixty-four per cent of the Finnish doctors considered information given by representatives to be useful, and only 14 per cent considered it useless [36]. Even greater satisfaction was expressed with the scientific journals published by drug firms and the courses arranged by drug firms. Advertising by journals and by post was not so highly appreciated. However, only 9 per cent of the Finnish doctors had refused to receive medical advertising post to their homes in the year 1972 even though it makes a heavy pile to receive [40]. The positive attitude towards advertising can be expected to influence prescribing [41, 42]. According to Becker *et al.*, the doctors with more appropriate prescriptions were more critical of drug firms [15].

Besides advertising doctors are also indirectly affected by drug firms in many other ways. Through finance and other support the drug firms exert a notable effect on medical journals, education, post-graduate education, research, and all affect prescribing [43–49]. Although some companies provide excellent educational services it ought not to be forgotten that drug firms are in business to sell drugs and many of these educational facilities are referred to by the industry as 'below the belt' [34].

Colleagues

According to Wilson *et al.*, the doctors announced that their therapeutical knowledge for prescribing was derived in 15 per cent of cases from another general practitioner or a consultant [7]. In the study made by Linn *et al.*, 37 per cent of the doctors answering the questionnaire considered other physicians as the most important way of finding out about new prescription drugs [10]. Coleman *et al.* found that doctors who maintained a variety of contacts with a large number of colleagues introduced the new drug before their relatively isolated colleagues [50]. It should be noted, however, that the effect of colleagues is always secondary to some other factors, such as advertising and education. For example, the following advertisements issued by the Advertising Department of the New England Journal of Medicine can be examined:

'What every medical media buyer should know about subscribers to the New England Journal of Medicine. This latest examination of NEJM readers reveals some startling statistics about their wide sphere of influence on the medical profession. It is a study that will give you a clear picture of why these key physicians are important to the success of many marketing efforts and the one best way to reach them.' [51]

Control and regulation measures

Literature on this subject is scanty. This may be partly because control measures are temperately and narrowly used by health authorities. For instance, official drug registration has been required in Finland only since 1964 [52]. An experiment was made in Norway on the effect of a tighter control on the sales of narcotics [53] which showed that drug consumption could be decreased by control measures, at least for short periods. In South Carolina too, where benzodiazepines were restricted, drug consumption decreased [54]. Another investigation in an Indian reservation showed that prescriptions for all minor tranquillisers could be reduced by a third by extensive propaganda directed at both staff and patients [54]. In Sweden the sale of drugs containing dipyrone was reduced after warnings of their side-effects were given by the Swedish Adverse Drug Reaction Committee [55]. During a study of psychotropic drug usage in a Danish hospital the high consumption was notably decreased in some drug groups [56]. Wolff reported that during a study in which peer-review was applied to doctors, the prescribing rates were very low (one prescription for every two office visits) [57]. Similarly a large prepaid group practice in Seattle has shown markedly lower prescribing costs than national averages in the USA, and part of this is due to control of the use of psychotropic drugs under their drug insurance benefit scheme [57]. These studies suggest a positive effect of control measures if used effectively. The drug industry seems to have understood this and consequently considers good relations with health authorities to be important [58].

It is often suggested that making drugs cheaper increases consumption. However in Great Britain, where the National Health Service has operated since 1948, the drug consumption is lower than in Western countries in general [22]. There prescription fees have been repeatedly abandoned and reintroduced since 1948. Such measures did not markedly affect drug use even though the numbers of prescriptions varied [22, 59]. This contradiction is mainly explained by the fact that imposition of charges makes doctors prescribe larger quantities to save their patients from paying the fixed charge frequently [22].

Demands from society and patients

It has been suggested that too little time for each patient might make doctors write more prescriptions [27]. So Stolley *et al.*'s observation that doctors who had hurried practices and more assistants and spent less time with each patient were better prescribers is somewhat astonishing, since the study also pointed out that more appropriate prescribing tended to be associated with a smaller percentage of office visits in which a prescription was written [60]. Accordingly, Dunnell and Cartwright found that doctors with relatively few patients wrote more prescriptions per patient than those with large lists [9], even though 52 per cent of the doctors thought that they would write fewer prescriptions if they had more time to spend with each patient. One plausible explanation for this is that doctors looking after small numbers of patients spend more time with them and in doing so find out about more conditions for which they prescribe medicines [9].

It is reasonable to expect that other circumstances besides the amount of work affect a doctor's prescribing. Families of the patients, employers, etc. impose their expectations on doctors and doctors have their role in keeping the system functioning [61]. The effects of these factors on prescribing remain to be established. Of old, magic is connected to the role of physician, and much of this magic has been transferred through drugs [62, 63]. Prescribing is essential to protect the image of the doctor's profession: 'The doctor may attempt to remain on the pedestal on which his patients and society at large have placed him, with a lavish supply of prescriptions' [62]. On the other hand, Muller [27] has seen prescribing as a common interest of both the doctors and the patients:

'Prescribing is, theoretically at least, a means of terminating the interview in a fashion that satisfies both doctor and patient. The prescribing is a signal for the approaching end of the encounter, it both summarizes and carries forward the relationship, it is an expression of concern, and it deals with the interests of both parties in a manner perceived as equitable.'

It is difficult to estimate which one of these explanations above is relevant. The relevance may differ greatly from one doctor-patient contact to another.

The idea that one of the main reasons for increased drug consumption is the demand from the patients is often put forward [62, 64], and the stress created by today's way of living is emphasized [65]. Health services are more available so more people consult the doctor for minor ailments. According to this view doctors are only passive distributors of drugs. In the case of psychotropic drugs apparently: 'We may see the doctor as helpless in the face of a population who have an overwhelming need to alter chemically their experience of the world in which they live' [62].

However, these opinions seem to be based more on personal views than on thorough studies. A study of Balter *et al.* [2] about the attitudes toward psychotropic drug use indicated that the American public remained generally conservative and most of those currently taking tranquillising drugs, or who had done so in the past, expressed a discomfort with their drug taking. So, at least in the case of psychotropic drugs, the claim that patient's demands were important was not supported.

Although convenience, ignorance and trust of the patients probably explains much of the consumption of drugs available without prescription, patient demand may have been exaggerated in the case of ethical drugs – particularly psychotropic drugs because psychic diseases are largely aversed and a request for psychotropic drugs might signify confession of psychic problems.

But once a doctor has prescribed psychotropic drugs and taught his patients an easy and acceptable way to handle their problems, perhaps on later visits the patients may again ask for these drugs. Or the patient may learn this method of solving problems from his relatives or friends. A study by Pernanen in Canada showed that in over half of the families someone had received psychotropic drugs during a year [66]. (If combination preparations containing psychotropic drugs were included, the proportion was much higher.) The doctors' prescribing habits might thus influence patients' expectations.

Doctor's characteristics

Menzel *et al.* found 'modernism' (readiness to try new drugs) to be a consistent trait in a doctor [67] and the more 'profession-orientated' doctors used a drug earlier than less 'profession-orientated' ones [68]. In England, where national records of drug prescriptions are available, Joyce *et al.* interviewed doctors and compared the records with the real prescription figures [69]. In their study no more than 15 per cent of the variation in individual patterns of prescribing could be explained by the personal factors studied. Besides higher educational qualifications, an 'orientation towards the whole person' was associated with lower prescribing of drugs of all kinds. Linn, studying the doctors' attitudes toward the appropriate use of psychotherapeutic drugs, found that the evaluations of such drugs' use were more likely to be related to characteristics reflecting values, social position or social background than characteristics reflecting medical or scientific background [10, 70]. Stolley *et al.* interviewed doctors about their characteristics and prescribing habits. Appropriateness of prescribing was determined by expert judges [60], and by checking the amount of chloramphenicol prescribed [71]. They found more appropriate prescribers to be younger, more cosmopolitan, modern and concerned with both the psycho-social and quality dimensions of medical care. They were more dissatisfied with their communities and their patients, and the pharmaceutical industry had a poorer image to them. They had a greater willingness to approve of government regulation of drug prices. No correlation was found with preventative orientation or political choice. Parish has reported prescribing of psychotropic drugs to be higher among younger doctors, even among doctors with a special interest in psychological disorders [72].

No generalizations can be drawn from all these studies. The aspects examined were different, and methods, materials and years of investigations varied. However, it is obvious that differences found in prescribing practices can be described also at the level of the individual doctor.

Suggestions for further work

As the above review shows, the knowledge on the factors affecting drug prescribing is limited, at least in the medical and other scientific literature. It is possible that more accurate knowledge exists in sources not freely accessible to investigators, e.g. in drug firms.

The factors affecting doctors' prescribing may be divided in two groups in respect to possibilities of intervention: (1) factors easily modified by administrative measures, such as advertising, education and extent of control: (2) factors not easily modified by administrative activities, such as the characteristics of patients and doctors, and the role of physicians. If the aim is to describe the *phenomenon* of prescribing, all of the aspects listed above are worth study, so limited is knowledge of them all. The nature of the factors may vary from country to country and national studies are therefore needed.

If the aim is to produce information for prompt improvement of the prescribing habits, only the factors which can be altered by administrative activities are worth study. Even though the relative importance of the different factors or their quantitive effects are unestablished, the available literature and common knowledge appear to suggest drug firms as one of the major factors in the Western countries. Drug firms influence doctors in many ways. So far the traditional advertising forms, journal and post advertising have been the most studied. The effect of other forms of advertising, such as detail-men, information services of drug firms (journals, booklets, abstracting services), and PR-activities, should be studied more thoroughly. The 'non-advertising' activities of drug firms and the effect of these activities on the prescribing of individual doctors should be additionally analysed. Such 'non-advertising' activities of drug firms are their effect on research policy, their relationships to medical trainees and health authorities, and the financial dependence of medical journals, societies and post-graduate education on drug firms.

The earlier studies suggest that education positively influences the quality of prescribing, as discussed above. The features, both intellectual and affectional, correlating to good prescribing should be unravelled in more detail. The nature of good prescribing should be defined.

The regulatory measures used by authorities probably greatly differ from one country to another. The collection of data on the effects of these measures on prescribing would be easiest in countries where drug sales statistics, an essential part of the result of controlling, are available for researchers. Particular attention should be paid to the object of control, e.g. whether it is more effective to control the prescriptional habits of individual doctors or the factors affecting him, such as advertising.

Note

This review is based on the author's thesis Prescription of Psychotropic Drugs in Outpatient Care [1].

References

1   Hemminki, E. Prescription of psychotropic drugs in outpatient care. *Acta Universitatis Tamperensis*, A, vol. 58. Tampereen Yliopisto, Tampere. 1974.
2   Balter, M.B. and Levine, J. The nature and extent of psychotropic drug usage in the United States. *Psychopharmacol. Bull.* 5:3. 1969.
3   Lee, J.A.H., Draper, P.A., and Weatherall, M. Prescribing in three English towns. *Millbank Mem. Fd Quart.* 43:285. 1965.
4   Maronde, R.F., Lee, P.V., McCarron, M.M., and Seibert, S. A study of prescribing patterns. *Med. Care* 9:383. 1971.
5   Schroeder, S.A., Kenders, K., Cooper, J.K., and Piemme, T.E. Use of laboratory tests and pharmaceuticals. Variation among physicians and effect of cost audit on subsequent use. *J. Am. Med. Ass.* 225:969. 1973.

6 Hemminki, E. (1975) The role of prescriptions in therapy. *Medical Care* 13(2): 150–59.

7 Wilson, C.W.M., Banks, J.A., Mapes, R.E.A., and Korte, S.M.T. Influence of different sources of therapeutic information on prescribing by general practitioners. *Brs. Med. J.* 3:599. 1963.

8 Jenssen, P.G. and Lunde, P.K.M. Legens avendelse og vurdering av legemiddel-informasjonen i Norge, Resultatet av en generell rundsporring hosten 1970 og en tilleggsundersokelse hosten 1971. *T. norske Laegeforen* 92:407. 1972.

9 Dunnell, K. and Cartwright, A. *Medicine takers, prescribers and hoarders.* Routledge & Kegan Paul, London. 1972.

10 Linn, L.S. and Davis, M.S. Physicians' orientation toward the legitimacy of drug use and their preferred source of new drug information. *Social Science and Medicine* 6:199. 1972.

11 Friebel, H. Drug safety in theory and practice. *WHO Chron.* 27:59. 1973.

12 Läkedelsförmånen. SOU 1966; **28**, Stockholm, 1966.

13 Norwood, G.J. and Smith, M.C. Market mortality of new products in the pharmaceutical industry. *J. Am. pharm. Ass.* 11:592. 1971.

14 Joyce, D. What was prescribed. In *Treatment or diagnosis. A study of repeat prescriptions in general practice,* (edited by Balint, M. *et al.*) p. 63. Tavistock Publications. London. 1970.

15 Becker, M.H., Stolley, P.D., Lasagna, L., McEvilla, J.D., and Sloane, L.M. Differential education concerning therapeutics and resultant physician prescribing patterns. *J. Med. Educ.* 47:118, 1972.

16 Bauer, R.A. and Wortzel, L.H. Doctor's choice: the physician and his sources of information about drugs. *J. Marketing Res.* 3:40. 1966.

17 Teeling-Smith, G. Advertising and the pattern of prescribing. *Proc. R. Soc. Med.* 61:748, 1968.

18 Cooper, M.H. *Prices and profits in the pharmaceutical industry.* Pergamon Press, Oxford. 1966.

19 Garai, P.R. Advertising and promotion of drugs. In *Drugs in Our Society,* (edited by Talalay, P.). Johns Hopkins. Baltimore. 1964.

20 Läkemedelsindustrin. SOU 1969: **36**, Stockholm, 1969.

21 *Report of the committee of enquiry into the relationship of the pharmaceutical industry with the National Health Service 1965–1967.* Chairman: Lord Sainsbury. HMSO. London. 1967.

22 Schicke, R.K. The pharmaceutical market and prescription drugs in the Federal Republic of Germany: Gross-national comparisons. *Int. J. Hlth Serv.* 3: 223. 1973.

23 Lääketeollisuus-ja apteekkilaitoskomitean mietintö. Komitea-mietintö 1970. A. 18, Helinski. 1970.

24 Yleinen terveyden ja sairaanhoito 1967–68. Suomen virallinen tilasto XI. 70. Helsinki. 1970.

25 Sjöström, H. and Nilsson, R. *Thalidomide and the power of the drug companies.* Penguin, Harmondsworth. 1972.

26 Bruun, K., Lynn, P., and Rexed, I. *The gentlemen's club. International control of drugs and alcohol.* (In press.)

27 Muller, C. The overmedicated society: forces in the marketplace for medical care. *Science* 16: 488. 1972.

28 Smith, M.C. *Principles of pharmaceutical marketing.* Lead Febiger, Philadelphia, 1968.

29 Abraham, R.E. *Analyse van de Geneesmiddelenreclame Door Middel van Advertenties in Medische Vakbladen*. De Erven F. Bohn N.V., Haarlem, 1970.

30 Pillard, R.C. Drug advertising and the prescribing physician. *New Physician* 20, 183, 1971.

31 Wilson, K.S. Analysis of a general practitioner's communications from the pharmaceutical industry. *Hlth Bull*. 27, 40, 1969.

32 Smith, M.C. Social barriers to rational drug therapy. *Am. J. Hosp. Pharm*. 29, 121, 1972.

33 Ingelfinger, F.J. Advertising: informative but not educational. *New Engl. J. Med*. 286, 1318, 1972.

34 Parish, P.A. What influences have led to increased prescribing of psychotropic drugs? *J.R. Coll. Gen. Practit*. 23, 49, 1973.

35 Worthen, D.B. Prescribing influences: an overview. *Br. J. med. Educ*. 7, 109, 1973.

36 Laitinen, A. Lääkäreiden asenteet ammattikuntaansa kohdistuvaan lääkemainontaan. *Suom. LääkL*. 28, 1907, 1973.

37 Ljödquist, J. Dags för mera selektiv information. *Läkartidningen* 69, (I), 35, 1972.

38 Stolley, P.D. and Lasagna, L. Prescribing patterns of physicians. *J. Chron. Dis*. 22, 395, 1969.

39 Barnes, C.J. and Holcenberg, J.S. Student reactions to pharmaceutical promotion practices. *Northw. med*. 70, 262, 1971.

40 Suhtautuminen mainospostiin. *Suom. LääkL*. 27, 2097, 1972.

41 Garb, S. Teaching medical students to evaluate drug advertising. *J. med. Educ*. 35, 729, 1960.

42 Shepherd, M. The use and abuse of drugs in psychiatry, *Lancet* 1, 31. 1970.

43 Barnhart, R. The medical profession-drug industry alliance. *New Physician* 20, 164, 1971.

44 Cooperstock, R. Some factors involved in the increased prescribing of psychotropic drugs. In: *Social aspects of the medical use of psychotropic drugs* (edited by Cooperstock, R.). Addiction Research Foundation of Ontario, Toronto, 1974.

45 Ingelfinger, F.J. Annual discourse – swinging copy and sober science. *New Engl. J. Med*. 281, 526, 1969.

46 May, C.D. Selling drugs by educating physicians. *J. med. Educ*. 36, 1, 1961.

47 Mintz, M. FDA and Panalba: A conflict of commercial, therapeutic goals. *Science*, 165, 875, 1969.

48 Mintz M. and Cohen, J.S. *America, Inc: Who owns and operates the United States*, pp. 34–35, 253–255. Dell P., New York, 1972.

49 Seidenberg, R. Advertising and abuse of drugs. *New Engl. J. Med*. 284, 789, 1971.

50 Coleman, J., Menzel, H., and Katz, E. Social processes in physicians' adoptation of drugs. *J. Chron. Dis*. 9, 1, 1959.

51 *Drug Trade News*, August 7, p. 8, 1972.

52 Mattila, M., Airaksinen, M.M., and Rautiainen, I. Viisi vuotta farmaseuttisten erikoisvalmisteiden rekisteröintiä Suomessa. *Suom. LääkL*. 24, 1098, 1969.

53 Norsk Medisinaldepot. Beretning og regnskap 1.1–31.12., 1971.

54 Benzodiazepines: use, overuse, misuse, abuse? *Lancet* **1**, 1101, 1973.
55 Böttiger, L.E. and Westerholm, B. Drug-induced blood dyscrasias in Sweden. *Br. med. J.* **3**, 339, 1973.
56 Jensen, F.F. and Bille, M. Forbruget af psykofarmaka og sovemidler på et central sygehus. *Arch. Pharmaci og Chemi* **126**, 675, 1969.
57 Wolff, S. The social responsibility of the physician in prescribing mind-affecting drugs. In: *Social aspects of the medical use of psychotropic drugs* (edited by Cooperstock, R.) Addiction Research Foundation of Ontario, Toronto, 1974.
58 Woodward, E.G. The development and future structure of the pharmaceutical industry. *Svensk. farm. T.* **77**. 356, 1973.
59 Dunlop, D. Drug control and the British Health Service. *Ann. intern. Med.* **71**, 237, 1973.
60 Stolley, P.D., Becker, M.H., Lasagna, L., McEvilla J.D., and Sloane, L.M. The relationship between physician characteristics and prescribing appropriateness. *Med. Care* **10**, 17, 1972.
61 Lennard, H.L., Epstein, L.J., Bernstein, A., and Ransom, D.C. *Mystification on Drug Misuse. Hazards in using psychoactive drugs*. Harper & Row, New York. 1972.
62 Marinker, M. The doctor's role in prescribing. *J.R. Coll. gen. Practit.* **23**, (2), 22, 1973.
63 Temkin, O. Historical aspects of drug therapy. In: *Drugs in our society* (edited by Talalay, P.). Johns Hopkins, Baltimore, 1964.
64 Fulton, W.W. Why do doctors prescribe psychotropic drugs? *J.R. Coll. gen. Practit.* **23**, (2), 22, 1973.
65 Balint, M., Hunt, J., Joyce, D., Marinker, M., and Woodcock, J. (eds) *Treatment or diagnosis. A study of repeat prescriptions in general practice*. Tavistock Publications, London, 1970.
66 Pernanen, K. Family patterns in prescriptions of psychotherapeutic drugs. In: *Social aspects of the medical use of psychotropic drugs* (edited by Cooperstock, R.). Addiction Research Foundation of Ontario, Totonto, 1974.
67 Menzel, H., Coleman, J., and Katz, E. Dimensions of being 'modern' in medical practice. *J. Chron Dis.* **9**, 20, 1959.
68 Coleman, J., Katz, E., and Menzel, H. The diffusion of an innovation among physicians. *Sociometry* **20**, 253, 1957.
69 Joyce, C.R.B., Last, J.M., and Weatherall, M. Personal factors as a cause of differences in prescribing by general practitioners. *Br. J. prev, soc. Med.* **22**, 170, 1968.
70 Linn, L.S. Physician characteristics and attitudes toward legitimate use of psychotherapeutic drugs. *J. Hlth Soc. Behav.* **12**, 132, 1971.
71 Becker, M.H., Stolley, P.D., Lasagna, L., McEvilla, J.D., and Sloane, L.M. Characteristics and attitudes of physicians associated with the prescribing of chloramphenicol. *HSMHA Health Rep.* **86**, 993, 1971.
72 Parish, P.A. The family doctor's role in psychotropic drug use. In: *Social aspects of the medical use of psychotropic drugs* (edited by Cooperstock, R.). Addiction Research Foundation of Ontario, Toronto, 1974.

8

Sex differences in the content and style of medical advertisements

Jane E. Prather and Linda S. Fidell

Abstract An analysis of drug advertisement from four leading American medical journals was performed to determine if content and style were related to the sex of the patient portrayed.

Content differences emerged in that advertisements for psychoactive drugs tended to show women while those for nonpsychoactive drugs showed men. Within the psychoactive drug category alone, women were shown with diffuse emotional symptoms while men were shown with anxiety because of pressures from work or from accompanying organic illness. Stylistic differences were also found. The parallel relationship between the advertising, physician attitudes and rates of psychoactive drug usage by women was discussed.

This study focuses on the relationship between sex differences in medical advertisements for drugs and physician attitudes as these attitudes are influenced by and/or reflected in drug advertisements. The sex of the patient is a salient variable because there are sex differences in the extent, type and source of drugs in use.

Women receive 60 per cent of the prescriptions for drugs in all categories, and 67 per cent of the prescriptions for psychoactive (mood-modifying) drugs [1]. A 1971 survey [2] indicated that 45 per cent of the women and 33 per cent of the men had taken psychoactive drugs in the preceding year. Chambers [3] concluded that women were the major users of barbiturates, non-barbiturate sedative-hypnotics, relaxants and minor tranquillisers, antidepressants, pep pills, diet pills, non-controlled narcotics and analgesics, and controlled narcotics (not including heroin). Men were the major users of marijuana/hashish, LSD, the inhalants, methedrine and heroin.

Reprinted, with permission, from *Social Science and Medicine* 9: 23–6. 1975.

Another sex difference in drug taking behaviour involves the source of the drug. Women are much more likely than men to obtain psychoactive drugs from a physician (primarily from their general practitioner or internist) while men obtain them from other (less legitimate) sources [2]. Obtaining psychoactive drugs from a physician rather than obtaining them from other sources has been shown to lead to longer term and more consistent usage of the drugs [2].

Because women tend to receive psychoactive drugs by prescription more frequently than men, it is relevant to inquire into the variables which encourage or discourage a physician from writing such a prescription.* Linn [6] found that physicians' attitudes about the legitimacy of prescribed psychoactive drug usage in a variety of settings were more strongly related to the social values and moral standards of the physicians than to their scientific backgrounds. Intervention of social values in judgements by physicians about legitimate drug use lends plausibility to the view that physicians' attitudes may be influenced by advertising techniques.

Physicians, in fact, report that drug advertisements are an important source of information. In a recent study [7], 73 per cent of physicians rated advertisements in medical journals as either somewhat or very important to them as sources of information about drugs. This source of information ranked behind only that of detailmen † (84 per cent) and other physicians (83 per cent) in importance for physicians. Although the exact extent of this influence has not been directly measured, the potential for influence is great. Any consistently developed view shown in the advertisements about characteristics of patients (male and female) may potentially influence the attitudes of physicians who consider this source of information important.

The present study involved in-depth content analysis of medical advertisements to determine which, if any, relationships exist between the sex of the patient shown in advertisements and the style and content of the advertisements.

Method

The sample of medical advertisements was taken from the *New England Journal of Medicine, California Medicine,* the *Journal of the American Medical Association,* and the *American Journal of Psychiatry*. These journals were selected because of their wide circulation as well as their prestige. One issue from each journal for each year between 1968 and 1972 was selected randomly from the complete set of issues for that year (see Appendix A for a list of issues sampled). All the advertisements from each issue of each journal were tabulated.

Advertisements were initially tabulated according to whether or not they included a specific reference to the sex of the patient for whom the drug was to be prescribed. Classification by sex was most often made according to the sex of the patient shown in accompanying photographs or sketches, although occasionally the sex was determined by display of sex-stereotyped paraphernalia (e.g. a purse or a wallet) or from a verbal description which specifically included reference to either a female or a male.

For advertisements for which the sex of the patient could be ascertained, information was collected as to the drug name, the drug company, the symptoms or disease for which the drug was advertised, the pictorial accompaniment and the verbal description of the complaint for which the drug was appropriate. In addition, the ages of the people displayed in the advertisements were estimated by the coders along with their race and social class.

For advertisements for which the sex of the patient could not be determined, information was collected as to whether the ailment was psychogenic (anxiety, depression or insomnia) or nonpsychogenic (all other conditions). Although we realize that certain other illnesses such as asthma, ulcers, hypertension and so forth, may have psychogenic origins, we felt that once a disease had progressed to the point that it could be identified by medical criteria such as X-rays or physiological disturbances, it was no longer strictly an emotional, as opposed to an organic illness.

Results and discussion

Sex-identifiable advertisements were tabulated according to whether the illness was psychogenic or nonpsychogenic and according to whether the patient was a female or a male. Of the 423 sex-identifiable advertisements, 48 per cent portrayed females as patients and 52 per cent males as patients. Of these 423 advertisements, 40 per cent were for alleviating primarily psychogenic symptoms and 60 per cent for primarily nonpsychogenic symptoms.

The sex-identifiable advertisements were further subdivided by type of illness (psychogenic and nonpsychogenic). For women, 59 per cent of the advertisements fell into the psychogenic category (41 per cent in the nonpsychogenic category) and for men the reverse was true (41 per cent psychogenic, 59 per cent nonpsychogenic). There was indeed, a strong relationship between type of illness and sex of patient; the χ^2-value (with 1 df) was 14.22 ($P < 0.001$). Expected frequencies for this χ^2 were calculated on the assumption that the sex of the patient was unrelated to the type of illness. The results indicate that more women (and fewer men) than would be expected by chance were associated with the psychogenic illness category.

However, because women use both psychoactive and nonpsychoactive drugs at rates greater than those for men [1] the distribution of

Table 1 *Analysis of drug advertisements for psychogenic and nonpsychogenic illnesses by sex of patient with expected frequencies calculated under assumptions of independence*

	psychogenic		nonpsychogenic		
female	101	(82)*	103	(122)	204
male	69	(88)	150	(131)	219
	170		253		423

* Expected frequency.

$\chi^2 = 14.22$, 1 df, $P < 0.001$.

advertisements may have been merely reflecting the actual frequency rates of usage of drugs in these categories. Another χ^2 was calculated, therefore, using as expected frequencies the rate with which women actually use psychoactive drugs (67 per cent of prescriptions) and nonpsychoactive drugs (60 per cent of prescriptions). The χ^2-value with these expected frequencies was 43.65, which is also significant at or beyond the 0.001 probability level. Surprisingly, the main source of the discrepancy between expected and observed frequencies did not appear in the psychoactive drug category (where, in fact, there were somewhat fewer women than predicted). The main source of the discrepancy was in the nonpsychoactive drug category where there were more male patients portrayed than had been predicted. The χ^2-value for the nonpsychoactive drug category alone was over 39 (see *Table 2*). This relationship indicates that women

Table 2 *Analysis of drug advertisements for psychogenic and nonpsychogenic illnesses by sex of patient using actual rates of drug usage among men and women as expected frequencies*

	psychogenic		nonpsychogenic		
female	101	(113.9; 67%)*	103	(151.8; 60%)	204
male	69	(56.1; 33%)	150	(101.2; 40%)	219
	170		253		423

* Expected frequency.

$\chi^2 = 43.65$, 1 df, $P < 0.001$.

tend to be shown as suffering from primarily emotional illness while men are shown as having primarily organic illness. If this reflects or influences the prevailing views of patients, physicians or both, then illness behavior and reactions to illness behavior may be sex related. That is, women may display (or be interpreted as displaying) emotional symptoms when the problem is organic, while men show (or are thought to show) organic symptoms when the 'cause' is emotional. The possibility for misdiagnosis for both sexes would appear, therefore, to be increased.† †

Table 3   *Reasons given for psychoactive drug usage by sex of patient*

	anxiety	insomnia	physical disability
female	54(45.6)*	13(13.8)	5(12.6)
male	22(30.4)	10(9.2)	16(8.4)

* Expected frequency under assumption of independence.
$\chi^2 = 15.39$. 2 df, $P < 0.001$.

The next analysis involved a breakdown of the reasons given for dispensing psychoactive drugs according to the sex of the patient. Hemminki [8] noted that the psychoactive drug advertisements, in general, showed greater appeal to emotion than advertisements for drugs in other categories. This relationship was confirmed in the present study, and particularly in those advertisements which showed a female as the patient. Advertisements in the psychoactive drug category alone were broken down by sex of patient and according to the type of symptom presented: (1) diffuse anxiety, tension or depression; (2) insomnia; or (3) tension accompanying physical disability or work. There was a strong relationship between these two variables (χ^2, with 2 df = 15.39, $P < 0.001$) with men portrayed as needing psychoactive drugs because of tension accompanying physical disability or work while women required them because of diffuse anxiety, tension or depression. One wonders whether or not the need for a prescription for a psychoactive drug would be recognized if the patient failed to present the symptoms in a sex-appropriate manner.

Advertisements also showed sex differences in both the ages of patients and the dispersions of ages. From estimates of the ages of patients portrayed in the advertisements, a Z-test of the mean differences in ages between men and women resulted in a value of 2.12 (significant at the 0.05 level). Male patients were shown as older than female patients by approximately 2 years. More meaningful, perhaps, was the significant difference in the dispersion of scores. An F-value of the ratio of variance in men's ages to variance in women's ages (with 186 and 189 df) was 1.48 which is significant at the 0.02 level. Women tended to be portrayed in the age range between 20 and 40 years while men were shown at a greater variety of ages. In addition, some of the advertisements showed young, attractive female patients in poses which might be considered alluring or provocative and with captions which might be considered suggestive. Consider the following examples:

'A very attractive young woman in a seductive pose wearing a smart outfit saying: "Dear Doctor, you made me what I am today – a whole lot slimmer".'

'A very pretty young woman in a negligee in a rather provocative pose in a bed without covers, and the caption: "Midnight Therapy. Waking hours are the best time for regular psychiatric treatment. At night her best therapy is sleep".'

Roughly one-fourth of the advertisements did not include a picture of a person of either sex although the illness could readily be categorized as either psychogenic or nonpsychogenic. Of the 423 advertisements which showed a person, 40 per cent were for psychoactive drugs. Of the 141 advertisements which did not show a person, 29 per cent were for psychoactive drugs. The ^{2}-value, under assumptions of independence, was 5.62 (with 1 df) which was significant at the 0.05 level of probability; there is a tendency to show people in advertisements for psychoactive drugs and a tendency not to show people in other advertisements.

No advertisements portrayed a woman as the physician despite the fact that women are 7 per cent of the physicians in the United States. Nurses, on the other hand, were always shown as women. These images are noteworthy because they reinforce the notion that different sex-linked qualifications exist for the two professions.

Many advertisements acknowledged that the role of housekeeper/housewife may be frustrating and suggested psychoactive drugs for relief of symptoms. Because many physicians endorse daily use of Librium by housewives [6] and since the advertisements strongly reinforced belief in the 'housewife syndrome', it is not surprising to find that usage of prescribed tranquillisers is especially high among suburban women [10]. However, whether this drug usage reflects a greater neuroticism among this group of people [11] or whether it stems from a self-fulfilling prophecy based on physician attitudes and expectations, or an interaction of the two, remains to be determined.

Another interesting sex difference involved the wording of the captions describing the illnesses for which drugs (psychoactive and nonpsycho-active) were required. Symptoms of female patients seemed frequently to be presented with a clever play on words while symptoms of males were announced in a grave and straightforward manner. For example, in an advertisement for a drug for hypertension, a female librarian was shown reshelving books and saying: 'Last week I felt woozy in fiction'. An advertisement for a minor tranquilliser showed a bride and groom at the altar with the bride in obvious distress and the caption: 'When diarrhea wrings the wedding belle. . .'. On the other hand, an advertisement for a minor tranquilliser for a male patient showed a distinguished looking grey haired man with his head in his hands and the caption: 'Sick, and worried sick'. This qualitative difference, together with the other differences noted above, seems further to reinforce the notion that women have less serious organic health problems than do men.

Lastly, the medical problems of women were sometimes shown as causing irritation to others – her family or her physician. Consider the following examples:

> 'A picture of a grotesque-looking man had the caption: "This 42-year old man actually looks like a Greek god and is good to his family and to his wife – but this is how SHE sees him: female climateric conjures phantoms of monsters".'

> 'A picture of a family gathering with focus on the woman "Treat one . . . six people benefit".'

> 'A carved wooden chair in which the back and arms fade into the head and hands of a woman. "Is this patient becoming a fixture in your office?" '

This difference in advertising is consistent with a sex difference in physician attitudes. Cooperstock [12] asked 68 internists and general practitioners to describe the typical complaining patient, sex unspecified. Of the physicians responding, 72 per cent spontaneously referred to a woman, 24 per cent to a person of neither sex, and 4 per cent to a man. If a physician shares the attitudes that the typical complaining patient is female, then the advertisements would appear to encourage him or her to prescribe tranquillisers to bring relief – to the physician.

Summary and conclusions

Advertisements for psychoactive drugs were strongly associated with showing a female as the patient, but not out of proportion to the rate of usage of these kinds of drugs by women. The correspondence between the rates with which women are depicted as needing the drugs in the advertisements and the rates with which they receive them by prescription was striking. Further research is needed to determine whether the advertising companies are adjusting to physician/patient behavior or the physicians (and patients) adjusting to expectations aroused by advertising.

Advertisements for nonpsychoactive drugs were strongly associated with showing a male as the patient, and out of proportion to the rate of usage of nonpsychoactive drugs by men. In this drug category, at least, advertising agencies were not reflecting the rates of usage of drugs. We suspect, rather, that the agencies are conforming to the cultural stereotype which holds that women tend to have emotional illnesses while men tend to have organic ones.

Moreover, within the psychoactive drug category alone, the reasons given for which women vs men required the drugs were different, with men needing them for illness or work related reasons and women having less specific symptoms.

The advertisements also tended to show women in restricted age ranges, in provocative situations, or as irritating patients. There were differences in both quantitative and qualitative aspects of the advertisements. Qualitatively, advertisements showing women as patients tended to use humor or a clever play on words while those depicting a man seemed to be more straightforward. Indirect evidence [13] indicates that the manner in which symptoms are presented is related to the seriousness with which symptoms are perceived by physicians (fewer symptoms presented stoically were seen as indicative of more serious illness).

Principles governing advertising in AMA journals as well as restrictions set by Federal Drug Administration guidelines indicate that the advertisements should not be deceptive or misleading. The different images of women and men created in the advertising literatures may, therefore, be given special credibility because they presumably conform to both sets of standards. Justification of these advertising techniques by appeal to scientific evidence (as opposed to clinical opinion which may derive partially from the advertisements) would appear to be in order.

Although it cannot be argued conclusively that drug advertisements cause physicians to prescribe differently for women and men, one can at least speculate upon the possible effects these advertisements may have upon both patient and physician. The images of the two sexes are (perhaps not surprisingly) very similar to the cultural stereotype: women tend to be shown as emotional, irrational and complaining while men tend to be shown as nonemotional, rational and stoic. Patients may tend to bring their illness behavior, as well as their everyday behavior, in line with cultural expectations. If a male or female patient desires a prescription for a certain drug, he or she may learn which behavior produces the results. The advertisements may also encourage physicians to interpret symptoms presented by women as reflecting emotional illness and those of men as reflecting organic illness, even though the actual symptoms and/or illness might be identical for the two patients. For whatever reason, the prescription rates for psychoactive drugs for the two sexes are quite different. These factors may combine to produce a higher incidence of misdiagnosis and treatment for members of both sexes than would otherwise be the case.

Notes

* Both Seidenberg [4] and Lennard *et al*. [5] have discussed the impact of drug advertising upon the physician's decision to write a prescription.
† Detailmen often leave the physician reprints of advertisements identical to those that appear in the journals.
† †Discrepancies such as this may be responsible, in part, for the conclusions

reached by the 1972 'Report of the Women's Action Program' for the US Department of Health, Education and Welfare that, 'Physicians may be more likely to dismiss women's symptoms as neurotic or as "normal" female problems, sometimes until physical diseases are beyond treatment.' [9, p. 48].

References

1   Balter, M. and Levine, J. (1969) The nature and extent of psychotropic drug usage in the U.S. *Psychopharmacological Bulletin* **5**: 3.
2   Mellinger, G.D., Balter, M.B., and Manheimer, D.I. (1971), Patterns of psychotherapeutic drug use among adults in San Francisco. *Archives of General Psychiatry* **25**: 385.
3   Chambers, C.D. (1971) *An Assessment of Drug Use in the General Population of New York State*. Monograph published by New York State Narcotic Control Commission.
4   Seidenberg, R. (1971) Drug advertising and perception of mental illness. *Mental Hygiene* **55**: 21.
5   Lennard, H.L., Epstein, L.J., Bernstein, A., and Ransom, D.C. (1971) *Mystification and Drug Misuse*. San Francisco: Jossey-Bass.
6   Linn, L.S. (1971) Physician characteristics and attitudes toward legitimate use of psychotherapeutic drugs. *Journal of Health and Social Behaviour* **12**: 132.
7   Linn, L.S. and Davis, M.S. (1972) Physicians' orientation toward the legitimacy of drug use and their preferred source of new drug information. *Social Science and Medicine* **6**: 199.
8   Hemminki, E. (1973) The quality of drug advertisements in two Finnish medical journals. A comparison between psychotropic and other drug advertisements. *Social Science and Medicine* **7**: 51.
9   Report of the Women's Action Program (1972) Washington, D.C.: U.S. Department of Health, Education and Welfare.
10   Mellinger, G.D. (1971) Psychotherapeutic drug use among adults: a model for young drug users? *Journal of Drug Issues* October, 274.
11   Bernard, J. (1972) *The Future of Marriage*. New York: World Publishing Co.
12   Cooperstock, R. (1971) Sex differences in the use of mood-modifying drugs: an explanatory model. *Journal of Health and Social Behaviour* **12**: 238.
13   Zola, I.K. (1966) Culture and symptoms – an analysis of patients' presenting complaints. *American Sociological Review* **31**: 615.

Appendix A

Sample of journals selected

	year	volume/issue
New England Journal of Medicine	1972	286 (5)
	1971	284 (22)
	1970	283 (10)
	1969	280 (1)
	1968	279 (5)
California Medicine	1972	116 (1)
	1971	115 (3)
	1970	112 (5)
	1969	110 (3)
	1968	109 (3)
Journal of the American Medical Association	1972	April 10
	1971	April 4
	1970	May 18
	1969	September 8
	1968	April 29
American Journal of Psychiatry	1972	March
	1971	February
	1970	September
	1969	March
	1968	December

9

Family roles, structure, and stressors in relation to sex differences in obtaining psychotropic drugs

Gail Lee Cafferata, Judith Kasper, and Amy Bernstein

Although it is well-documented that women are more likely than men to use prescribed psychotropic drugs, there are conflicting explanations of this pattern. The purpose of this paper is to examine this sex difference in relation to three theoretical perspectives: (1) the sex-role theory, (2) social support theory, and (3) stress theory. Data from the National Medical Care Expenditure Survey confirm that women were more likely than men to obtain a psychotropic drug. The data also showed that for both men and women, the likelihood of obtaining a psychotropic drug is influenced by family role responsibilities, family structure, and stressful events. However, women had a significantly higher likelihood of use than men under similar family circumstances. When sociodemographic and health-status/access-to-care variables were controlled, the association for men between family circumstances and obtaining a psychotropic drug disappeared. For women, however, certain family role responsibilities, structures, and stressful events significantly affected the likelihood of obtaining a psychotropic drug even when sociodemographic and health-status/access-to-care variables were controlled.

It is well-documented that women are more likely than men to use prescription drugs and, in particular, psychotropic drugs – a class of drugs that includes antidepressants, sedatives and hypnotics, antipsychotics, and antianxiety agents. Community studies in the U.S. and Canada (Cooperstock 1971, 1978; Guttman 1978; Lech *et al.* 1975; Shapiro and Baron 1961; Stolley *et al.* 1972; Uhlenhuth *et al.* 1978); national studies in the U.S. (Chambers and Griffey 1975; Cohen 1979; National Commission on

Reprinted, with permission, from the *Journal of Health and Social Behavior* 24: 132–43, 1983.

Marijuana and Drug Abuse 1973; Parry 1968; Parry *et al*. 1973); and studies in other nations (Balter *et al*. 1974; Cooperstock 1979) all support the observation that women are more likely than men to use psychotropic drugs. This pattern is of concern as a public health issue because of evidence that such drugs are often abused (U.S. Congress 1979). It also is of interest theoretically as a behavioural measure of a sex difference in mental health status or psychological distress. The purpose of this paper is to explore how this sex difference in the use of psychotropic drugs might be explained in the light of three theoretical perspectives. In particular, we attempt to understand how family role responsibilities, family structure, and exposure to family stressors affect the probability of obtaining a psychotropic drug.

Literature review

The variety of perspectives that can be used to explain why women use psychotropic drugs more than men can be classed under three major headings: (1) 'sex-role' theories, (2) 'social support' theories, and (3) 'stress' theories.

Sex-role theories

Studies that draw on sex-role theories to explain male/female differences, for example, Cooperstock (1971); Bush and Osterweis (1978); Nathanson (1977, 1978); and Verbrugge (1976a, 1976b, 1978), suggested that society permits women to perceive more morbidity and use more services than it permits men, who are expected to be stoic in the face of illness. For example, Kessler *et al*. (1981:60) showed that:

> 'men are less likely than women to interpret symptoms associated with depression and low general well-being as signs of emotional problems. As a consequence, men are considerably less likely than women to obtain professional help voluntarily for psychiatric problems.'

This sex difference has been associated with the concept of female 'learned helplessness' (Radloff and Monroe 1978). According to Cooperstock (1971), females use more drugs than do males because society permits them (1) to express feelings, such as anxiety; (2) to perceive emotional problems in self; and (3) to use medical care for emotional problems.

Sex-role theories also reflect the observation that society has historically permitted women more time to become ill, i.e. women have fewer fixed role obligations (Marcus and Seeman 1981). Although the labor force participation rates of women have more than doubled from 22 per cent in 1948 to 48 per cent in 1977 (Hayghe 1978), they remain lower than male rates. In 1977, for example, nearly 40 per cent of never-married women between the ages of 16 and 65 did not work (Hayghe 1978:52). Another aspect of the time argument proposes that women with more children, or with preschool children, may have less time to engage in sick-role behavior (Woods and Hulka 1979).

In sum, sex-role theories suggest that the greater likelihood of women's obtaining a psychotropic drug may be explained by women's greater willingness to recognize and express emotional problems and the greater availability of time to engage in sick-role behavior.

Social support theories

Social support theories attribute differences in health status and use of health services to the adequacy or inadequacy of a person's integration into social support networks (Antonovsky 1979; Berkman and Syme 1979; Brown and Rawlinson 1977; Cumming *et al.* 1975; Glenn 1975; Gove 1978; Kaplan *et al.* 1977; LaRocco *et al.* 1980; Liem and Liem 1978; Linn and Davis 1971; McCubbin *et al.* 1980; Nathanson 1980; Scanzoni and Fox 1980). Consistent with Emile Durkheim's (1951) theory of egoistic suicide, work in this tradition asserts that the absence of social supports can cause mental and physical illness. This may occur in the absence of (other) family stressors.[1] Factors found to affect the degree of social support a family can provide include (1) the family's economic structure, (2) whether the family has stayed intact, and (3) whether the family is nuclear or extended.

Economic structure. There are conflicting theories about the effects of a family's economic structure on its ability to provide social supports. Some researchers theorize that a nontraditional work arrangement such as both husband and wife work and there are children under six years of age, or only the wife works and there are children under six years of age, undermines family cohesion. Croog (1970:30), for example, called these 'quasi-broken family forms.' Others argue that nontraditional arrangements provide economic and social rewards that far outweigh these 'disruptions' (Bernard 1973). Empirical evidence is inconclusive. One study has shown the health status of men to be negatively affected by nontraditional economic arrangements (Rosenfield 1980), but another has shown the opposite (Booth 1979). While several studies have indicated that the health of women is negatively affected by employment under certain conditions (Haynes and Feinleib 1980; Welch and Booth 1977), there is other evidence that working women are in better health than housewives (Nathanson 1980; Welch and Booth 1977). Cumming *et al.* (1975), for example, demonstrated that female suicide rates, an indicator of mental health, vary inversely with employment in all types of marital situations at nearly every age.

Intactness. Nonintact families are expected to provide less support to family members. Croog (1970) argued that mental illness is more likely when a family is no longer intact through an event such as death of a spouse or divorce, separation, or desertion. Divorce, separation, and widowhood are also associated with other indicators of health status (National Institute of Mental Health 1975; Verbrugge 1979).

Extended or nuclear. Although empirical evidence is scant, several theorists have contrasted the social support available to members of extended and nuclear families. The nuclear family, as characterized by Parsons and Fox (1952), is ill-equipped to cope with illness in the home setting. Hill (1949) and, more recently, Burr (1973) suggested that an extended family offers more social support than a nuclear one to family members. According to Croog (1970: 25):

'The autonomy, independence and freedom that characterize nuclear family systems also have their costs. For example there tends to be high emotional commitment between members of the small relatively isolated nuclear family and when disruption occurs because of death or divorce, the consequences may be severe for individual members.'

In sum, social support theories suggest that greater likelihood of psychotropic drug use is associated with membership in a family that offers less social support. Women may use more psychotropic drugs either because they are more likely than men to live in a less supportive type of family or because they are more senstive to lack of family social support.

Stress theories

Stress theories (Berkman and Syme 1979; Booth 1979; Dohrenwend and Dohrenwend 1974, 1976, 1977, 1978: Haynes and Feinleib 1980; Holmes and Rahe 1967; McCubbin *et al.* 1980; Pleck 1977; Radloff 1975; Rosenfield 1980; Scanzoni and Fox 1980) would explain the higher female use of psychotropic drugs similarly; they suggested that either women are subject to more stresses than are men (Gove 1978; Gove and Hughes 1979) or the same stressors affect men and women differently (Dohrenwend and Dohrenwend 1977; Kessler 1979).

McCubbin *et al.* (1980:857) defined a family stressor as 'those life events or occurrences of sufficient magnitude to bring about change in the family system.' These events, such as unemployment or the death of a spouse, have profound impact on the family and have been linked to stress and health status among women and men. There are basically two classes of stressors: those associated with true psychiatric or physical illnesses and injuries and those which 'are independent of either the subject's physical health or his psychiatric condition,' such as the death of a spouse

(Dohrenwend and Dohrenwend 1978:10; Thoits 1981). The variety of life events of the second type that have appeared in studies of health status and health services use include: unemployment (Brenner 1979; Gore 1978; Roghmann and Haggerty 1972); death in the family (Dohrenwend and Dohrenwend 1974; Holmes and Rahe 1967); migration (Holmes and Rahe 1967; McCubbin *et al.* 1980); divorce or separation (Radloff 1975; Verbrugge 1979); job change (Ruch 1977); serious illness in the family (Woods and Hulka 1979); temporary absence of spouse (Snyder 1978); and traffic accidents (Roghmann and Haggerty 1972).

The consequences of family stressors include changes in health status, such as the reporting of symptoms (Welch and Booth 1977; Woods and Hulka 1979); mental illness (Warheit *et al.* 1976); depression (Radloff 1975); psychosomatic complaints (Snyder 1978); coronary heart disease (Haynes and Feinleib 1980); problem-drinking (Parry *et al.* 1974); and mortality (Brenner 1979), as well as the incidence of many other diseases. Researchers also have shown increased utilization of health services among persons experiencing family stressors, including outpatient physician visits (Snyder 1978) and use of psychotropic medicines (Pflanz *et al.* 1977; Welch and Booth 1977). With regard to sex difference in response to stress, Parry *et al.* (1974) have suggested that alcohol use and psychotherapeutic drugs are alternative coping mechanisms for anxiety and depression. Men are more likely than women to become coping drinkers in response to anxiety and depression, while women are more likely to become users of prescription psychotherapeutic drugs.

There also is evidence that stress interacts with social support. The effects of stressful events may be mediated or enhanced by the social support resources available to an individual. Nuckolls *et al.* (1972) showed that complications of pregnancy and childbirth are negatively related to levels of social support. A study of unemployed men by Gore (1978) demonstrated that within a population experiencing the stress of unemployment, differences existed in serum cholesterol levels in relation to the availability of a social network involving friends, family, and community.

This paper focuses on family roles, family structure, and stress events as they affect the likelihood of men's and women's obtaining psychotropic drugs. Accordingly, the analysis first shows the zero-order association for the total population, men and women, of phychotropic drug use with variables suggested by the three theoretical perspectives discussed in the foregoing. It is known from earlier studies that a number of individual characteristics are important predictors of the probability of using health services in general (Andersen 1968). These include age, education, race, family income, insurance coverage, and measures of health status and access to care. To examine the relative importance of family circumstances in the presence of these other characteristics, they are introduced as control variables in separate regressions for men and women.

Data and methods

Data for this paper were supplied by the National Medical Care Expenditure Survey (NMCES).[2] The NMCES was a national survey of health care use and expenditures for calendar year 1977. In the survey, 14,000 randomly selected households in the civilian noninstitutionalized population were interviewed six times over an 18-month period during 1977–78. The population of interest in this paper is a subset of (1) all persons between 18 and 65 years of age who were heads of a family, excluding those who were the only person in their family, and (2) all spouses. The 7,039 men and 8,465 women in this population resided in 11,083 separate households.

The sampling unit in this survey was the household. Interviewers routinely assigned married males as household 'head' and their wives as 'spouse'. In some respects, the inclusion of spouses created a violation of the assumption of independent observations necessary for logit analyses, since heads and spouses often were drawn from the same household. However, requiring that women and men be drawn from a separate household would restrict the analysis of women to those living in a nonintact family, a biased representation of women as a group. Further, since men and women were analyzed separately here, the problem of nonindependent observations due to marriage seemed minimal.

The dependent variable in this analysis was whether or not a person ever bought or obtained a psychotropic drug, including medicines received from a doctor or clinic at no charge. Over-the-counter products such as Nytol were excluded. Psychotropic drugs were those appearing in *AMA Drug Evaluations* (1973) as sedatives and hypnotics (Chapter 27), antianxiety drugs (Chapter 28), antipsychotic drugs (Chapter 29), and antidepressants (Chapter 32). For each family member, all prescribed medicines obtained were recorded by name, along with conditions for which the drug was obtained and expenditure data. For all prescribed medicines, the question was asked, 'Who was (this medicine) obtained for?' Only medicines obtained for household heads and spouses 18 to 65 years old were included in this analysis. The expression 'use of psychotropic drugs' occasionally appears as a synonym for 'obtaining psychotropic drugs.' However, it should be remembered that these data pertain to obtaining a psychotropic drug, not whether it was ever taken or how much of the drug was taken.

Variables concerning the family were grouped into three categories corresponding to the theoretical perspectives examined in this paper.[3] The first group of variables reflects levels of fixed family role responsibilities. These are: (1) employment status – anyone who never had a job for pay during the year is in the 'never worked' category, (2) number of children, and (3) presence of a child under five years of age.

The second set of variables was constructed to explore the usefulness of social support theories. Three dimensions of family structure were combined to form eight family types; the three dimensions were: (1) whether the family was intact (consisting of a head and spouse) or not (head only); (2) whether the family was nuclear or extended (relatives other than a spouse or children lived with the family); and (3) whether the family had a traditional economic structure (male head was employed, and wife, if present, was not employed or, if employed, had no children under six years of age) or a nontraditional one (male head was unemployed, or wife with children under six years of age was employed). The extensive literature on structural effects (Blau 1960; Campbell and Alexander 1968; Tannenbaum and Backman 1964) suggests family structure as a plausible measure of social support.

The third group of variables indicated whether a stressful event occurred during the year. These events were: a death in the family; moving (measured by a change in zip code); departure of a family member (any family member leaving for any reason including marital breakup; a child leaving for college or going into the military; anyone entering a nursing home, mental hospital, or other institution); unemployment of male spouse (person was unemployed but reported they were looking for work); hospitalization of a family member; birth of a child; and illness of a spouse or child (measured by a response of 'poor' to the question, 'Compared to other people your age, would you say your health is excellent, good, fair, or poor?').

Several control variables are introduced in *Table 2*; these consist of age, education, race, family income, insurance coverage (Medicaid, private or uninsured), health status of individual (excellent, good, fair, or poor), and presence of a health problem that limits activity. These are variables known to affect patterns of obtaining health care (Andersen 1968). Also included are physician visits, hospital stays, and whether the person had a usual source of care, since the probability of obtaining any prescribed medicine increases as contact with physicians increases.

Results

Confirming previous studies, use of a psychotropic drug in 1977 by adult heads of household and their spouses was highly correlated with sex. Nearly twice as many women as men obtained psychotropic drugs at least once in 1977 (15.9 per cent compared with 8.1 per cent). *Table 1* shows the per cent of the total population and of men and women who ever purchased a psychotropic drug, in relation to family characteristics for which significant sex differences are suggested by the sex-role, social support, and stress theories.

Table 1 *Percent of household heads and spouses 18 to 65 years of age who obtained at least one psychotropic drug by sex and selected family characteristics* [a]

family characteristics	per cent total	men	women	standard error total	men	women
total	12.3	8.1	15.9	0.4	0.3	0.6
family role responsibilities						
employment status						
never worked	18.7*	17.7**	18.9***	0.8	1.6	0.8
worked part year	14.9*	11.6**	16.1	1.0	1.5	1.2
worked all year	9.3*	6.7**	13.3***	0.3	0.3	0.7
number of children						
none	15.2*	10.2**	19.6**	0.6	0.6	1.0
1	11.1	6.7**	14.7	0.6	0.6	0.9
2	10.4*	7.4	13.1***	0.6	0.8	0.9
3 or more	9.0*	5.7*	11.8***	0.7	0.6	1.0
presence of child under 5 years of age						
yes	6.3*	4.4**	8.0***	0.4	0.5	0.6
no	13.7*	9.0	17.8***	0.4	0.4	0.6
family structure						
traditional	12.1	7.2**	16.5	0.4	0.3	0.6
nontraditional	12.9	11.3**	14.2	0.7	0.9	0.9
intact	11.9	8.1	15.4	0.4	0.3	0.6
nonintact	18.1*	7.5****	19.4***	1.3	2.8	1.5
nuclear	12.3	8.1	15.9	0.4	0.3	0.6
extended	12.5	8.2	15.8	1.1	1.4	1.5
traditional nuclear intact	11.6	7.2	16.0	0.4	0.4	0.6
traditional extended intact	10.6	6.7	14.4	1.2	1.4	1.9
traditional nuclear nonintact	19.1*	8.9****	20.3***	1.4	3.6	1.6
traditional extended nonintact	18.0*	—[d]	20.4	3.4	—[d]	3.8
nontraditional nuclear intact	12.7	11.1**	14.1	0.8	0.9 ·	0.9
nontraditional extended intact	15.6	14.5****	16.6	3.3	4.3	4.0
nontraditional nuclear nonintact	14.8	—[d]	15.3	3.2	—[d]	3.5
nontraditional extended nonintact	—[d]	—[d]	—[d]	—[d]	—[d]	—[d]
family stressors						
death in family	27.0*	26.2**	27.7***	3.7	4.5	5.0
family moved from one residence to another	11.9	7.5	15.6	0.6	0.6	0.7
departure of family member[b]	12.5	6.5	17.5	0.9	0.9	1.4
unemployment of spouse	NA	NA	22.8***	NA	NA	2.4
hospitalization in family	10.9	6.1**	17.3	0.7	0.6	1.3
birth of child	7.2*	3.2**	10.8***	1.0	1.0	1.5
spouse in poor health[c]	22.2*	14.0**	28.5***	1.8	2.6	2.4
child in poor health[c]	18.4*	12.6	22.2	2.4	3.3	3.4

[a] Excludes single, never-married individuals.

[b] Head or spouse moved out of the family; child over 17 moved out other than to attend college.

[c] Person appraised health as 'poor' in response to question, 'Compared to other people your age, would you say your health is excellent, good, fair, or poor.'

[d] Fewer than 50 cases in the cell.

  * Significantly different from estimate for total population at .05 level using Z-scores.

  ** Significantly different from estimate for all men at .05 level using Z-scores.

  *** Significantly different from estimate for all women at .05 level using Z-scores.

  **** Relative standard error > 30 per cent.

The data in *Table 1* (column 1) shows that for the total population, the use of psychotropic drugs was inversely related to family role responsibilities, such as full-time employment and number and presence of young children. Persons who never worked in 1977 were twice as likely to purchase a psychotropic drug as those who worked the whole year (18.7 versus 9.3 per cent). Likelihood of use decreased as number of children increased and with the presence of young children. The pattern among men and women followed that of the population as a whole. However, significant differences in drug use remained between men and women with similar role responsibilities. Psychotropic drugs were more frequently obtained by women than men, regardless of number of children or presence of a child under age five. Only for men and women who never worked was the difference in likelihood of having a psychotropic drug eliminated.

Social support theory suggests that psychotropic drug use will be lower in intact or extended families than in nonintact or nuclear families. This theory does not suggest any clear prediction about the effects of living in a family with a traditional or nontraditional economic structure. Both social support and stress theories suggest that one explanation for a sex difference may be that more women are exposed to a less supportive family structure or to more stress events. Examining the impact of these variables within the male and female populations controls for effects of different rates of exposure to a less supportive family structure or to more stressful events. However, these data showed men and women generally were equally at risk, with the exception of intact versus nonintact families; 98.3 per cent of the men in our sample were in intact families versus 88.0 per cent of the women (data not shown).

Table 1 shows that for the population as a whole (column 1), the only significant difference in obtaining a psychotropic drug was for persons in a nonintact household; the latter had a higher likelihood of use compared to the population as a whole (18.1 versus 12.3 per cent). However, for men, the only significant difference occurred between those in a traditional economic family and those in a nontraditional family. Women in a nonintact household were significantly more likely than women as a whole to obtain a psychotropic drug. Cross-classification of family structure characteristics confirmed these findings. Among women, the likelihood of obtaining a psychotropic drug was greatest in a traditional, nuclear, nonintact household (women with no spouse who, if working, had no children under six, or had children under six and did not work). As before, among men, the only significant difference in the cross-classification was the higher rate of use among men in a nontraditional, nuclear, intact household. The difference between men and women in obtaining a psychotropic drug was significant within the three family structure types, although family structure appeared to affect men and women differently.

Among the family stress variables, a death in the family and a spouse or child in poor health resulted in a higher likelihood of psychotropic drug use than was the case for the population as a whole. The birth of a child resulted in lower use. In addition, among men, a hospitalization in the family also was associated with lower psychotropic drug use. For women, an unemployed spouse was associated with a higher likelihood of psychotropic drug use.

Only one family stress variable, i.e. death in the family, eliminated the difference in psychotropic drug use between men and women. Under other circumstances of stress, psychotropic drug use was nearly twice as likely for women as for men. Interestingly, even the birth of a child had as much impact on patterns of use by men as by women.

In sum, *Table 1* shows that the likelihood of obtaining psychotropic drugs was generally higher among women than men, regardless of family role responsibilities, social support provided by family structure, or family stressors. Only among persons who never worked; who lived in a nontraditional, extended, intact family; or who experienced a death in the family did differences in use by sex disappear. Under other circumstances, women were still more likely to obtain psychotropic drugs than were men. This suggests that simple additive or unconditional theories of psychotropic drug use, i.e., models predicting no interactions with sex, are inappropriate. While both men and women were affected by role responsibilities, women appeared to be affected more. For instance, women were significantly more likely to obtain these drugs in the absence of young children; men were not similarly affected.

Logit analysis confirms the existence of interactions associated with sex. Due to the violation of the continuity assumption one encounters when using traditional regression analysis with dichotomous data, a logistic regression analysis was used; this satisfies the assumption through a variable transformation (Pindyk and Rubinfeld 1976). Since the logit procedure used here does not produce a statistic such as an R^2, stepwise regression-equivalent R's are shown. These are likely to underestimate the fit of the model. To facilitate interpretation of the coefficients, we performed a linear transformation of dichotomous variables into a $(1,-1)$ format. Therefore, a positive coefficient for a group with a value of $+1$ indicates that the log odds for that group relative to its opposite is increased, whereas a negative coefficient indicates a decrease. *Table 2* shows the results of logistic regressions of ever obtaining a psychotropic drug (never $= 0$, ever $= 1$) for family role responsibilities, structure, and stress (*Table 1* variables), controlling for sociodemographic and health-status/access-to-care variables.

Among women, the family role responsibility that affected psychotropic drug use when other variables were controlled was the presence of young children. The presence of children under age five decreased the likelihood

Table 2 *Logit estimate of the probability a psychotropic drug was purchased for household heads and spouses 18 to 65 years of age[a] (NMCES: United States, 1977)*

independent variables	women B-value	t-value	men B-value	t-value
constant	−1.55**	4.63	−2.31**	4.12
family role responsibilities				
number of children	−0.01	0.32	0.02	0.53
presence of children under 5 years (1, −1)	−0.15*	2.16	−0.07	0.70
never worked[b] (1, −1)	0.05	1.18	−0.19	1.54
worked part year (1, −1)	0.03	0.48	−0.01	0.16
family structure				
traditional	0.11*	2.11	−0.07	0.77
nuclear	0.12	1.76	0.10	0.94
intact	−0.16**	2.76	−0.11	0.55
family stressors				
death in family (1, −1)	0.16	1.09	0.50	1.82
family moved (1, −1)	−0.00	0.06	−0.02	0.36
departure of family member (1, −1)	0.06	1.05	−0.20*	2.09
unemployment of spouse (1, −1)	0.15	1.94	NA	NA
hospitalization in family (1, −1)	0.09	1.76	0.06	0.83
birth of a child (1, −1)	−0.36**	3.44	−0.12	0.66
spouse in poor health (1, −1)	0.20*	2.26	−0.25	1.92
child in poor health (1, −1)	0.07	0.62	0.06	0.29
demographic/socioeconomic				
age	0.02**	4.23	0.02**	3.19
education	−0.01	0.90	−0.00	0.24
race (1 = white, −1 = all others)	0.13*	2.35	0.12	1.28
family income	0.00	1.02	0.00	0.39
medicaid[c] (1, −1)	0.00	0.03	−0.07	0.49
private insurance (1, −1)	−0.01	0.15	−0.08	0.74
uninsured (1, −1)	−0.03	0.27	−0.26	1.71
health status/access to care				
'good' health[d] (1, −1)	0.20**	4.63	0.34**	5.32
'fair' health (1, −1)	0.54**	10.05	0.60**	7.58
'poor' health (1, −1)	0.58**	7.07	0.98**	9.54
limitation of activity (1, −1)	0.24**	5.44	0.36**	5.64
physician visits	0.05**	12.80	0.03**	6.35
hospital stays	0.26**	5.59	0.41**	6.37
regular source of care (1, −1)	0.31**	4.81	0.45**	4.98
regression equivalent R^2	0.15		0.14	

[a] Excludes single, never-married individuals.
[b] Worked all year omitted.
[c] Persons covered only by Medicare or CHAMPUS/CHAMPVA omitted.
[d] 'Excellent' omitted.
 * $p < .05$.
** $p < .01$.

of psychotropic drug use, even when variables such as age, access to care, and number of physician visits were controlled. For men, none of the family role responsibilities remained significantly related to likelihood of psychotropic drug use once these other factors were taken into account.

Similarly, none of the family structure variables was significant for men. But for women, obtaining a psychotropic drug was significantly and positively related to a traditional and to a nonintact family structure. Among family stress variables, a spouse in poor health remained positively associated with psychotropic drug use for women, while the birth of a child was negatively related. For men, departure of a family member was negatively associated with use.

As expected, many of the sociodemographic and health-status/access-to-care variables known to affect the use of health services also affected the likelihood of obtaining psychotropic drugs. The likelihood of obtaining a psychotropic drug was positively related to age for men and women and to race for women. The health-status/access-to-care variables – perceived health, limitation of activity, having a regular source of care, and the number of physician visits and hospital stays – also were significantly related to obtaining a psychotropic drug.

Discussion

Three theoretical perspectives – sex-role theory, social support theory, and stress theory – have been examined in an effort to understand the relationship between sex and psychotropic drug use. Sex-role theory suggests that the difference in obtaining a psychotropic drug occurs because the female role leads either to more illness or to a greater willingness to recognize or indulge whatever illness exists. Social support theory hypothesizes that certain circumstances that leave an individual less socially integrated, such as a nonintact family, a family with a nontraditional economic structure, or a nuclear family, have a negative impact on health. Similarly, stress theory suggests that certain life events are sufficiently important and stressful to affect health. Both social support and stress theory also suggest, however, that women may be more sensitive than men to the effects of less supportive or more stressful family circumstances.

The first table shows that while psychotropic drug use by both men and women was affected by family role responsibilities, the difference in likelihood of use remained significant by sex. Of course these role responsibilities have different implications for men and women. The presence of a child under age five is much more likely to affect a woman's participation in the labor force than a man's, for example. In fact, the finding of higher use of psychotropic drugs among men in a nontraditional family (a family in which the male does not work or in which both parents work and there are children under five years) suggests that men who more closely approximate the 'female' role with regard to work status or childcare may have the same tendency as women toward higher levels of psychotropic drug use.

Although men in a traditional family were less likely than men in a nontraditional family to use a psychotropic drug, regardless of the family's economic structure, women had a higher likelihood of use. Women also appeared to feel the effects of a nonintact family more than men; however, the number of men in this type of family was quite small, so the estimate is subject to considerable variation. The relationship between social integration and psychotropic drug use is supported by these findings, but the sex difference in use is not explained. Neither is it completely explained by stress theory. Both men and women were affected by stressful events with regard to obtaining a psychotropic drug. But only in the extreme occurrence of a death in the family did the sex difference disappear.

Table 2 shows that regardless of the apparent effects of family circumstances on whether men obtain psychotropic drugs, these effects disappear when sociodemographic and health-status/access-to-care variables are controlled; an exception was the anomalous finding of lower use on the departure of a family member. For women, however, the impact of family circumstances remained. The presence of a child under five years of age, the birth of a child, or living in an intact family significantly reduced the likelihood of women's obtaining a psychotropic drug. Women whose spouse was in poor health or who lived in a traditional family were significantly more likely to obtain such a drug. These findings lend credence to the social support and stress theories, which suggest that women may be more sensitive than men to the effects of less supportive or more stressful family circumstances. However, this conclusion must be viewed in relation to Parry *et al.*'s (1974) suggestion that men are more likely than women to become coping drinkers in response to anxiety and depression, while women are more likely to become users of psychotropic drugs.

Two other explanations of the differential impact of family circumstances on men and women can be drawn from sex-role theory. One is that women may be more likely than men to seek medical assistance in certain family circumstances. In *Table 2*, number of visits and having a regular source of care were controlled, thus removing the impact of women's greater access to and use of physician services. However, the reason for seeing a doctor could not be taken into account here. It is possible that a greater proportion of visits by women are initiated for reasons that derive from family circumstances. If physicians perceive these visits as less clearly tied to an organic physical cause, they may be more likely to prescribe a psychotropic drug as treatment. Mechanic (1972), among others, has suggested that a substantial proportion of physician visits cannot be clearly tied to an organic physical cause. Kessler *et al.* (1981:49) suggested that women 'translate nonspecific feelings of distress into conscious recognition that they have an emotional problem more readily than men do.' To the extent that women see physicians and express these feelings as the reason for their visit while men do not, a psychotropic drug prescription may be more likely.

The other explanation, also from sex-role theory, is that regardless of the similarity of presenting symptoms, physicians may be more likely to prescribe psychotropic drugs for women. Linn and Davis (1971) found that 84 per cent of psychotropic-drug-using women mentioned that a physician had first recommended the particular drug to them. Cooperstock and Sims (1971) asked a sample of Canadian physicians to describe why they wrote more mood-modifying prescriptions for women than men; their responses ranged from biological vulnerability, to differential life stress, to self-indulgence, to male reluctance to seek help.

Regardless of whether women more often present their symptoms to physicians in ways that elicit a psychotropic drug prescription or physicians are simply more inclined toward this type of treatment for women, a clear relationship between some aspects of family circumstances and psychotropic drug use by women exists. Although some of these same family circumstances appear to influence the use of psychotropic drugs by men, when health-status, access-to-care, and sociodemographic variables are taken into account, their impact disappears.

Notes

The views expressed in this paper are those of the authors and no official endorsement by the National Center for Health Services Research is intended or should be inferred. The authors gratefully acknowledge the useful criticism of Ronald M. Andersen, Samuel Meyers, Lawrence Stern, Thomas T.H. Wan, and Daniel C. Walden, and the clerical assistance of John Carrick, Martha Hartley, and Jane Schmidt.

1 The literature on social supports and crisis extends back to Hill's (1949) model of family response to wartime separation and reunion, widely known as the A-B-C-X model (Burr 1973; McCubbin *et al.* 1980). In this formulation:

A (the event and related hardships) – interacting with B (the family's crisis-meeting resources) – interaction with C (the definition the family makes of the event) – produce X (the crisis).

Recent research on Hill's B factor, the family's crisis-meeting resources, confirms that families vary in their ability to provide social supports to each other.

2 NMCES was funded by the National Center for Health Services Research and

cosponsored by the National Center for Health Statistics. Data collection for the survey was done by Research Triangle Institute, NC, and its subcontractors, National Opinion Research Center for the University of Chicago, and Abt. Associates, Inc., of Cambridge, MA under contract HRA 230-76-0268. For more information about NMCES and other publications from these data write to: U.S. Department of Health and Human Services, Public Health Service, Office of Health Research, Statistics and Technology, National Center for Health Services Research, 3700 East-West Highway, Hyattsville, Maryland 20782.

3   Since NMCES was designed primarily to collect information on health services use and expenditures, measures of family role responsibilities, family structure, and stress are necessarily limited. No subjective measures of these concepts were available.

References

American Medical Association (1973) *AMA Drug Evaluations*, 2nd ed. Chicago: American Medical Association.

Andersen, Ronald (1968) *A Behavioral Model of Families' Use of Health Services*. Chicago: Center for Health Administration Studies, University of Chicago.

Antonovsky, Aaron (1979) *Health, Stress and Coping*. San Francisco: Jossey-Bass.

Balter, M.B., Levine, J., and Manheimer, D.J. (1974) Cross-national study of the extent of anti-anxiety/sedative drug use. *New England Journal of Medicine* 290:769–74.

Berkman, L. and Syme, S.L. (1979) Social networks, host resistance and mortality: A nine-year follow-up study of Alemeda County residents. *American Journal of Epidemiology* 109:186–204.

Bernard, Jessie (1973) *The Future of Marriage*. New York: Bantam Books.

Blau, Peter M. (1960) Structural effects. *American Sociological Review* 25:178–93.

Booth, A. (1979) Does wives' employment cause stress for husbands? *The Family Coordinator* 28:445–49.

Brenner, M.H. (1979) Mortality and the national economy: A review and the experience of England and Wales, 1936–76. *Lancet* 8142:568–73.

Brown, J. and Rawlinson, M. (1977) Sex differences in sick role rejection and in work performance following cardiac surgery. *Journal of Health and Social Behavior* 18:276–92.

Burr, Wesley R. (1973) *Theory Construction and the Sociology of the Family*, New York: John Wiley.

Bush, P.A. and Osterweis, M. (1978) Pathways to medicine use. *Journal of*

Health and Social Behavior 19:179-89.

Campbell, E.Q. and Alexander, C.N. (1968) Structural effects and interpersonal relationships. *American Journal of Sociology* 73:284-89.

Chambers, C.D. and Griffey, M.S. (1975) Use of legal substances within the general population: The sex and age variables. *Addictive Diseases: An International Journal* 2:7-19.

Cohen, R. (1979) Drug abuse applications: Some regression explorations with national survey data. National Institute of Drug Abuse Research Monograph Series 24:194-213.

Cooperstock, R. (1971) Sex differences in the use of mood modifying drugs: An explanatory model. *Journal of Health and Social Behavior* 12:238-44.

(1978) Sex differences in psychotropic drug use. *Social Science and Medicine* 12B:179-86.

(1979) A review of women's psychotropic drug use. *Canadian Journal of Psychiatry* 24:29-33.

Cooperstock, R. and Sims, M. (1971) Mood-modifying drugs prescribed in a Canadian city: Hidden problems. *American Journal of Public Health* 61:5.

Croog, S.H. (1970) The family as a source of stress. Pp. 19-53 in Sol Levine and Norman A. Scotch (eds) *Social Stress*. Chicago: Aldine.

Cumming, E., Lazer, C., and Chisholm, L. (1975) Suicide as an index of role strain among employed and not employed married women in British Columbia. *Review of Canadian Sociology and Anthropology* 12:462-70.

Dohrenwend, Barbara and Dohrenwend, Bruce P. (eds) (1974) *Stressful Life Events: Their Nature and Effects*. New York: Wiley.

(1976) Sex differences and psychiatric disorders. *American Journal of Sociology* 81:1447-454.

(1977) Reply to Gove and Tudor's comment on 'Sex differences and psychiatric disorders.' *American Journal of Sociology* 81:1336-345.

(1978) Some issues in research on stressful life events. *Journal of Nervous and Mental Disease* 66:7-15.

Durkheim, Emile (1951) *Suicide*. New York: Free Press.

Glenn, N.D. (1975) The contribution of marriage to the psychological well-being of males and females. *Journal of Marriage and the Family* 37:594-99.

Goldberg, E.L. and Comstock, G.W. (1976) Life events and subsequent illness. *American Journal of Epidemiology* 104:146-58.

Gore, S. (1978) The effect of social support in moderating the health consequences of unemployment. *Journal of Health and Social Behavior* 19:157-65.

Gove, W.R. (1978) Sex differences in mental illness among adult men and women. *Social Science and Medicine* 12B:187-98.

Gove, W. and Hughes, M. (1979) Possible causes of the apparent sex differences in physical health: An empirical investigation. *American Sociological Review* 44:126–46.

Gove, W.R. and Tudor, J. (1977) Sex differences in mental illness: A comment on Dohrenwend and Dohrenwend. *American Journal of Sociology* 82:1327–336.

Guttman, D. (1978) Patterns of legal drug use by Americans. *Addictive Diseases* 3:337–56.

Hayghe, H. (1978) Marital and family characteristics of workers, March 1977. *Monthly Labor Review* 101:51–4.

Haynes, S. and Feinleib, M. (1980) Women, work and coronary heart disease: Prospective findings from the Framingham Heart Study. *American Journal of Public Health* 70(2): 133–41.

Hill, Reuben (1949) *Families under Stress*. New York: Harper and Row.

Holmes, T.H. and Rahe, R.H. (1967) The social readjustment rating scale. *Journal of Psychosomatic Research* 11:213–18.

Kaplan, B.H., Cassel, J.C., and Gore, S. (1977) Social support and health. *Medical Care* 15:47–58.

Kessler, R.C. (1979) Stress, social status, and psychological distress. *Journal of Health and Social Behavior* 20:259–72.

Kessler, R.C., Brown, R.L., and Broman, C.L. (1981) Sex differences in psychiatric help-seeking: Evidence from four large scale surveys. *Journal of Health and Social Behavior* 22:49–64.

LaRocco, J.M., House, J.S., and French, J.R.P. (1980) Social support, occupational stress, and health. *Journal of Health and Social Behavior* 21:202–18.

Lech, S.V., Friedman, G.D., and Ury, H.K. (1975) Characteristics of heavy users of outpatient prescription drugs. *Clinical Toxicology* 8:599–610.

Liem, R. and Liem, J. (1978) Social class and mental illness reconsidered: The role of economic stress and social support. *Journal of Health and Social Behavior* 19:139–56.

Linn, L. and Davis, M.S. (1971) The use of psychotherapeutic drugs by middle-aged women. *Journal of Health and Social Behavior* 12:331–40.

McCubbin, H.I., Joy, C., Cauble, A.E., Comeau, J., Patterson, J., and Needle, R. (1980) Family stress and coping: A decade review. *Journal of Marriage and the Family* 42:855–71.

Marcus, A.C. and Seeman, T.E. (1981) Sex differences in reports of illness and disability: A preliminary test of the 'fixed obligations' hypothesis. *Journal of Health and Social Behavior* 22:174–82.

Mechanic, D. (1972) Social psychologic factors affecting the presentation of bodily complaints. *New England Journal of Medicine* 28:1132–139.

Nathanson, C.A. (1977) Sex, illness and medical care. *Social Science and Medicine* 11:13–25.

——(1978) Sex roles as variables in the interpretation of morbidity data: A methodological critique. *International Journal of Epidemiology* 7:253–62.

——(1980) Social roles and health status among women: The significance of employment. *Social Science and Medicine* 14A:463–71.

National Commission on Marijuana and Drug Abuse (1973) *Drug Use in America: Problem in Perspective.* Washington, DC: Government Printing Office.

National Institute of Mental Health (1975) *Marital Status and Mental Disorders: An Analytical Review.* DHEW Publication No. (ADM) 75-217. Washington, DC: Government Printing Office.

Nuckolls, K.B., Cassel, J., and Kaplan, B.H. (1972) Psychosocial assets, life crisis and the prognosis of pregnancy. *American Journal of Epidemiology* 95:431–41.

Parry, H.J. (1968) Use of psychotropic drugs by U.S. adults. *Public Health Reports* 83:799–810.

Parry, H.J., Balter, M., Mellinger, G.D., Cisin, I., and Manheimer, D. (1973) National patterns of psychotherapeutic drug use. *Archives of General Psychiatry* 28:769–83.

Parry, H.J., Cisin, I., Balter, M., Mellinger, G., and Manheimer, D. (1974) Increasing alcohol intake as a coping mechanism for psychic distress. Pp. 119–44 in Ruth Cooperstock (ed.) *Social Aspects of the Medical Use of Psychotropic Drugs.* Toronto: Alcoholism and Drug Addiction Research Foundation of Ontario.

Parsons, T. and Fox, R. (1952) Illness, therapy and the modern urban American family. *Journal of Social Issues* 8:31–44.

Pflanz, M., Basler, H., and Schwoon, D. (1977) Use of tranquilizing drugs by a middle-aged population in a West German city. *Journal of Health and Social Behavior* 18:194–205.

Pindyk, Reuben S. and Rubinfeld, Daniel L. (1976) *Econometric Models and Economic Forecasts.* New York: McGraw-Hill.

Pleck, J.H. (1977) The work-family role system. *Social Problems* 24:417–27.

Radloff, L. (1975) Sex differences in depression: The effects of occupation and marital status. *Sex Roles* 1:249–65.

Radloff, L.S. and Monroe, M.K. (1978) Sex differences in helplessness – with implications for depression. Pp. 199–221 in L. Sunny Hansen and Rita S. Rapoza (eds) *Career Development and Counseling of Women.* Springfield, IL: Charles C. Thomas.

Roghmann, K.J. and Haggerty, R.O. (1972) Family stress and the use of health services. *International Journal of Epidemiology* 1:279–86.

Rosenfield, S. (1980) Sex differences in depression: Do women always have higher rates? *Journal of Health and Social Behavior* 21:33–42.

Ruch, L. (1977) A multidimensional analysis of the concept of life change. *Journal of Health and Social Behavior* 18:71–83.

Scanzoni, J. and Fox, G.L. (1980) Sex roles, family and society: The seventies and beyond. *Journal of Marriage and the Family* 42:743–56.

Shapiro, S. and Baron, S.H. (1961) Prescriptions for psychotropic drugs in a non-institutionalized population. *Public Health Reports* 76:481–88.

Snyder, A.I. (1978) Periodic marital separation and physical illness. *American Journal of Orthopsychiatry* 48:637–43.

Stolley, P.D., Becker, M., McEvilla, J.D., Lasagna, L., Gainor, M., and Sloane, L. (1972) Drug prescribing and use in an American community. *Annals of Internal Medicine* 76:537–40.

Tannenbaum, A.S. and Bachman, J.G. (1964) Structural versus individual effects. *American Journal of Sociology* 69:585–95.

Thoits, P. (1981) Undesirable life events and psychophysiological distress. *American Sociological Review* 46:97–109.

Uhlenhuth, E.H., Balter, M.B., and Lipman, R. (1978) Minor tranquilizers: Clinical correlates of use in an urban population. *Archives of General Psychiatry* 35:650–55.

U.S. Congress, Senate Committee on Labor and Human Resources (1979) *Use and Misuse of Benzodiazepines.* 96th Congress, 1st session. Washington, DC: Government Printing Office.

Verbrugge, L.M. (1976a) Females and illness: Recent trends in sex differences in the United States. *Journal of Health and Social Behavior* 17:387–403.

—— (1976b) Sex differentials in morbidity and mortality in the United States. *Social Biology* 23:275–96.

——(1978) Sex and gender in health and medicine. *Social Science and Medicine* 12:329–33.

——(1979) Marital status and health. *Journal of Marriage and the Family* 41:267–85.

Warheit, G.J., Holtzer, C.E., Bell, R.A., and Arey, S. (1976) Sex, marital status, and mental health: A reappraisal. *Social Forces* 55:459–70.

Welch, S. and Booth, A. (1977) Employment and health among married women with children. *Sex Roles* 3:385–97.

Woods, N. and Hulka, B. (1979) Symptom reports and illness behavior among employed women and homemakers. *Journal of Community Health* 5:36–45.

10

A preliminary study of search procedures and patient management techniques in general practice

Norma V. Raynes

Summary A record of one in three consultations occurring in 10 general practice surgeries in two evening sessions was made by an observer. The results showed marked variation in the frequency of the general practitioners' use of different means of eliciting information about the patient and in forms of management. These activities were further analysed within subgroups of the patients' symptoms and some activities were shown to be influenced by patients' presenting symptoms whilst others were not. I discuss how much general practitioners' behaviour is responsive to patients' presenting symptoms and also some of the practical implications of these findings for general practice.

Introduction

There is now a large literature on general practitioners' workloads, their activities in the consultation, and how these vary. Several studies from individual practices or partnerships have contributed to our knowledge of the content of general practice consultations. Reports have indicated how often general practitioners refer patients or recall them, prescribe drugs for them, or physically examine them (Backett *et al*. 1954; Scott *et al*. 1960; Morrell 1971; Floyd and Livesey 1975; Marsh and Kaim-Caudle 1976). Buchan and Richardson (1973) in Scotland analysed in a major comparative study the activities in which the general practitioner is involved during the consultation. They showed how much general

Reprinted, with permission, from the *Journal of the Royal College of General Practitioners* 30: 166–72, 1980.

practitioners vary in what they do in consultations. This has also been noted by others. Morrell (1971), in his comparison of three general practitioners, reported variations in a whole range of consultation-based activities. Parish (1971) and Shepherd and colleagues (1966) showed large variation between general practitioners in the number of psychotropic drugs prescribed and psychiatric diagnoses made. Byrne and Long (1976) recently showed how doctors vary in their style of eliciting and imparting information to the patient. Floyd and Livesey (1975) indicated that there is consistency in the amount of time a general practitioner spends on various activities in the consultation, which suggests that interpractice differences could reflect consistent patterns in any given practice.

A recent editorial in this *Journal* (1977), reviewing practice content studies, argues that we should change our focus from quantity to quality. If we are to do this and begin to understand why general practitioners do what they do, we must first describe the different parts of their activities and then try and discover which factors influence behaviour. Bloor's work (1976, 1978), carried out in a different medical context, is a useful starting point and his conceptual framework has influenced me in this study.

Part of Bloor's research sought to identify factors which might account for the variation in adenotonsillectomy rates, which are as marked in ENT clinics as are prescribing and referral rates in general practice. Sitting in on ENT consultations he recorded the ways in which the surgeons obtained information about the children referred to them for possible adeno-tonsillectomy and the bases for their decisions on whether to operate or not. He noted that the consultants tended consistently to use certain procedures for obtaining information and certain criteria for making their decisions, which he called 'routine ways'. In other words, their actions and decisions followed a regular course and were more or less unvarying within their own consultations. However, differences existed between the consultants in the kinds of routines they adopted. Bloor argued that the use of different routine practices by different consultants contributed to the observed differences in adenotonsillectomy rates.

Goffman's (1961) concept of the encounter is also useful in studying the consultation in general practice. He identified as 'encounters' those social situations which occur when two or more people are in one another's immediate physical presence and when there is a 'single visual and cognitive focus of attention' (p.18). He pointed out that what occurred in such a situation was determined largely, but not exclusively, by the roles and events peculiar to that situation. Attributes of the parties to the encounter which are externally based may also influence what occurs in the specific social situation. This distinction is helpful in thinking about consultations in general practice because it enables one to differentiate between features of it which are generated in the consultation itself and those which exist independently of it but which nevertheless may influence what occurs within it.

I define the features which are characteristic of the consultation as 'situation specific characteristics'. These would include the patients' symptoms and the doctors' actions. The attributes of the patients and doctors which exist independently of the consultation I call 'non-situation specific factors', and these include the age and sex of the patient or doctor, the length of time they have known each other, and the doctor's attitudes. The choice of non-situation specific factors to be studied as possible influences on what occurs within the consultation is influenced by research which has identified particular doctor and patient characteristics as important.

Aims

I wish to establish which of the general practitioners activities can be classed as routines and which are responsive to differences in the patient's presenting symptoms. The activities discussed are:
1. The general practitioner's questions.
2. The general practitioner's use of physical examination.
3. The general practitioner's use of patients' notes.
4. The general practitioner's prescribing practices.
5. The general practitioner's referral of patients.
6. The general practitioner's recall of patients.
7. The general practitioner's writing of certificates.
The first three activities are referred to collectively as the general practitioner's search procedures, being the means by which he elicits information about his patient's condition. The last four activities are referred to collectively as the general practitioner's patient management techniques, which are all ways in which he deals with the patient's condition, having defined it for himself. All of these behaviours are situation specific, as defined above.

I hope to discuss the influence on these behaviours of non-situation specific factors such as the general practitioner's attitudes, age, sex, type of practice, as well as the patient's age, sex, occupation, and marital status, in future papers.

Method

Ten general practitioners gave permission for me to sit in on two of their morning and afternoon surgeries. The sample is not random but I tried to seek the co-operation of general practitioners who were representative of all general practitioners in terms of age, sex, practice size, and location of practice. The extent to which this was achieved is discussed in another paper (Raynes 1979). A verbatim record of one in three of the consultations occurring in these surgeries was made. Details of data collection techniques have been described elsewhere (Raynes 1978).

The general practitioner's search procedures I analysed were his questions, his use of physical examination, and his reference to the patient's notes. His questions were classified in terms of their focus. They could be physical, social, emotional, or administrative.

Thus, a general practitioner could ask questions about the location or duration of the patient's physical pain, or about social issues, such as his work, or about his emotional state perhaps relating to his depression, and finally, he could also ask questions of an administrative nature such as his age or address. Obviously, there could be some overlap of categories and for analytical purposes I distinguished between the questions which focussed exclusively on the physical characteristics of the patient's problem (P questions) and those which combined physical, social, and emotional elements (PSE questions).

A second search precedure used by the general practitioner to elicit information about the patient's problem is, of course, physical examination. No attempt was made to distinguish the locus of the examination as did Buchan and Richardson (1973). Its occurrence was simply recorded as being present or absent.

Patients' notes provide a third source of information for the doctor. Their contents are known to be variable but in so far as they contain a medical history, they constitute a potentially useful way of helping the general practitioner to complete his picture of the patient's problem so that he can begin to move towards patient management. Thus, the general practitioner's reference to notes was observed as a third search procedure used to elicit information.

Patient management was defined in terms of:
(a)   The writing of a prescription.
(b)   The writing of a prescription for a psychotropic drug.
(c)   Referrals for either evaluation or treatment.
(d)   A request for a patient to return for further consultation.
(e)   The writing of a certificate.
I recorded all of these activities during the course of the consultation.

I had the same difficulties over classification of presenting problems as others (Parish 1971; Howie 1972; Buchan and Richardson 1973). Since no standard system could be applied to the problems I saw, I devised a system whereby I was able to classify presenting symptoms in nine categories (*Table 1*) derived essentially from the data. The presenting symptoms in each consultation were classified independently by two raters and a high coefficient of concordance was obtained, the raters agreeing on the classification of 96 per cent of the symptoms.

In order to clarify a complex situation, I refer only to three of the nine

Table 1 *Patient presenting symptom categories*

1. physical symptoms
2. psychological symptoms (mood, behaviour, depression, anxiety, marital problems, delusions, phobias)
3. social problems (housing, leisure, work or family problems, excluding marital problems)
4. patient feels unwell but is unable to identify specific symptoms
5. problems relating to pregnancy
6. improvement in condition being treated
7. no change in, or worsening of, condition being treated
8. physical symptom with psychological symptoms superimposed
9. no symptoms

categories in this paper. The first of these, referred to as subgroup 1, is the category comprising all those consultations in which the patient presented with a physical symptom. The second category comprises those patients who presented with a psychological symptom (that is, one concerned with mood, behaviour, depression, anxiety, marital problems, delusions, or phobias). The third comprises all those consultations in which the patients presented with a social problem (housing, leisure, work, or familial problems other than marital problems). The second and third categories were combined to become subgroup 2 (psychosocial).

All of the consultations in subgroup 1 were patient-initiated episodes. Thirteen (68.4 per cent) in subgroup 2 were patient-initiated episodes and six (31.6 per cent) were consultations initiated by the general practitioner. There is no evidence to show that in subgroup 2 general practitioner-initiated consultations were any different from patient-initiated consultations in terms of the general practitioners' behaviours discussed here.

Results

The group of ten general practitioners not unexpectedly showed variance in their search procedures as well as in their patient management techniques (*Tables 2 and 3*).

Three of the general practitioners (C, D, and H) asked PSE questions in over half of their consultations. Physical examination was used in over four fifths of the consultations of general practitioners G and J, compared with just over half of the consultations of general practitioners H and I. General practitioner D referred to his patients' notes in all consultations whereas general practitioner F made reference to them in less than 40 per cent of his consultations. Similar variation is apparent in the patient management techniques (*Table 3*). Individual profiles were developed for

Table 2   *Frequency of search procedures used in all consultations*

general practitioner	physical no.	%	physical, social, and emotional no.	%	physical examination no.	%	reference to patient's notes no.	%
			focus of questions					
A	17	70.8	6	25.0	12	66.7	11	64.7
B	23	67.9	11	32.4	19	70.4	18	69.2
C	24	39.3	37	60.7	30	63.8	42	89.4
D	10	30.3	23	69.7	17	68.0	25	100.0
E	14	51.9	11	40.7	17	70.8	19	79.2
F	22	51.2	19	44.2	25	75.8	13	39.4
G	25	50.0	24	48.0	29	87.9	32	97.0
H	11	32.4	22	64.7	12	54.5	20	95.2
I	8	53.3	6	40.0	11	55.0	17	85.0
J	14	58.3	10	41.7	13	86.7	13	86.7
Total	168	46.9	169	48.9	185	70.1	210	80.5

Table 3   *Frequency of patient management techniques used in all consultations*

general practitioner	writing of prescription no.	%	prescription of psycho-tropic drug no.	%	referral of patient no.	%	recall of patient no.	%	issuing of certificate no.	%
A	11	61.1	3	16.7	3	16.7	5	27.8	1	5.6
B	18	72.0	4	16.0	6	22.2	12	44.4	2	7.4
C	20	43.5	1	2.2	9	19.1	19	40.4	9	19.1
D	24	96.0	6	24.0	1	4.0	13	52.0	5	20.0
E	15	62.5	0	0	9	37.5	14	58.3	1	4.2
F	22	66.7	2	6.1	8	24.2	18	54.5	3	9.1
G	21	63.6	7	21.2	8	24.2	23	69.7	2	6.1
H	15	75.0	6	30.0	1	4.8	15	68.2	2	9.1
I	9	45.0	2	10.0	3	15.0	7	35.0	2	10.0
J	11	73.8	3	20.4	6	40.0	12	80.0	1	6.7
Total	166	64.1	34	13.1	54	20.5	138	52.3	28	10.6

their search procedures (*Figure 1*) and for their patient management techniques (*Figure 2*).

When these same behaviours were examined within the patients' symptom-presenting subgroups, there were differences in some search procedures and patient management techniques used by the general practitioners when confronted by patients with physical problems on the one hand and emotional and social problems on the other. It is also clear that some behaviours in the consultation were not affected by these differences in the patients, the latter group containing behaviours which have been described by Bloor (1976) as routines. They are 'tried and tested

Figure 1 Search procedures: all consultations

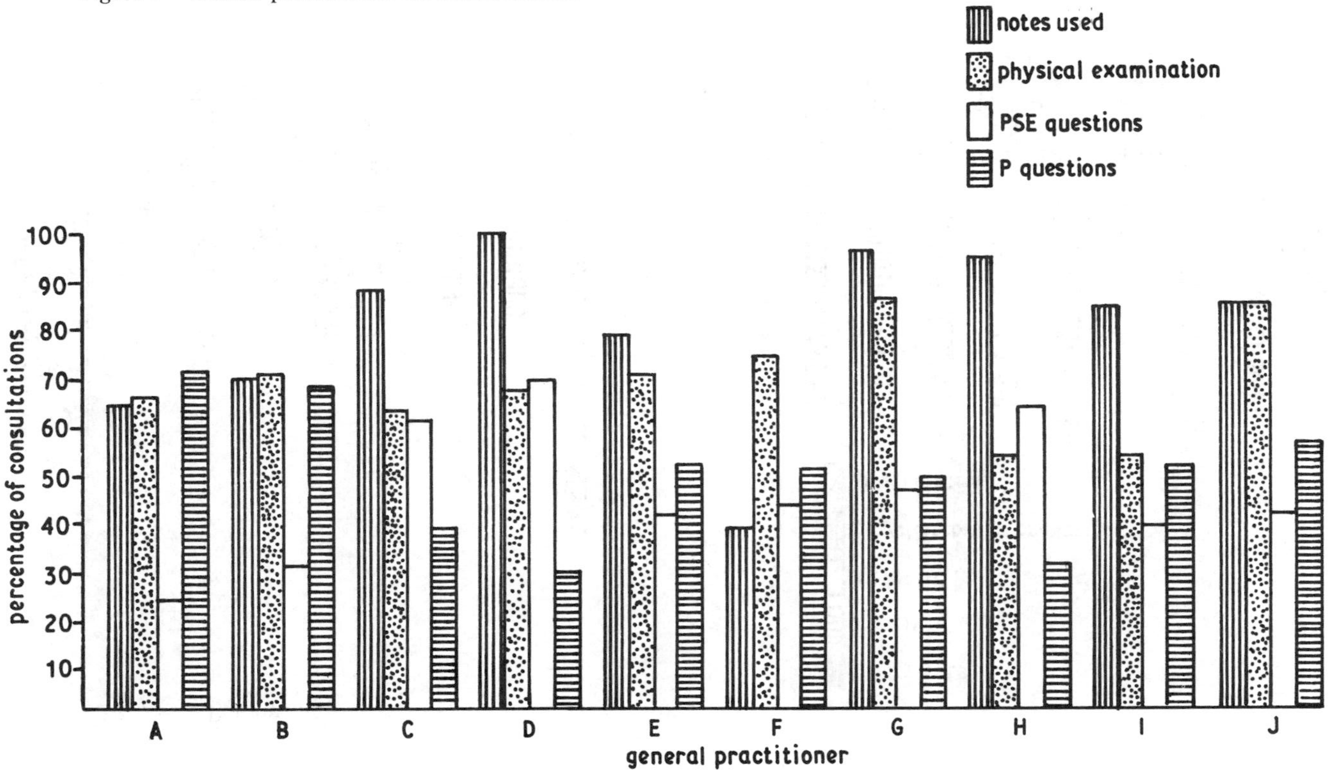

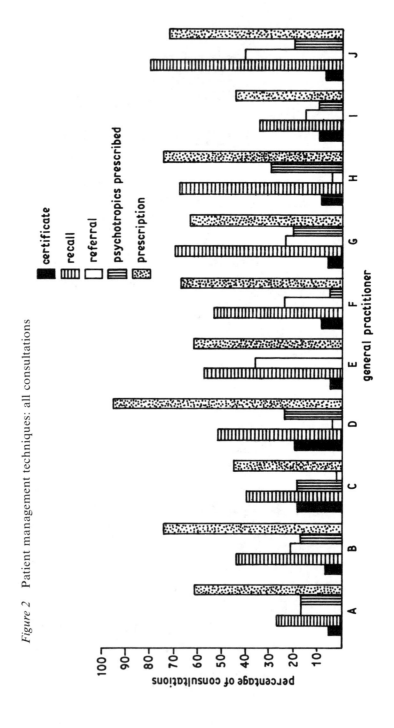

Figure 2 Patient management techniques: all consultations

certificate
recall
referral
psychotropics prescribed
prescription

percentage of consultations

general practitioner

recipes' employed to investigate familiar complaints and to manage them in familiar ways (Bloor 1978; p. 53). *Table 4* summarizes the effect of the patients' presenting symptoms on the general practitioners' search procedures and patient management techniques.

Among the general practitioner's search procedures only the focus of his questions was affected by differences in the patients' presenting symptoms. More PSE questions were asked by all the general practitioners in subgroup 2 than in subgroup 1. The use of patients' notes and physical examinations were unaffected by the patients' presenting symptoms (*Table 4*). In so far as the general practitioners' patient management techniques were concerned, a similar routine quality characterized the general level of prescribing, referral and recall of patients, and writing of certificates. For each general practitioner, these practices were unaffected by patients' presenting symptoms (*Table 4*). However, the prescribing of psychotropic drugs was affected by patients' symptoms, considerably more being prescribed in subgroup 2 than in subgroup 1.

Table 4 *Effect of symptoms on general practitioner search procedures and patient management techniques*

	direction of change between subgroup 1 and 2
search procedures	
P questions	fewer asked in subgroup 2*
PSE questions	more asked in subgroup 2**
physical examination	no change
reference to patients' notes	no change
management techniques	
general prescribing level	no change
prescribing of psychotropic drugs	more prescribed in subgroup 2**
referral of patients	no change
recall of patients	no change
certificate written	no change

*p < .05   **p < .01.

On examination it was found that none of the search procedures was related to each other. Amongst the patient management techniques frequency of prescribing and patient recall were found to be unrelated in subgroups 1 and 2. High prescribing levels, however, were found to be inversely related to patients' referral in both subgroups 1 and 2, which meant that the general practitioners who often prescribed seldom referred their patients. High referral rates were found to be related to high recall rates in subgroup 1, but not in subgroup 2. Thus the general practitioners who often referred patients presenting with physical symptoms also often recalled such patients. These techniques are not statistically significantly associated when patients with social and emotional symptoms are being treated.

Discussion

The research I have described has several limitations. The first is the small size and non-random nature of the sample of doctors studied. Thus, though it can be argued that the findings have implications for patient care in general practice, it is clear that a larger randomly selected data base is needed against which they can be tested.

Secondly, whilst the routines which were observed can themselves have consequences for patient care, as well as implications for training general practitioners, their relative importance to these matters compared with that of patient socio-economic status, general practitioner attitudes, or location of practice, for example, needs to be explored. Such factors as the patient's age or occupation may well have a greater influence on the general practitioner's behaviour than patient symptoms, particularly when considering patient management, for example. An analysis of the contribution of these factors (categorized as non-situation specific) to the general practitioner's behaviour in the consultation is under way.

A third limitation is the failure to tap the stored knowledge about the patient which all general practitioners have. This knowledge may well explain some of the differences in question focus used by general practitioners. For example, a general practitioner who has known a patient for 10 years may well not need to ask questions which we have called PSE questions, but it is equally arguable that be cannot rely on his stored knowledge without consistently updating it in aspects which are more volatile, say, than the presence of an inflamed throat.

Despite these limitations the findings of the study raise some important questions relevant to general practice and the training of general practitioners.

Although they reiterate the existence of the variance in general practitioners' prescribing practices, particularly of psychotropics, and other activities in the consultation observed by other workers, they suggest that some of it is a function of the general practitioner's response to an important situation specific factor, namely, recognition of the patients' presenting symptoms. Such factors were ignored by Byrne and Long (1976) in their study of doctors interacting with patients. In this study both the nature of the general practitioner's questions and his prescribing of psychotropic drugs were influenced by the patient's presenting symptoms. However, it is clear that some activities in the consultation, perhaps most important, the general level of prescribing practised by the general practitioner and his use of referral, are routines not significantly influenced by the patient's presenting problem.

Much criticism has been levelled at the ever increasing size of the drug bill which extends the cost of general practitioners' own income and professional expenses combined (*Journal of the Royal College of General*

Practitioners 1978). This study suggests that the use, or lack of use, of the prescription pad is a routine behaviour for general practitioners. Again, in this study this routine behaviour is inversely associated with referring patients for evaluation or treatment (another routine). Perhaps low referral rates limit fuller scrutiny of prescribing practices and thus one possible source of change in this routine behaviour. The prescribing of psychotropics is, however, for eight of the 10 general practitioners an activity responsive to patients' symptoms. Most of the prescriptions for psychotropic drugs written by these were given to patients in consultations in which the patients presented with social and emotional symptoms. It should not be forgotten, however, that two of the highest prescribers of this type of drug had no patients presenting with such symptoms. The situation responsive activity of asking more PSE than P questions may or may not produce better care. If this practice is thought to be worth encouraging, then teaching it will have to be linked to its relevance to specific kinds of pathology or uncertainty about patient disorder. On the other hand, the modification of routines, if thought desirable, needs different kinds of techniques.

Conclusion

The research has identified some of the components of the general practitioner's behaviour in the consultation and has demonstrated the feasibility of doing this. The findings suggest that some of the observable behaviour of the general practitioners is best understood as the implementation of familiar and trusted techniques by means of which they seek to impose order on the world in the consulting room. The data cannot be accepted as proof of this argument; the size of the sample alone precludes that. The findings, however, at least indicate the need to examine this line of reasoning further, over a wide range of general practice morbidity and using a more detailed identification of pathological signs and symptoms than was feasible in this study.

What influences the choice by a general practitioner of one routine method of assessment or patient management rather than another is another issue which deserves further research, especially if one approach is considered to be more effective in the identification of pathology or its management. It has been argued that general practitioners do remain ignorant of potentially treatable conditions in their patients (Williamson *et al.* 1964; Cartwright *et al.* 1976) and some factors which contribute to this situation may well be elucidated by further research into which of those behaviours of the doctors are routine responses and which are not. It would also be useful to identify those factors which contribute to the emergence and implementation of particular routines. If such research is carried out it should then become possible to assess the appropriateness of the routine techniques in specified clinical contexts, which could in turn lead to the development of practical guidelines for the general practitioner and vocational trainee.

Acknowledgements

I am indebted to Professor Michael Shepherd, Director of the General Practice Research Unit at the Institute of Psychiatry, under whose auspices the study was carried out. The work was supported by a grant from the Department of Health and Social Security. None of the work would have been possible without the collaboration of the 12 general practitioners involved in the study: Dr Bruce Armstrong, Dr Steven Curson, Dr David Finer, Dr John Fry, Dr Graeme Jupp, Dr Thomas Madden, Dr Sheila O'Hara, Dr Beryl Palmier, Dr Aaron Rapoport, Dr Peter Sowerby, Dr Keith Thompson, and Dr Julian Tower, to whom I am particularly indebted. I am also grateful to Ms Victoria Cairns, who did the computing, and to Ms Gillian Andrews for her patient assistance with the collation of data.

References

Backett, E.M., Heady, J.A., and Evans, J.C.G. (1954) Studies of a general practice. *British Medical Journal* 1:109–15.

Bloor, M. (1976) Bishop Berkeley and the adenotonsillectomy enigma. *Sociology* 10:43–61.

Bloor, M. (1978) On the routinised nature of work in people processing agencies. In A. Davis (ed.) *Relationships between Doctors and Patients*. London: Saxon House.

Buchan, I.C. and Richardson, I.M. (1973) *Time Study of Consultations in General Practice*. Edinburgh: Scottish Home and Health Department.

Byrne, P.S. and Long, B.E.L. (1976) *Doctors Talking to Patients*. London: HMSO.

Cartwright, A., Lucas, S., and O'Brien, M. (1976) Some methodological problems in studying consultations in general practice. *Journal of the Royal College of General Practitioners* 26:894–906.

Floyd, C.B. and Livesey, A. (1975) Self-observation in general practice – the bleep method. *Journal of the Royal College of General Practitioners* 25: 425–31.

Goffman, E. (1961) *Encounters*. New York: Bobbs-Merril.

Howie, J.G.R. (1972) Diagnosis – the Achilles heel? *Journal of the Royal College of General Practitioners* 22:310–15.

Journal of the Royal College of General Practitioners (1977) How many patients? Editorial **27**:3.

Journal of the Royal College of General Practitioners (1978) Prescribing in general practice. Editorial **28**:515–16.

Marsh, G. and Kaim-Caudle, P. (1976) *Team Care in General Practice.* London: Croom Helm.

Morrell, D.C. (1971) Expressions of morbidity in general practice. *British Medical Journal* **2**: 454–58.

Parish, P.A. (1971) The prescribing of psychotropic drugs in general practice. *Journal of the Royal College of General Practitioners* **21**: suppl. 4.

Raynes, N.V. (1978) General practice consultation study. *Social Science and Medicine* **12**:311–15.

Raynes, N. (1979) Factors affecting the prescribing of psychotropic drugs in general practice consultations. *Psychological Medicine* **9**:671–79.

Scott, R., Anderson, J.A.D., and Cartwright, A. (1960) Just what the doctor ordered. *British Medical Journal* **2**: 293–99.

Shepherd, M., Cooper, B., Brown, A.C., and Kalton, G. (1966) *Psychiatric Illness in General Practice.* London: Oxford University Press.

Williamson, J., Stokoe, I.H., Gray, S., Fisher, M., Smith, A., McGhee, A., and Stephenson, E. (1964) Old people at home. *Lancet* **1**:1117–120.

PART 4

Alternatives to tranquilliser use

11
Introduction

The various concerns about the extent of tranquilliser use, discussed in Part 1, indicate the need to consider alternative therapeutic approaches. Such alternatives may be considered in three groups, depending on who is the therapist. First, there are those therapeutic strategies which the general practitioner him/herself initiates and carries out; second are approaches which involve other members of, or other workers attached to, the primary care team, and third, an approach in which the therapists are the patients themselves: self-help groups.

Alternatives to tranquillisers will consist largely of treatments loosely classified as 'psychotherapy' and/or 'counselling'. While the definition of these terms is problematic, it is useful to distinguish between dynamic psychotherapy (treatment derived from, and developed within, a particular theoretical formulation of personality structure and its development), behavioural psychotherapy (treatment based on principles of learning theory and aimed at direct modification of behaviour), and other, less theoretically circumscribed forms of psychotherapy/counselling based on listening and advice-giving.

Apart from the general practitioner him/herself, a range of professionals have provided such treatments within the primary care setting. For example, a number of reports have documented the work of psychologists in general practice, mostly using behavioural methods (Koch 1979; Earll and Kincey 1982; Freeman and Button 1984; Robson, France, and Blanch 1984), while others have described the activities of social workers (Clare and Corney 1982; Corney 1983) and marriage guidance counsellors (Waydenfeld and Waydenfeld 1980; Martin and Mitchell 1983) in primary care. In general, the available outcome research shows that such activities are associated with a reduction in tranquilliser prescribing, although these studies have not always been adequately controlled and the follow-up period has sometimes been short (see Martin (1985) for a recent review).

Such treatments may not be suitable for all patients, and not all doctors may have the experience or inclination to carry them out, or the personnel to whom to refer. In such circumstances self-help groups are of particular

135

importance. They can provide people trying to stop taking tranquillisers who feel isolated with sympathetic support and understanding, help them to realize that the withdrawal symptoms they might experience are not unique, and strengthen their resolve to achieve their goal of a tranquilliser-free life.

It should be borne in mind that most of these therapeutic approaches will cost more than tranquillisers. As Joyce (1985) has observed, 'Talking goes deeper but drugging is cheaper.' Thus, in any cost-effectiveness analysis (an economic comparison in which the different treatments are assumed to be equally beneficial), tranquillisers will almost invariably emerge as the superior treatment (although the same will not necessarily apply in a cost–benefit analysis – an economic comparison which takes differential cost *and* differential benefit into account).

Alternatives to tranquilliser treatment may be considered either at the initial consultation – that is, before tranquilliser treatment is initiated – or during the course of pre-existing drug treatment. The controlled evaluation of tranquilliser treatment by Catalan and his colleagues is an example of the former. This study is unique and unrepeatable: as indicated by the evidence discussed in Part 1 (decreasing tranquilliser prescriptions; constant prevalence with increasing duration of treatment), the rate at which tranquilliser treatment is initiated has decreased substantially. Recent attempts by one of the editors to recruit a sample of patients receiving tranquillisers for the first time had to be abandoned because too few patients could be found.

The second paper in this section, by Hopkins and his colleagues, investigates the effect of a programme of planned withdrawal in patients already established in treatment with benzodiazepines. Although the withdrawal programme proved successful (in terms of continued abstinence from benzodiazepines) for a majority of patients, no 'alternative treatment' (other than the withdrawal regime itself) was offered. One such alternative, the self-help group, is discussed by Ettore in the third paper in this section. She summarizes the literature on this subject and considers its implications for the study of tranquilliser self-help groups. This provides a basis for a descriptive analysis and assessment of one of the first tranquilliser self-help groups to be set up in Britain.

One important aspect of any alternative therapeutic initiative is the extent to which it is accepted by, and taken up by, doctors and their patients. Further evaluation of the non-drug approaches to the management of psychological ill-health described in this section should ideally include consideration of this issue and, if necessary, the exploration of ways in which it could be improved.

References

Clare, A.W. and Corney, R.H. (eds) (1982) *Social Work and Primary Health Care*. London: Academic Press.

Corney, R.H. (1983) Social work in general practice. In J. Lishman (ed.) *Collaboration and Conflict: Working with Others*. Research Highlights 1983, Department of Social Work, University of Aberdeen.

Earll, L. and Kincey, J. (1982) Clinical psychology in general practice: A controlled trial evaluation. *Journal of the Royal College of General Practitioners* 32(234): 322-37.

Freeman, J.K. and Button, E.J. (1984) The clinical psychologist in general practice. *Journal of the Royal College of General Practitioners* 32(264): 377-80.

Joyce, C.R.B. (1985) Review of 'Psychopharmacology and Psychotherapy'. *Psychological Medicine* 15(1): 205-06.

Koch, G.C.H. (1979) Evaluation of behaviour therapy intervention in general practice. *Journal of the Royal College of General Practitioners* 29(203): 337-40.

Martin, E. (1985) Counselling in general practice. *Journal of the Royal Society of Medicine* 78(3): 186-88.

Martin, E. and Mitchell, H. (1983) A counsellor in general practice: a one-year survey. *Journal of the Royal College of General Practitioners* 33(251): 366-67.

Robson, M.H., France, R., and Blanch, M. (1984) Clinical psychologist in primary care: controlled clinical and economic evaluation. *British Medical Journal* 288(1): 1805-809.

Waydenfeld, D. and Waydenfeld, S.W. (1980) Counselling in general practice. *Journal of the Royal College of General Practitioners* 30(220): 671-77.

12

The effects of non-prescribing of anxiolytics in general practice

Jose Catalan, Dennis Gath, Gillian Edmonds, John Ennis, Alison Bond, and Pauline Martin

I. CONTROLLED EVALUATION OF PSYCHIATRIC AND SOCIAL OUTCOME

Summary Ninety-one patients with new episodes of minor affective disorder were selected by their general practitioners as suitable for anxiolytic medication. Half the patients were allocated randomly to a drug group (anxiolytic medication), and half to a non-drug group (brief counselling without anxiolytics). Psychiatric and social assessments were made (i) at initial consultation when treatment was started; (ii) one month later; (iii) seven months later. Before treatment the two groups were similar on all main variables. On the General Health Questionnaire, 85 per cent of patients were psychiatric cases before treatment, 40 per cent at one month and 30 per cent at seven months. Similar improvements were found with other measures of psychiatric state (Profile of Mood States; Present State Examination) and social functioning (SAS-M). Improvements were similar and parallel in the two groups. Neither group of patients increased their consumption of alcohol, tobacco or non-prescribed drugs. The non-drug group did not make increased demands on the doctors' time.

It is established that minor affective disorders are common amongst patients consulting general practitioners (Goldberg and Blackwell 1970; Goldberg *et al*. 1976). These disorders present mainly with symptoms of anxiety or depressed mood and often a mixture of the two (Goldberg and Huxley 1980; Shepherd *et al*. 1981). In many cases social problems appear to have been important in aetiology (Kedward 1969; Cooper 1972; Cooper

Reprinted, with permission, from the *British Journal of Psychiatry* 144:593–610. 1984.

and Sylph 1973). Such disorders usually improve within six to twelve months (Kedward 1969; Goldberg and Blackwell 1970; Mann *et al*. 1981).

General practitioners commonly prescribe psychotropic drugs for these minor affective disorders. During the 1960s, there was a steep increase in general practice prescriptions for these drugs, particularly the minor tranquillisers, non-barbiturates and antidepressants (Trethowan 1975). During the 1970s such prescriptions continued to increase, but more slowly (Williams 1980). In a recent survey of five group general practices in Oxford, Skegg *et al*. (1977) found that psychotropic drugs were the type of drugs most frequently prescribed in general practice. Amongst registered patients, in the course of one year more than 20 per cent of women and about 10 per cent of men received at least one prescription for a psychotropic drug. Amongst women aged 45, more than 30 per cent received at least one prescription for psychotropic medication in the course of a year.

Views are divided on this large scale prescribing of psychotropic medication. Some writers believe such prescribing is justified, others deplore it. Three main arguments are usually put forward to justify the widespread prescribing of psychotropic drugs in general practice. The first and commonest argument is that general practitioners usually lack the time to provide counselling as an alternative treatment (Edwards 1974). The second argument is that some widely used drugs, notably benzo-diazepines, are safer than alcohol or other drugs which patients might obtain for themselves (*Lancet* 1978). Thirdly, it is argued that drugs such as benzodiazepines are safer than many other drugs when taken in overdosage.

Considerable doubts have been expressed about the value of certain psychotropic drugs in general practice, especially the benzodiazepines (*Lancet* 1973, 1978; Trethowan 1975; Grahame-Smith 1975; Edwards 1979). There are three main arguments against benzodiazepines:– (a) they are not known to be effective for the symptoms seen in general practice, (b) they may be dangerous, (c) they are costly.

The evidence for the effectiveness of benzodiazepines is mixed. Some writers have reported that they may be valuable in general practice for minor affective disorders (Wheatley 1972; Priest 1980). On the other hand, studies of psychiatric out-patients and in-patients have suggested that a placebo may be as effective as anxiolytic medication, especially for patients with moderate or low levels of anxiety (Rickels and Downing 1967; Dasberg and van Praag 1974; Johnstone *et al*. 1980). There is little evidence that long-term use of benzodiazepines is effective for insomnia or anxiety (Committee on the Review of Medicines 1980).

Several possible dangers of benzodiazepines have been reported, includ-ing: increased proneness to road traffic accidents (Betts *et al*. 1972; Seppala *et al*. 1976; Skegg *et al*. 1979); physical dependence and withdrawal reactions

(Covi *et al*. 1973; Winokur *et al*. 1980; Petursson and Lader 1981); hostility and paradoxical reactions (Gardos *et al*. 1968; Hall and Joffe 1972; Salzman *et al*. 1974; *British Medical Journal* 1975; Goldney 1977); interaction with alcohol (Hayes *et al*. 1977); contribution to self-poisoning (Hawton and Blackstock 1976). With regard to cost, Trethowan (1975) drew attention to the substantial cost to the health service, whilst Leach and White (1978) pointed out that prescribed psychotropic drugs were often wasted.

Apart from these three arguments, it has been reported that the prescribing of psychotropic drugs is often incorrect pharmacologically (Tyrer 1978). It is also argued that it can be illogical (and possibly unethical) to prescribe drugs for emotional disorders that appear to be largely caused by social factors.

For all these reasons, it is important to ask whether it would be helpful or harmful to try to reduce the prescribing of psychotropic drugs in general practice. There is evidence that prescriptions for sedatives can be reduced by advertisements directed to doctors and patients (Keeler and McCurdy 1975), but the effect of this reduction on patients is not known. In one general practice it has been reported that barbiturate hypnotics could be withheld from patients and the prescribing of all hypnotic medication reduced by half, without causing any apparent harm to patients (Wells 1973). Apart from these two reports, little is known about the effects of withholding psychotropic medication from patients with minor affective disorders.

This paper reports a study of the effects of reducing the prescribing of anxiolytic medication in two group practices. The main aim was to study the effects of withholding anxiolytic drugs from patients to whom the general practitioner would usually prescribe them. In particular, it was intended to discover how far withholding drugs in this way would lead to the following undesirable effects: (1) prolongation of psychological distress that might have been relieved by anxiolytic medication; (2) increased consumption by patients of other substances, for example, drugs other than anxiolytics, non-prescribed drugs, alcohol, or tobacco; (3) failure to fulfil the patients' expectations at initial consultation; (4) unreasonable increases in demands on general practitioners' time. These questions are dealt with in this paper.

The design of the study also enabled us to examine a separate question: in patients to whom anxiolytics are usually prescribed in general practice what factors are associated with a poor outcome in terms of psychiatric status or long-term prescribing? This question is dealt with in the second paper.

Method

The study was designed as a prospective trial in which patients were allocated randomly to one of two treatments: anxiolytic medication; or brief counselling without anxiolytic medication. Psychiatric and social assessments of the patients were made on three occasions: at the initial consultation with the general practitioner, when treatment was started; one month after the initial consultation; seven months after the initial consultation.

Selection of patients
In the course of their normal work, the general practitioners identified all those patients to whom they would normally prescribe anxiolytic medication at the time of presentation. Within this group, patients were eligible for the trial if they fulfilled two conditions:–
(1) They were presenting with a new episode of psychiatric disorder. (For this condition 'new' meant that the patient had not consulted the general practitioner for a psychiatric disorder during the preceding three months.)
(2) They were not currently taking psychotropic drugs and had not done so during the preceding three months.

Patients were excluded from the trial either if they refused treatment, or the general practitioner judged the psychiatric disorder to be so severe that withholding medication was not justifiable.

Allocation to treatment groups
Patients were randomly allocated to one of the two treatments as soon as the general practitioner had decided they were suitable for inclusion in the trial, and before he had given any advice, reassurance, or other form of treatment. It is emphasised that the general practitioner always decided whether or not to admit a patient to the trial without knowledge of which treatment would be given. Random allocation was achieved by drawing cards sequentially from a random pack (unknown to the patient).

The two treatment groups

Anxiolytic medication
This group will be referred to as the 'drug group'. The general practitioner prescribed anxiolytic medication of his choice for up to two weeks. Thereafter the doctor was free to prescribe further anxiolytic medication as long as it was judged necessary. For the purpose of the investigation, the general practitioners agreed that anxiolytic medication would consist of minor tranquillisers, such as diazepam or chlordiazepoxide, to be taken for their calming effect by day, or as hypnotics at night. In this treatment group the general practitioner gave such reassurance and advice as he would usually give when prescribing anxiolytic medication.

Brief counselling without anxiolytic medication
This group will be referred to as 'the non-drug group'. The general practitioner was to give brief counselling without attempting any specialized counselling or psychotherapy. It was stipulated that this brief counselling could include:– explanation of the nature of any symptoms and why they had occurred; exploration of underlying personal or other problems, and ways of dealing with them; and reasons for not prescribing drugs (if appropriate). The general practitioners were given guidance and written information about the use of these techniques during the pilot stage of the investigation.

In both treatments, the general practitioners carried out any necessary physical examinations.

Methods of assessment
At the end of the initial consultation, the general practitioner explained to the patient that an investigation was being made into emotional problems and methods of treatment. The general practitioner then invited the patient to take part in the assessment procedures described below. The assessment procedures and their timing are shown in *Table I*. As already explained, assessments were made on three occasions:– at the initial consultation; one month later; and seven months after the initial consultation. The information collected was of three main kinds:– self-ratings by the patients; observations recorded by the general practitioners; observations made by three interviewers from the research team.

Table 1   *Timing of assessments*

	initial contact with GP	one month follow-up	seven months follow-up
patients' self-ratings			
GHQ	+	+	+
POMS	+	+	+
SAS-M	+	+	+
expectations/satisfaction	+	+	+
consumption of other substances	+	+	+
GPs' observations			
duration of interview with GP; presenting complaint	+	–	–
information from GP records	–	–	+
researchers' observations			
PSE	+ (⅓ of patients)	+ (⅓ of patients)	+ (all patients)
life events	–	–	+

Patients' self-ratings

At all three stages of assessment the patients completed the following self-ratings:–

(a) Mental state measured by the General Health Questionnaire, or GHQ (Goldberg 1972; Goldberg and Hillier 1979), and by the Profile of Mood States, or POMS (McNair and Lorr 1964).

(b) Social adjustment measured by the Social Adjustment Scale in the version modified by Cooper *et al.* (1982) from the original by Gurland *et al.* (1972). This scale is referred to as SAS-M.

(c) Views of treatment: expectation and satisfaction with the treatment after the initial consultation, and satisfaction and compliance with treatment at the two follow-up stages.

(d) Extent to which prescribed drugs had been taken.

(e) Consumption of non-prescribed medication, alcohol and drugs.

The questionnaires were handed to patients by the general practitioner at the end of the initial consultation and were returned to the research team by post. At the two follow-up assessments, the questionnaires were sent out and returned by post.

Observations by general practitioners

At the initial interview, the general practitioners used standard forms to record the following:– the nature, severity and duration of the psychiatric problem; any physical disorder; any social problems; all medication prescribed at the initial consultation, and any other help given; the duration of the initial consultation. At the end of the study, members of the research team examined the practice records of all patients in the study, and abstracted information on GP-patient contacts and any prescription of psychotropic medication during the seven month follow-up.

Observations by research assistants

It was thought important to avoid as far as possible any therapeutic effects that might occur through extended contact between patients and research assistants. For two thirds of the patients, therefore, during the initial and the one-month assessments, the research assistants made contact only to give out or collect self-administered questionnaires. For a randomly selected one third of patients, contact at these two assessments included an interview using the Present State Examination, or PSE (Wing *et al.* 1974). On completion of the study at seven months, all patients in the trial were assessed with the PSE. The PSE was used to provide an outcome measure and to check the findings with the self-administered questionnaires (GHQ and POMS). At the final follow-up, the research assistants also administered an inventory of life events (Paykel *et al.* 1969), covering the six months before the interview.

Most interviews were held in the patients' homes but a few were held (at the patient's request) in the health centre. Interviews were carried out by a research psychiatrist (JC) and two research assistants (AB and GE), all of whom had extensive experience in psychiatric interviewing and particularly the use of the PSE.

The practices
Patients were selected from those attending two health centres sited in towns within a few miles of Oxford City. Patients were admitted to the study over a period of twelve months in one health centre, and four months in the other. Six general practitioners participated, three from each health centre.

Results

Requests were made to 124 patients to enter the study of whom 33 (27 per cent) were excluded because they were unwilling to complete the questionnaires. These excluded patients did not differ from the remaining patients in their sex, age and presenting complaints as rated by the general practitioners. On entering the study, all 91 patients completed the first set of questionnaires and 31 (34 per cent) of them were interviewed by the research assistants (this was in accordance with the research plan outlined above). At the one-month follow-up, two of the 91 patients declined to participate (one of whom was from the previously interviewed group). At the seven-month follow-up, two patients declined to participate, whilst a further three completed questionnaires but declined to be interviewed. At this final follow-up, therefore, questionnaire data were available from 87 (96 per cent), and interview data from 84 (92 per cent) of the initial sample.

Of the patients admitted at the initial consultation, 42 (46 per cent) were allocated to the drug group, and 49 (54 per cent) to the non-drug group. At the first assessment, the two treatment groups were comparable on virtually all measures. As shown in *Table 2*, the groups were comparable in demographic characteristics, and also in the general practitioners' assessments of their presenting complaints, social difficulties, and associated physical disorders (see below). As shown in *Table 3*, at the initial assessment there were only minor differences between the two treatment groups in the standardized measures of mental state. The same also held for the measures of social functioning (not shown in *Table 3*). Both of these sets of measures are described in detail later.

The characteristics of the two samples are given in *Table 2*; the social class distribution of the patients did not differ significantly from the general population. As shown in *Table 2*, the general practitioners' findings were much the same for the two treatment groups. According to the GPs

Table 2 *Comparison of the two treatment groups at the initial consultation*

	drug group (n = 42)		non-drug group (n = 49)	
	no.	(%)	no.	(%)
sex females	29	(69)	36	(73)
age mean (SD)	35	(11)	33	(11)
marital status				
single	5	(12)	9	(18)
married	31	(74)	37	(75)
wid., div., or sep.	6	(14)	3	(6)
social class				
I	—	—	1	(2)
II	14	(33)	13	(27)
III	21	(50)	21	(43)
IV	5	(12)	12	(24)
V	1	(2)	1	(2)
unclassified	1	(2)	1	(2)
general practitioner's assessments				
presenting complaints:				
tension	24	(57)	21	(43)
misc. physical symptoms	10	(24)	15	(30)
(palpitations, breathing diff.)				
headaches	7	(17)	7	(14)
marital problems	6	(14)	8	(16)
depression	6	(14)	8	(16)
insomnia	4	(10)	9	(18)
duration of presenting complaint:				
less than 1 week	6	(14)	10	(20)
1–4 weeks	18	(43)	19	(39)
5–12 weeks	12	(29)	13	(27)
13–24 weeks	3	(7)	5	(10)
over 24 weeks	3	(7)	2	(4)
concurrent social difficulties:				
family (other than marital)	18	(43)	21	(43)
work	14	(34)	15	(31)
marital	17	(40)	15	(31)
financial	2	(5)	2	(4)
concurrent physical disorder:	15	(36)	13	(27)

There were no significant differences between treatment groups.

the main presenting complaint was tension; other common complaints were palpitations, breathing difficulties, headaches, depressed mood, and insomnia. Over half of these complaints had started less than a month previously.

Concurrent social difficulties in family, marriage or work were each reported by over a third of the patients. Concurrent medical conditions were diagnosed by the general practitioner in about a third of the patients. Most of these conditions were minor physical ailments or chronic disorders.

Treatment given

1. At initial consultation
(a) Duration of consultation: According to records kept by the general practitioners, the durations of initial consultations were: drug group 3–20 minutes (mean 10.5; SD 4.2); non-drug group 3–25 minutes (mean 12; SD 4.7); the difference is not significant.

(b) Psychotropic medication: At the initial consultation the non-drug group received no psychotropic medication. In the drug group, the numbers of patients receiving anxiolytic drugs were:- diazepam by day, 33 (78 per cent); chlordiazepoxide by day, 5 (12 per cent); nitrazepam at night, 2 (5 per cent). In addition, two (5 per cent) patients received minor tranquillisers combined with an antidepressant, prescribed specifically for their anxiolytic effects. All drugs were prescribed in the dose recommended in the National Formulary. All initial prescriptions were for two weeks' supply.

(c) Non-psychotropic drugs: These were prescribed to nine patients (21 per cent) in the drug group, and 16 patients (32 per cent) in the non-drug group (difference not significant). The drugs prescribed most commonly were analgesics and preparations acting on the alimentary and cardio-vascular systems.

(d) Counselling by the general practitioners: According to the practitioners, advice on coping with difficulties was given to more patients in the non-drug group (66 per cent) than in the drug group (35 per cent) ($\chi^2 =$ 6.78; df $=$ 1; P $<$ 0.01). No significant differences were found in the frequency, as reported by the practitioners, of the following:- listening to the patients (98 per cent in both groups); explaining symptoms (50 per cent in the non-drug group, and 67 per cent in the drug group); reasurrance (33 per cent in the non-drug group, and 35 per cent in the drug group). It is interesting that the patients generally perceived their doctors' actions in the same way. Thus, according to the patients, the frequencies were: advice on coping with difficulties – non-drug group 41 per cent, drug group 17 per cent ($\chi^2 =$ 4.44; df $=$ 1; P $<$ 0.05); listening to the patient – drug group 96 per cent, non-drug group 93 per cent; explaining cause of symptoms – drug group 41 per cent, non-drug group 51 per cent.

2. One-month follow-up
In the *drug group*, 19 patients (46 per cent) were still taking anxiolytic medication; of the 22 patients (54 per cent) who were not doing so, three (7 per cent) never took the prescribed medication (one losing the prescription, two recovering rapidly before using it), nine (22 per cent) stopped taking the prescribed drug within one week and 10 (24 per cent) within one to two weeks. In the *non-drug group*, one patient returned to the practitioner a

Table 3 Psychiatric status by treatment group at initial consultation and both follow-ups

measure of psychiatric status	initial assessment		1/12 follow-up		7/12 follow-up	
	drug	non-drug	drug	non-drug	drug	non-drug
case status						
GHQ	36 (86%)	39 (80%)	16 (38%)	22 (46%)	12 (28%)	12 (26%)
PSE*	12 (80%)	12 (75%)	6 (43%)	7 (44%)	11 (29%)	15 (33%)
	mean (sd)		mean (sd)		mean (sd)	
GHQ: total score	26.4 (13.8)	24.2 (13.5)	11.3 (13.7)	13.7 (11.2)	7.6 (10.8)	7.2 (12.5)
sub-scores:						
somatic	4.0 (2.2)	3.4 (1.9)	1.3 (1.8)	1.9 (1.8)	1.0 (1.8)	1.3 (1.6)
anxiety	4.0 (2.1)	3.6 (2.2)	1.7 (1.8)	2.0 (2.2)	1.3 (1.9)	1.0 (1.8)
social	2.5 (2.1)	2.5 (2.1)	1.3 (2.0)	1.3 (1.9)	0.5 (1.3)	0.7 (1.6)
depression	1.5 (1.1)	1.5 (1.1)	0.5 (1.2)	0.7 (1.3)	0.4 (1.0)	0.5 (1.1)
PSE* total score	15.2 (7.0)	14.7 (8.5)	9.5 (7.4)	10.3 (10.1)	7.8 (6.7)	7.5 (7.2)
POMS: total score	55.5 (2.0)	52.7 (2.0)	40.9 (17.6)	39.7 (21.0)	35.0 (22.0)	31.5 (21.9)
sub-scores:						
anger	7.2 (4.7)	5.0 (4.8)	4.4 (3.4)	4.1 (3.4)	5.1 (4.0)	3.7 (3.1)
tension	14.0 (5.0)	14.0 (6.0)	9.1 (4.6)	8.6 (5.5)	7.9 (6.2)	7.3 (5.8)
depression	10.0 (7.3)	9.6 (8.1)	6.7 (6.1)	6.1 (6.0)	6.0 (5.6)	4.3 (3.4)
fatigue	14.0 (3.7)	16.0 (6.4)	13.1 (3.6)	13.5 (3.7)	11.4 (4.1)	11.5 (3.9)

Lower scores indicate less severity.
*PSE results apply to a subsample at initial assessment (N = 31) and one-month follow-up (N = 30), and 84 patients at the seven-month follow-up.

week after the initial consultation and was given a prescription for a hypnotic.

3. Seven-month follow-up

In the *drug group*, information was available on 40 patients. Of these, 13 (32 per cent) had received at least one prescription for psychotropic drugs in the six months since the one month follow-up. These patients included five who had received a single prescription and eight who had received two to six prescriptions; nine of these patients were given anxiolytics, and four antidepressants. In the *non-drug group*, information was available on 47 patients. Of these, seven (15 per cent) had received at least one prescription; they included four patients who had received one prescription for psychotropic medication and three who had received two to four such prescriptions. Three of these had received antidepressants.

There was thus a trend for the non-drug group to receive fewer prescriptions but the difference was not significant.

4. Further contacts with the general practitioner

Between the initial interview and the seven-month follow-up, the mean numbers of further contacts with the practitioner were:- drug group, 4.6; non-drug group, 4.5 (N.S.). According to the practitioners' records, psychological symptoms were mentioned in significantly more re-visits by the drug group (55 per cent) than by the non-drug group (35 per cent; $\chi^2 =$ 15.4; df = 1; P < 0.001).

5. Consumption of other substances

According to the patients' reports, during the study period there were no increases in the numbers of patients consuming alcohol or tobacco, or in the amounts consumed by individual patients. No differences were found between the two treatment groups in the use of these substances. Similarly, there was no significant change in consumption of non-prescribed drugs over time or by treatment group.

Psychiatric status

The information given in the following section is summarized in *Table 3*.

General Health Questionnaire (GHQ)

(a) GHQ cases: There were no significant differences between the drug group and the non-drug group on any GHQ measure at any stage of the enquiry. Patients were classed as psychiatric cases if they had a total score of 12 or more on the GHQ (60 item version). On this definition, at the initial consultation, there were 36 cases (86 per cent) in the drug group and 39 (80 per cent) in the non-drug group.

Figure 1   Proportions of GHQ cases by treatment group at the three assessments

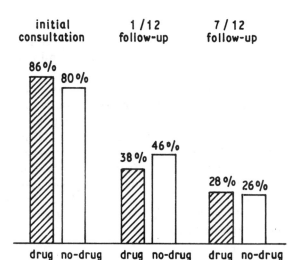

At the one-month follow-up, the numbers of cases had fallen to 16 (38 per cent) in the drug group, and 22 (46 per cent) in the non-drug group. Both reductions were significant at the 0.001 level.

At the seven-month follow-up, the numbers of cases were again smaller, 12 (28 per cent) in the drug group, and 12 (26 per cent) in the non-drug group; again these proportions were lower than those at initial consultation at the one in a thousand level of significance. The proportions of cases by treatment groups at the three stages of assessment are shown in *Figure 1*.

(b) GHQ mean total score: The above findings for GHQ cases were reflected in the mean total scores of the two treatment groups. At the initial consultation, the means were: drug group 26.4 (sd 13.8), non-drug group 24.2 (sd 13.5). At one-month follow-up the means were: drug group 11.3 (sd 10.1), non-drug group 13.7 (sd 11.2); and at seven month follow-up: drug group 7.6 (sd 10.8), non-drug group 7.2 (sd 12.5). Compared with the initial consultation, the mean total scores were significantly reduced at both follow-ups (P < 0.001).

(c) GHQ sub-scores: The main finding was that, at all three stages of assessment, sub-scores for anxiety and for somatic symptoms were considerably higher than for depression. GHQ sub-scores showed improvements at the one-month and seven-month follow-ups, with no significant difference between treatment groups. Taken together, the GHQ findings suggest that the general practitioners had initially identified a group of patients who had high levels of psychiatric morbidity, which mainly took the form of anxiety.

Profile of mood states (POMS)
(a) Total score: There was no difference between the two treatment groups at any stage of assessment. Compared with initial consultation, there were significant reductions (improvement) in the POMS total score both at the one-month follow-up (P < 0.001 for both treatment groups), and at the seven-month follow-up (P < 0.001 for both treatment groups).

(b) Sub-scores: At the initial consultation, the drug group had a higher mean score than the non-drug group on one of the five sub-scores, – anger ($t = 2.09$, P < 0.05). At the one-month follow-up, both treatment groups showed significant improvements in three of the sub-scores, – tension, depression and fatigue (P < 0.001). Only the drug group showed a significant improvement in 'anger' (P < 0.001) but analysis of covariance showed no significant difference between the two treatment groups in this respect ($t = 1.20$, NS). Analysis of covariance showed that the non-drug group had improved significantly more in 'vigour' ($t = 4.03$; P < 0.01). At the seven-month follow-up, all the POMS sub-scores showed significant reductions when compared with the initial consultation; there were no significant differences between the two treatment groups.

Present state examination (PSE)
Patients were counted as PSE cases if they were at level 5 or higher on the PSE Index of Definition (Wing *et al.* 1974). At the initial consultation, interviews were held with 15 patients in the drug group and 16 in the non-drug group. The numbers of PSE cases were 12 (80 per cent) and 12 (75 per cent) respectively. At the one-month follow-up, 15 patients from each treatment group were interviewed. The numbers of PSE cases were six (43 per cent) in the drug group and seven (44 per cent) in the non-drug group. At the seven-month follow-up, 84 patients were interviewed. The numbers of PSE cases were 11 (29 per cent) in the drug group, and 15 (33 per cent) in the non-drug group. Twenty eight patients were assessed with the PSE at all three assessments. Analysis of the change scores showed significant reductions at one month (drug group, P < 0.05; non-drug group, P. < 0.001) and at seven months (drug group, P < 0.001; non-drug group, P < 0.001). Analysis of covariance showed no significant difference between the two treatment groups in this respect.

Relationships between GHQ and PSE findings
Highly significant correlations (Pearson) were found between PSE total scores and GHQ total scores at the initial consultation (P < 0.001), at the one-month follow-up (P < 0.001) and at the seven-month follow-up (P < 0.001). On comparison of psychiatric cases v. non-cases identified by the PSE Index of Definition and those identified by the GHQ, agreement was found to be 80 per cent at initial consultation, 80 per cent at one-month follow-up and 87 per cent at seven-month follow-up.

Table 4 *Patients' ratings of changes in presenting complaints at the two follow-up assessments*

| | one month follow-up | | | | seven month follow-up | | | |
| | drug group | | non-drug group | | drug group | | non-drug group | |
	no.	(%)	no.	(%)	no.	(%)	no.	(%)
recovered	4	(10)	8	(17)	9	(22)	13	(28)
better	29	(71)	28	(58)	19	(48)	28	(60)
no change	8	(19)	12	(25)	10	(25)	3	(6)
worse	—	—	—	—	2	(5)	3	(6)
total	41	(100)	48	(100)	40	(100)	47	(100)

Patients' self-assessment of psychiatric status
The patients' ratings of changes in their presenting problems are shown in *Table 4*. It can be seen that over three quarters of the patients rated themselves as better or recovered at both follow-ups. There were no significant differences between treatment groups.

Deliberate self-harm
No patients deliberately took overdoses or injured themselves during the study period.

Social adjustment
(a) SAS-M total score: Compared with the initial assessment, there were significant improvements in SAS-M total scores both at the one-month follow-up (drug group, $P < 0.01$; non-drug group, $P < 0.01$) and at the seven-month follow-up (drug group, $P < 0.001$; non-drug group, $P < 0.01$). There were no significant differences between the two treatment groups in degree of improvement at either follow-up.

(b) SAS-M sub-scores: The SAS-M includes the sub-scores: work, housework, social and leisure, extended family, marriage, children, and family unit. At both the one-month and the seven-month follow-ups, the two treatment groups showed significant improvements on most of the sub-scores. At the seven-month follow-up, analysis of covariance showed significant differences between the two treatment groups in just one sub-score, – social and leisure ($t = 7.44$, $P < 0.01$), in favour of the drug group.

Patients' expectations and satisfaction
(a) Satisfaction with duration of initial consultation: Of the 91 patients entering the study, only five (four drug group and one non-drug group) expressed dissatisfaction with the duration of the initial consultation.

(b) Expectations of receiving drugs: Of the 91 patients, 47 (52 per cent) said they expected to receive a prescription for psychotropic drugs. There

Table 5   *Patient's satisfaction with prescribing/non-prescribing of psychotropic drugs at the initial interview and both follow-up assessments*

	initial interview drug group		non-drug group		one month drug group		non-drug group		seven months drug group		non-drug group	
	no.	(%)	no.	(%)	no.	(%)	no.	(%)	no.	(%)	no.	(%)
glad	15	(36)	22	(45)	14	(34)	21	(44)	19	(47)	25	(53)
don't mind	14	(33)	16	(33)	14	(34)	19	(40)	11	(28)	12	(26)
reluctant	13	(30)	6	(12)	11	(27)	7	(14)	10	(25)	10	(21)
against	—	—	5	(10)	2	(5)	1	(2)	—	—	—	—
	42	(100)	49	(100)	41	(100)	48	(100)	40	(100)	47	(100)

were no significant differences between the two treatment groups in these expectations. Thirteen patients in the drug group (31 per cent) and 11 in the non-drug group (22 per cent) said they had asked the practitioner to prescribe drugs for their 'nerves'.

(c) Patients' satisfaction with prescribing/non-prescribing: The patients' satisfaction with the prescribing/non-prescribing of psychotropic drugs is shown in *Table 5*. There were no significant differences between the two treatment groups at any stage, although the non-drug group tended to give more extreme responses. At the seven-month follow-up patients were asked whether they thought the practitioner might have done anything else to help. Affirmative responses were given by 19 patients in the drug group (66 per cent) as against 15 in the non-drug group (37 per cent; $x^2 = 3.92$; df = 1, P < 0.05). Amongst these patients giving affirmative responses, most would have welcomed referral to a psychiatrist or marriage guidance counsellor.

Discussion

Before discussing the findings, it is important to consider the sample of patients and the treatments they received.

The first point to stress about the sample is that patients were selected by the general practitioners and not by the research team. The general practitioners were asked to select all those patients to whom they would normally prescribe anxiolytic medication. It was hoped that this method of selection would make the investigation more realistic. The only limitations were that the patients must be presenting with a new episode of psychiatric disorder and must have taken no psychotropic medication in the preceding three months.

According to the general practitioners, the patients' initial complaints were mainly of tension, bodily symptoms typical of anxiety, and insomnia. About half the patients had experienced their symptoms for less than a month and 85 per cent for less than three months, during the present episode of illness. General Health Questionnaires completed at the initial interview showed that over 80 per cent of the patients were psychiatric cases. The sub-scores of the GHQ showed that symptoms of anxiety and somatic symptoms were more common than depressive symptoms. These findings suggested that the general practitioners had identified a group of patients with substantial psychiatric morbidity, mainly in the form of anxiety.

Two thirds of the patients were women. For patients of both sexes the mean age was in the early thirties and their social class was typical of the background population. Of the 91 patients initially admitted to the study, 42 (46 per cent) were allocated to the drug treatment group, and 49 (54 per cent) to the non-drug group. These two treatment groups were comparable in their demographic characteristics, presenting complaints, assessments by the general practitioners, and scores on all standardized measures of mental state (GHQ; POMS; PSE) and of social functioning (SAS-M).

The medication given to the drug group seemed typical of general practice prescribing for minor affective disorders. The drugs prescribed were diazepam, chlordiazepoxide, nitrazepam, and antidepressant combined with minor tranquillisers. Most of these drugs were taken for a short period, although at the one-month follow-up, 19 of the original 42 patients were still on psychotropic medication. At the seven-month follow-up, the figure was 13.

As judged by the general practitioner's reports of the content and duration of the initial interview, the treatment given to the non-drug group was certainly not intensive or specialised. The main treatment was advice, which was given to two thirds of the non-drug group (as against one third of the drug group). Other techniques included listening, explanation and reassurance, but these were given to the non-drug group no more frequently than to the drug group. After the initial interview there was some prescribing of medication to the non-drug group; by the one-month follow-up, one non-drug patient had received a prescription, and by the seven-month follow-up seven non-drug patients had done so.

Turning now to the findings, the purpose of the study was to answer four questions, which will be considered in turn. The first question was: *Does withholding anxiolytic drugs prolong psychological distress that might have been relieved by anxiolytic medication?* All the findings pointed to a negative answer to this question. Thus in the drug group the proportions of psychiatric cases on GHQ were: 86 per cent initially, 38 per cent at one month, and 28 per cent at seven months. For the non-drug group, the corresponding proportions were:- 80 per cent, 46 per cent and 26 per cent. For both treatment groups, there were significant improvements at one month and at seven months compared with their initial status. There were no significant differences between the two groups at any stage of assessment.

Similarly, when the POMS and PSE were used to measure psychiatric status, no significant differences were found between the drug group and the non-drug group at any stage of assessment. Again there were significant improvements at one month and at seven months, by comparison with the initial interview. The same observations held for social adjustment as measured by the SAS-M, – there were significant improvements at both follow-ups, and no significant differences between the two treatment groups. Finally, at both follow-ups over three quarters of the patients rated themselves as better or improved, and there were no significant differences between the treatment groups. Taken together, these findings point strongly to the conclusion that the prescribing of anxiolytic drugs made no significant difference to the psychiatric or social outcome.

The second question was: *Does withholding anxiolytic medication increase the comsumption by patients of other substances?* Here again the findings pointed to a negative answer. There were no reported increases in the use of alcohol, tobacco, or non-prescribed drugs. This was true both for the numbers of patients using the substances and for the amounts consumed by individuals. Nor was there any difference between treatment groups in these measures. It is of course possible that the patients' self-reports were not always dependable but the available evidence does not point to any increase in consumption of these substances.

The third question was: *Does withholding anxiolytic medication fail to fulfil the patients' expectations?* Several questions were asked about this possibility, and all the responses pointed to a negative answer. For example, when patients were asked to rate their satisfaction with the prescribing/non-prescribing of drugs, no significant difference was found between the two treatment groups.

The final question was: *Does withholding anxiolytic medication make unreasonable demands on the general practitioners' time?* Once again the answer appeared to be in the negative. The mean duration of the initial interview was 10.5 minutes for the drug group, and 12 minutes for the non-drug group. During the entire follow-up period, the mean rate of further consultations with the practitioner after the initial consultation was 4.6 consultations for the drug group, and 4.5 for the non-drug group.

In this particular sample of patients, therefore, all the findings suggested that withholding anxiolytic drugs did not have harmful effects. An important question is: *How far can the findings be generalised to other patients, and to other GPs?* In their demographic and psychiatric characteristics, the patients seemed similar to patients with new episodes of psychiatric disorder described in other general practice studies (Cooper and Sylph

1973; Shepherd *et al.* 1981). The general practitioners were perhaps unusual in their willingness to participate in the study, but they were typical in having no specialised experience or training in psychological methods of treatment. It therefore seems reasonable to suppose that the findings of the study may be widely applicable to patients and general practitioners in the United Kingdom.

Two main conclusions can be drawn from this part of the study. The first is that anxiolytic medication can be withheld without causing harmful effects to patients who have minor affective disorders and somatic complaints of recent onset, as diagnosed by the GP, and confirmed by standardized tests of mental state. If no medication is prescribed to them, such patients seem to recover as quickly and as much as patients who receive anxiolytic medication. The second conclusion is that managing patients without anxiolytic medication does not make unreasonable demands on the doctors' time. For most patients, the only requirements are brief discussion of their symptoms, explanation of family and social difficulties, and advice on dealing with problems. In some cases referral to other agencies, such as marriage guidance or social services, may be suitable.

Although patients allotted to the non-drug group were no more disturbed than patients allotted to the drug group at the one month follow-up, we do not know whether this was so in the days immediately following the initial consultation. It is possible that the main indication for anxiolytics is to tide the patient over these first few days by reducing acute distress. Whilst most of the patients in the trial recovered from the initial disorder, about one third were still unwell at the seven-month follow-up. Moreover, as many as 20 (24 per cent) patients received prescriptions for psychotropic medication between the one-month and seven-month follow-up. It is important to examine the characteristics of these patients, and to discover what factors were associated with a poor outcome.

II FACTORS ASSOCIATED WITH OUTCOME

Summary Factors associated with psychiatric outcome were examined in a series of 87 patients who had presented in general practice with new episodes of minor affective disorder. Two outcome measures were used: (i) Status on Present State Examination (PSE) seven months after initial consultation; (ii) prescribing of psychotropic medication between one-month and seven-month follow-up assessments. Outcome according to the PSE was significantly associated with: worse measures of psychiatric state (General Health Questionnaire, Profile of Mood states) and of social functioning (SAS-M) at initial consultation and one month later; and with persistent anxious or depressed mood during the follow-up period; but not with life events. During the follow-up period 20 patients received at least one psychotropic prescription; they were significantly associated with worse initial GHQ scores, consumption of tobacco and non-prescribed medication, and initial anxiety. A sub-group of 11 patients received multiple psychotropic prescriptions; they were significantly associated with the same initial measures, and also with poor outcome measures (psychiatric and social).

As reported above, a trial was carried out in general practice to evaluate psychiatric outcome in a series of patients who presented initially with minor affective disorders, and who were treated either with anxiolytic medication or with brief counselling but no medication. A large proportion of the patients recovered within one month of the initial consultation and a few more within seven months, irrespective of the type of treatment. This finding of rapid recovery for most patients agrees with findings from other studies in general practice (Kedward 1969; Goldberg and Blackwell 1970). Although such findings are encouraging, the third of patients who were still unwell at seven-month follow-up give cause for concern. If such longer-term patients are to be helped, it is important to know more about them and particularly whether they can be identified at an early stage.

Amongst the 87 patients, as many as a quarter received one or more psychotropic prescriptions between the one-month and the seven-month follow-ups. In view of the increasing evidence that repeated prescribing of anxiolytic medication may lead to dependence (Covi *et al.* 1973; Winokur *et al.* 1980; Petursson and Lader 1981), it is important to look for distinctive characteristics of patients who present with a new episode of minor affective disorder and who still need psychotropic medication one to seven months later.

This paper deals with these questions, which can be summarised thus:- In patients to whom anxiolytic medication is usually prescribed in general practice, what factors are associated with (i) a poor psychiatric outcome, (ii) prescribing of psychotropic medication more than a month later? The design and methods of the study are described earlier.

Results

The findings will be presented under two main headings: (i) PSE status at the seven month follow-up; (ii) The prescribing of psychotropic medication between the one-month and seven-month follow-ups.

1. PSE status at the seven month follow-up

Amongst the 84 patients examined with the Present State Examination at the seven-month follow-up, 26 (31 per cent) were psychiatric cases as defined by levels 5 and above of the PSE Index of Definition. Of the 24 men examined, six (25 per cent) were PSE cases; and of the 60 women examined, 20 (33 per cent) were PSE cases, the difference between sexes being non-significant.

In using these PSE findings as outcome measures, the first step was to examine their relationships to other findings at the same follow-up.

(a) *PSE status at the seven-month follow-up in relation to other psychiatric and social measures at the same follow-up*: There were highly significant associations ($P < 0.001$) between PSE case status and the following psychiatric and social measures at the seven-month follow-up:- GHQ total score and all four sub-scores; POMS total score and three of the five sub-scores; SAS-M total score and five of six sub-scores. These findings suggested that it was reasonable to use the PSE as the main measure of psychiatric outcome.

(b) *PSE status at the seven-month follow-up in relation to psychiatric and social status at initial consultation*: In *Table 1* are shown the significant relationships between PSE status at seven months and various pre-treatment (initial interview) measures of psychiatric and social functioning. The pre-treatment PSE findings were not included in this analysis because only one third of the patients were examined with the PSE at the initial interview, as explained in paper I.

From *Table 1*, it can be seen that the significant associations varied with sex. Considering first the main pre-treatment measures of GHQ, POMS and SAS, it was found for the combined sexes that patients who were PSE cases at seven-month follow-up had had significantly worse pre-treatment scores on: GHQ total score and all four sub-scores; POMS total score and three of the five sub-scores, SAS total score and four of the six sub-scores. When the women were examined separately, similar associations were found except that some were at a lower level of significance, and one (family unit) was non-significant. For the men, however, there was only one significant association (family unit).

For the combined sexes, a significant association was also found (not shown in *Table 1*) between PSE case status at seven months and GHQ case status at initial consultation (Fisher's exact test, $P < 0.01$). Turning to the other initial interview factors, three of them were weakly associated ($P < 0.05$) with PSE status at seven-month follow-up, but only for the combined sexes. These factors were:-longer duration of initial interview; patients' dissatisfaction with duration of initial interview; and less likelihood of receiving a prescription for a medical condition. For the men alone, another pre-treatment factor – initial complaint of depression – was significantly associated with PSE status at seven-month follow-up.

Table 1 *Factors at initial interview associated with PSE case status at 7 months follow-up*

	both sexes (n = 84)	males (n = 24)	females (n = 60)
GHQ – total score	**	NS	**
somatic	**	NS	**
anxiety	**	NS	*
social	**	NS	*
depression	**	NS	**
POMS – total score	**	NS	*
tension	**	NS	*
depression	***	NS	**
fatigue	*	NS	*
SAS-M – total score	**	NS	**
housework	**	NS	**
social/leisure	*	NS	*
extended family	*	NS	*
family unit	*	*	NS
– longer duration of initial interview	*	NS	NS
# – dissatisfaction with length of initial interview	*	NS	NS
# – less likely to receive prescription for medical condition	*	NS	NS
# – presenting complaint 'depression'	NS	*	NS

[2] was used for the items marked #; for the other listed items *t*-tests were used. For P values: *** = $P < 0.001$; ** = $P < 0.01$; * = $P < 0.05$.

In summary, PSE status at seven-month follow-up was strongly associated with pre-treatment mental state and social functioning for the combined sexes and for women, but not for men alone.

Despite these associations, measures of mental state at initial consultation did not discriminate strongly between PSE cases and non-cases at seven-month follow-up. Thus, amongst initial GHQ cases, only 35 per cent were PSE at seven months; whilst amongst initial GHQ non-cases, 5 per cent were PSE cases at seven months. When an initial POMS total score of 46 + (the best cut-off) was used, the corresponding figures were 35 per cent and 7 per cent. In other words, both initial measures identified an at-risk group which included most future PSE cases, but also a substantial proportion of future non-cases.

Linear discriminant function analysis: By using this statistical technique, it was found that two pre-treatment variables together gave the best discrimination between PSE cases and non-cases amongst patients of both sexes at the seven-month follow-up. These variables were: (i) the social and leisure sub-score of the SAS; (ii) patient's lack of satisfaction with the duration of the initial interview with the general practitioner. Together these two variables discriminated between PSE cases and non-cases with 71 per cent accuracy.

(c) *PSE status at the seven-month follow-up in relation to psychiatric and social status at the one-month follow-up*: Since levels of psychiatric morbidity fell substantially between the initial consultation and the one-month follow-up, it was important to discover whether any psychiatric or social factors detectable at one month would discriminate between PSE cases/non-cases at the seven month follow-up.

PSE outcome at seven months was significantly associated with scores at one month for GHQ total score ($t = 2.53$, P < 0.05), and the depression ($t = 3.43$, P < 0.01) and social ($t = 2.46$; P < 0.05) sub-scales; contrary to expectation, PSE outcome was not significantly associated with GHQ caseness, or with the somatic and anxiety sub-scales. There were highly significant associations between PSE outcome at seven months and scores at one month for POMS total score, ($t = 3.57$, P < 0.001); depression, ($t = 4.78$, P < 0.001) and fatigue ($t = 3.09$, P < 0.01). Similarly there were highly significant associations between PSE outcome at seven months and scores at one month for the SAS-M total score ($t = 3.72$, P < 0.001), and five of the sub-scores (P < 0.001 in four cases, and < 0.01 in one).

Measures of mental state at one month varied in the extent to which they discriminated between PSE cases and non-cases at seven months. Amongst GHQ cases at one month, only 35 per cent were PSE cases at seven months, whilst among GHQ non-cases at one month, as many as 24 per cent were PSE cases at seven months. When a POMS total score at one month of 46+ (the best cut-off) was used, the corresponding figures were considerably better, i.e. 50 per cent and 17 per cent. For the sub-group of 30 patients who had been interviewed at one month, the PSE provided the best discrimination. Thus amongst patients with a PSE total score of 12 or above at one month, as many as 63 per cent were PSE cases at seven months; amongst those with a total score below 12, only 10 per cent were PSE cases at seven months.

(d) *PSE status at the seven-month follow-up in relation to persistent symptoms of anxiety and depression*: During the administration of the PSE at seven months, patients were asked whether they had experienced anxious or depressed moods in the one-month to seven-month follow-up period, and for how long. For the combined sexes, PSE cases at seven months had experienced:- (i) anxious mood for a mean period of 5 months, as against 2.6 months for PSE non-cases ($t = 2.22$, P < 0.05); and (ii) depressed mood for a mean period of 4.5 months, as against 2.1 months for non-cases ($t = 3.11$, P < 0.01). Similarly significant associations were found when the sexes were examined separately.

(e) *PSE status at the seven-month follow-up in relation to life events*: As explained in paper 1, at the seven-month follow-up a life events inventory

(Paykel *et al.* 1969) was used to enquire about life events occurring in the six months preceding the interview. For the combined sexes, it was found that one or more events were reported by a somewhat larger proportion of PSE cases (92 per cent) than of PSE non-cases (74 per cent) at the seven-month examination, but the difference was not significant (Fisher's exact test). When the sexes were examined separately, similar trends were found, but again the differences were non-significant.

2. Prescribing of psychotropic medication between the one-month and seven-month follow-ups

Amongst the 87 patients for whom information was available, 20 (23 per cent) had received at least one prescription for psychotropic drugs between the one-month and the seven-month follow-up. This group will be referred to as the 'prescription group'. It included eight (32 per cent) men and 12 (19 per cent) women. In *Table 2* are listed the 20 patients who received prescriptions, together with the number of presciptions, timing of prescriptions, and nature of drug prescribed. Seven of them had belonged to the original non-drug group. It can be seen from the table that the prescription group included 11 patients (13 per cent of all those examined) who had received two or more prescriptions between the one-month and the seven-month follow-up. This sub-group will be referred to as the 'multiple prescription' group. It included six (24 per cent) men and five (8 per cent) women, the difference by sex being non-significant. It also included three patients who had belonged to the original non-drug group. When analysing the findings for the 'prescription' and 'multiple prescription' groups, no distinction will be made between patients from the original drug and non-drug groups, because of small numbers.

(a) *Prescription status in relation to initial interview factors*: As reported earlier in this paper, PSE status at the seven-month follow-up was strongly associated with pre-treatment mental state and social functioning (although not for men alone). It was therefore interesting to see whether prescription status at seven months showed similar associations with these or other pre-treatment factors. The findings were examined for the prescription group and the multiple prescription group separately.

(b) *Prescription group*: In *Table 3* are listed the pre-treatment factors that were significantly associated with the prescription group. By comparing this table with *Table 1*, it can be seen that the patterns of association for the prescription group (*Table 3*) and for PSE status at seven-months (*Table 1*) showed little overlap. For the combined sexes, the prescription group showed significant associations with GHQ total score and one sub-score (social), but not with the POMS or SAS-M. However, there were significant associations with a presenting complaint of anxiety (as recorded by the practitioner), and with the use of tobacco and non-prescribed medicines. For women alone, there were significant associations with several of these

Table 2 (I) Number, timing, and nature of prescribing between one-month and seven-month follow-up; and (II) PSE status at seven months for individual patients

patient no.	original treatment group	number of pre-scriptions	follow-up month						PSE status at 7-month follow-up
			1–2	2–3	3–4	4–5	5–6	6–7	
1	non-drug	1		DIAZ					non-case
2	drug	1		DIAZ					case
3	non-drug	1	DIAZ						non-case
4	drug	1	DIAZ						non-case
5	drug	1						NITRAZ	non-case
6	non-drug	1					NITRAZ		non-case
7	drug	1			NITRAZ				non-case
8	non-drug	1						DIAZ	non-case
9	drug	1	CDIAZ						non-case
'multiple prescription group'									
10	drug	2	NORTR			CLORAZ			non-case
11	drug	2					AMITR	AMITR	case
12	drug	2	DIAZ				NITRAZ		case
13	non-drug	2					MIANS	MIANS	case
14	drug	2	NITRAZ			DOTH			non-case
15	drug	3	AMITR	AMITR	IMIPR				non-case
16	non-drug	4		NORTR	NORTR	NORTR	NORTR		case
17	drug	4	DIAZ	DIAZ	DIAZ			DIAZ	case
18	non-drug	4	AMITR	AMITR	AMITR		DIAZ		case
19	drug	6	DIAZ	DIAZ	DIAZ	DIAZ	DIAZ	DIAZ	case
20	drug	6	DIAZ	DIAZ	DIAZ	DIAZ	DIAZ	DIAZ	case

AMITR = amitriptyline; CLORAZ = clorazepate; C-DIAZ = chlordiazepoxide; DIAZ = Diazepam; DOTH = dothiepin; MIANS = mianserin; NITRAZ = nitrazepam; NORTR = nortriptyline.

Table 3   *Factors at initial interview associated with the 'prescription group'*

	both sexes (n = 87)	males (n = 25)	females (n = 62)
GHQ – total score	**	NS	*
somatic	NS	NS	*
social	*	NS	NS
patient report			
# practitioner did not give advice	*	NS	*
tobacco (quantity)	*	NS	NS
# cough/cold medicines in previous week	*	NS	*
# vitamins/tonics in previous week	*	NS	NS
# complaints of psychological symptoms	NS	*	NS
# patient expected to be referred elsewhere	NS	*	NS
general practitioner's report			
# prescribed cardiovascular drugs by practitioner	NS	NS	*
# presenting complaint of anxiety	***	NS	*

χ^2 was used for the items marked #; for other listed items t-tests were used.
For P values: *** = $P < 0.001$; ** = $P < 0.01$; * = $P < 0.05$.

variables but for men there were only two significant associations (initial complaint of psychological symptoms; patient expecting referral elsewhere).

Linear discriminant function analysis: When this technique was applied to the prescription group and the rest of the patients, findings varied with sex. For the combined sexes, three pre-treatment variables together discriminated best between the two groups:- (i) having taken non-prescribed vitamins or tonics in the previous week; (ii) having taken non-prescribed cold and cough medicines in the previous week; (iii) GHQ total score. These three variables allocated 84 per cent of the patients correctly to the prescription/non-prescription groups.

For men alone, a combination of two factors discriminated best between the prescription group and the rest of the patients:- (i) the patient's expectation of referral elsewhere; (ii) the patient complaining of psychological symptoms. These two variables allocated 79 per cent of the men correctly. For women alone, a combination of three factors discriminated best:- somatic sub-scale of GHQ; patient having taken non-prescribed cold and cough medicines in the previous week; general practitioner reporting that cardiovascular drugs were prescribed to the patient.

Table 4 *Factors at initial interview associated with the multiple prescription group (both sexes)*

presenting complaint of anxiety (general practitioner)	$\chi^2 = 3.90$	*
GHQ – total score	$t = 2.20$	**
alcohol (quantity)	$t = 2.29$	*
tobacco (quantity)	$t = 2.23$	*

* $P < 0.05$.
** $P < 0.01$.

These three variables allocated 89 per cent of the women correctly.

(c) *Multiple prescription group*: in *Table 4* are listed the four pre-treatment factors that were significantly associated with the multiple prescription group. Three of the factors were shared with the prescription group; the fourth factor – quantity of alcohol used – was specific to the multiple prescription group.

Linear discriminant function analysis: When this technique was used, three treatment variables discriminated best between the multiple prescription group and the rest of the patients: (i) anxiety as presenting complaint; (ii) higher alcohol intake; (iii) cardiovascular drugs prescribed by the practitioner. These three variables allocated 78 per cent of the patients correctly.

In summary, of the main psychiatric and social pre-treatment variables, only the GHQ total score was associated with the prescribing of medication between the one-month and seven-month follow-ups. However certain other factors, such as consumption of tobacco, alcohol and non-prescribed medication, were significantly associated with such prescribing.

(d) *Prescription status in relation to outcome factors*

(i) *PSE at seven-month follow-up*: From *Table 2*, it is clear that PSE status at seven months was unlikely to be significantly related to the 'prescription' group, but more likely to be significantly related to the 'multiple prescription' group. The table shows that the proportion of PSE cases increased with increasing number of prescriptions. This impression was confirmed by statistical analysis. In the 'prescription' group (combined sexes), nine patients (45 per cent) were PSE cases, as against 18 patients (27 per cent) in the non-prescription group (difference not statistically significant). When the sexes were examined separately, there was still no significant difference. However, in the 'multiple prescription' group (combined sexes), eight patients (73 per cent) were PSE cases, as against 18 patients (25 per cent) of the remaining patients (Fisher's exact test, 2-tailed, $P < 0.01$). When the sexes were examined separately, the association was significant only for men (Fisher's exact test, 2-tailed, $P < 0.05$).

(ii) *Other psychiatric and social measures at seven months*: Here again there were the expected differences between the 'prescription' group and the 'multiple prescription' group. In the prescription group (combined sexes), the only significant association was with the outcome measure social adjustment. For men alone, there were significant associations with worse scores on two GHQ sub-scores, i.e. social impairment ($t = 2.14$, P $<$ 0.05) and depression ($t = 2.41$, P $<$ 0.05); and worse scores on the 'fatigue' sub-scale of POMS ($t = 2.44$, P $<$ 0.05). Men were also more likely to have had symptoms of depression over the preceding six months ($t = 2.75$, P $<$ 0.01). Women in the prescription group were not significantly associated with any other psychiatric or social measure. By contrast, the 'multiple prescription' group (combined sexes) showed significant associations with worse scores on considerably more measures:- GHQ total score ($t = 2.62$, P $<$ 0.01), and sub-scores for anxiety ($t = 2.68$, P $<$ 0.01), social impairment ($t = 2.92$, P $<$ 0.01) and depression ($t = 2.33$, P $<$ 0.05); POMS total score ($t = 2.44$, P $<$ 0.05) and sub-score for tension ($t = 2.35$, P $<$ 0.05); and SAS-M total score ($t = 3.19$, P $<$ 0.01) and sub-scores for work ($t = 2.20$, P $<$ 0.05), social and leisure ($t = 2.73$, P $<$ 0.01) and family unit ($t = 2.62$, P $<$ 0.05).

In summary, at the seven-month follow-up, psychiatric and social measures (including the PSE) were strongly associated with the multiple prescription group, but not with the prescription group as a whole.

Discussion

In this part of the study, the main aim was to examine patients presenting in general practice with minor affective disorders, and to discover how far long-term outcome was related to factors detectable at the initial consultation and subsequently. Two measures of long-term outcome were of particular interest – psychiatric outcome at the seven month follow-up, and the prescribing of psychotropic medication between the one-month and the seven-month follow-ups.

For the first of these outcome measures (psychiatric outcome), PSE case status at seven months was used. This choice seemed reasonable because PSE status was based on interview and because it was strongly associated with other outcome measures at seven months, both psychiatric (GHQ and POMS) and social (SAS-M). PSE outcome was found to be strongly associated with the initial interview measures of psychiatric status (GHQ and POMS) and social functioning (SAS-M). These associations held for the combined sexes and for women, but not for men alone. The explanation for this difference is probably that the sample included numerous women (20 PSE cases and 40 non-cases) but few men (six PSE cases and 18 non-cases). Despite these strong associations, these initial measures of mental state did not discriminate accurately between PSE cases and non-cases at seven months.

When a linear discriminant function analysis was carried out, two variables measured at initial interview discriminated well between patients who turned out to be PSE cases/non-cases at the seven month follow-up. Unfortunately these two factors (social and leisure score on the SAS-M; patient's dissatisfaction with duration of initial interview), would not help much in clinical practice.

PSE outcome at seven months was found to be significantly associated with several measures made at the earlier one-month follow-up, including GHQ total score, two GHQ sub-scales, and several of the POMS and SAS-M scores. Amongst measures of mental state at one month, the self-administered measures did not discriminate accurately between PSE cases and non-cases at seven months, but the PSE total score did discriminate well. As would be expected, PSE case status at the seven month follow-up was significantly associated with patients' reports that their symptoms of anxiety and/or depression had persisted throughout most of the follow-up period. However, there was no association between PSE outcome and life-events during the follow-up period.

In contrast with these findings for PSE outcome, the second outcome measure (prescribing of psychotropic medication) showed different patterns of association with variables measured at the initial consultation. Twenty patients (the 'prescription' group) received one or more prescriptions for psychotropic medication between the one-month and the seven-month follow-up. By contrast with PSE outcome, membership of the 'prescription' group was significantly associated only with initial GHQ total score, and not with initial POMS or SAS-M scores. Another difference was that the 'prescription' group was significantly associated with a presenting complaint of anxiety, consumption of tobacco, and the use of non-prescribed medicines in the week before consultation.

When a discriminant analysis was carried out, a combination of three factors discriminated well between the prescription group and the other patients. These factors were: use of non-prescribed vitamins and tonics; use of non-prescribed cough and cold medicines; and GHQ total score. Analysis for the sexes separately yielded good discriminators, but they would be of little value in clinical practice.

The 'prescription' group contained a sub-group of 11 patients who had received multiple prescriptions between the one-month and seven-month follow-up (the 'multiple prescription' group). This sub-group, like the 'prescription' group as a whole, was significantly associated with GHQ total score at initial interview, a presenting complaint of anxiety, and consumption of tobacco. It was also significantly associated with consumption of alcohol. A discriminant analysis showed that three factors discriminated best between the multiple prescription group and other patients, i.e. presenting complaint of anxiety, alcohol consumption, and prescription of cardiovascular drugs. Not surprisingly the 'prescription' group as a whole was only weakly associated with psychiatric outcome but the 'multiple prescription' group was strongly associated with all the main

The findings of this study point to three sets of conclusions.

First, the long-term outcome of minor affective disorders is related to their severity at the initial consultation and one month after the initial consultation. This conclusion agrees with other reports in the literature (Huxley *et al.* 1979; Corney 1981; Tennant *et al.* 1981; Williams *et al.* 1982).

Second, initial measures of mental state can be used to identify patients at risk of being psychiatric cases seven months later. Self-administered measures of mental state (notably the POMS) discriminate fairly well between future long-term cases and non-cases, but the PSE provides far the best discrimination. Such measures would be useful discriminators for research purposes, but would be of little value in the general practitioner's clinical work. It would be interesting to discover how far general practitioners, using their clinical skills, could distinguish as effectively as these standardised measures between future psychiatric cases and non-cases.

Third, it appears that patients who receive at least one psychotropic drug prescription during long-term follow-up (between one month and seven months) are distinguished not so much by initial intensity of psychiatric disorder as by use of tobacco and alcohol and by self-medication. Presumably this reflects personality factors. The sub-group of patients who receive multiple prescriptions show similar associations, but are significantly more likely to be psychiatrically disturbed at the seven-month follow-up.

Acknowledgements

This study was supported by a grant to one of the authors (D.G.) from the Department of Health and Social Security.

Warm thanks are expressed to the general practitioners who participated in the study: Doctors Iwan Hughes, Robert Pinches, Doreen Shewan, Wayne Smith, Simon Street, and Peter Tate.

The authors also wish to thank Miss Elizabeth Campbell, Dr Peter Cooper, Professor Michael Gelder, and Dr Keith Hawton for much helpful advice.

References

Betts, T.A., Clayton, A.B., and MacKay, G.M. (1972) Effects of four commonly used tranquillisers on low speed driving performance tests. *British Medical Journal* 4: 580–84.
British Medical Journal (1975) Tranquillisers causing aggression. 113–14.

Committee on the Review of Medicines (1980) Systematic review of the benzodiazepines. *British Medical Journal* 1: 910–12.

Cooper, B. (1972) Clinical and social aspects of chronic neurosis. *Proceedings of the Royal Society of Medicine* 65:19–22.

—— and Sylph, J. (1973) Life events and the onset of neurotic illness: an investigation in general practice. *Psychological Medicine* 3:421–35.

Cooper, P., Osborn, M., Gath, D., and Feggetter, G. (1982) Evaluation of a modified self-report measure of social adjustment. *British Journal of Psychiatry* 141: 68–75.

Corney, R. (1981) Social work effectiveness in the management of depressed women: a clinical trial. *Psychological Medicine* 11:417–23.

Covi, L., Lipman, R.S., Pattison, J.H., Derogatis, L.R., and Uhlenhuth, E.H. (1973) Length of treatment with anxiolytic sedatives and response to their sudden withdrawal. *Acta Psychiatrica Scandinavica* 49:51–64.

Dasberg, H. and Van Praag, H.M. (1974) The therapeutic effect of short-term oral diazepam treatment on acute clinical anxiety in a crisis centre. *Acta Psychiatric Scandinavica* 50:326–40.

Edwards, J.G. (1974) Doctors, drugs and drug abuse. *The Practitioner* 212:815–22.

—— (1979) Overprescribing of psychotropic drugs. In R.N. Gaind and B.L. Hudson (eds) *Current Themes in Psychiatry*. London: Macmillan.

Gardos, G., Dimascio, A., Salzman, C., and Shader, R.I. (1968) Differential actions of chlordiazepoxide and oxazepam on hostility. *Archives of General Psychiatry* 18:757–60.

Goldberg, D. (1972) *The Detection of Psychiatric Illness by Questionnaire*. London: Oxford University Press.

—— and Blackwell, B. (1970) Psychiatric illness in general practice. A detailed study using a new method of case identification. *British Medical Journal* 2:439–43.

—— and Hillier, V.F. (1979) A scaled version of the General Health Questionnaire. *Psychological Medicine* 9:139–45.

—— and Huxley, P. (1980) *Mental Illness in the Community*. London: Tavistock Publications.

——, Kay, C., and Thompson, L. (1976) Psychiatric morbidity in general practice and the community. *Psychological Medicine* 6:565–9.

Goldney, R.D. (1977) Paradoxical reaction to a new minor tranquilliser. *Medical Journal of Australia* 1: 139–40.

Grahame-Smith, D.G. (1975) Self-medication with mood-changing drugs. *Journal of Medical Ethics* 1:132–7.

Gurland, B.J., Yorkston, N.J., Stone, A.R., *et al.* (1972) The Structured and Scaled Interview to Assess Maladjustment (SSIAM): I. Description, rationale, and development. *Archives of General Psychiatry* 27:259–64.

Hall, R.C.W. and Joffe, J.R. (1972) Aberrant response to diazepam: a new syndrome. *American Journal of Psychiatry* 129:738–42.

Hawton, K.E. and Blackstock, E. (1976) General practice aspects of self-poisoning and self-injury. *Psychological Medicine* 6:571–5.

Hayes, S.L., Pablo, G., Radomski, T., and Palmer, R.F. (1977) Ethanol and oral diazepam abortion. *The New England Journal of Medicine* 296: 186–9.

Huxley, P., Goldberg, D., Maguire, G., and Kincey, V. (1979) The prediction of the course of minor psychiatric disorders. *British Journal of Psychiatry* 135:535–43.

Johnstone, E.C., Owens, D.C.G., Frith, C.D., McPherson, K., Dowie, C., Riley, G., and Gold, A. (1980) Neurotic illness and its response to anxiolytic and antidepressant treatment. *Psychological Medicine* 10:321–8.

Kedward, H. (1969) The outcome of neurotic illness in the community. *Social Psychiatry* 4:1–4.

Keeler, M.H. and McCurdy, R.L. (1975) Medical practice without anti-anxiety drugs. *American Journal of Psychiatry* 132:654–5.

Lancet (1973) Benzodiazepines: use, over-use, misuse, abuse? 1:1101–102.

—— (1978) Stress, distress and drug treatment. 1:1347–348.

Leach, R.H. and White, P.L. (1978) Use and wastage of prescribed medicines in the home. *Journal of the Royal College of General Practitioners* 28: 32–6.

McNair, D.M. and Lorr, M. (1964) An analysis of mood in neurotics. *Journal of Abnormal and Social Psychology* 69:620–27.

Mann, A., Jenkins, R., and Belsey, E. (1981) The twelve-month outcome of patients with neurotic illness in general practice. *Psychological Medicine* 11:535–50.

Paykel, E.S., Myers, J.K., Dievelt, M.N., Klerman, G.L., Lindenthal, J.L., and Pepper, M. (1969) Life events and depression. *Archives of General Psychiatry* 21:753–60.

Petursson, H. and Lader, M.H. (1981) Withdrawal from long-term benzodiazepine treatment. *British Medical Journal* 283:643–5.

Priest, R.G. (1980) The benzodiazepines: a clinical review. In R.G. Priest, U.V. Filho, R. Amrein, and M. Skreta (eds) *Benzodiazepines Today and Tomorrow*. Lancaster: MTP Press.

Rickels, K. and Downing, R.W. (1967) Drug and placebo treated neurotic out-patients. *Archives of General Psychiatry* 16:369–72.

Salzman, C., Kochansky, G.E., Shader, R.I., Porrino, L.J., Harmatz, J.S., and Swett, C.P. (1974) Chlordiazepoxide-induced hostility in a small group setting. *Archives of General Psychiatry* 31:401–5.

Seppala, T., Korttila, K., Hakkinen, S., and Linnoila, M. (1976) Residual effects and skills related to driving after a single oral administration of diazepam, medazepam or lorazepam. *British Journal of Clinical Pharmacology* 3:831–41.

Shepherd, M., Cooper, B., Brown, A.C., and Kalton, G. (1981) *Psychiatric*

Illness in General Practice. Second edition, London: Oxford University Press.

Skegg, D.C.G., Doll, R., and Perry, J. (1977) Use of medicines in general practice. *British Medical Journal* 1:1561–563.

——, Richards, S.M., and Doll, R. (1979) Minor tranquillisers and road accidents. *British Medical Journal* 1:917–19.

Tennant, C., Bebbington, P., and Hurry, J. (1981) The short term outcome of neurotic disorders in the community: the relation of remission to clinical factors and to 'Neutralizing' life events. *British Journal of Psychiatry* 139:213–20.

Trethowan, W.H. (1975) Pills for personal problems. *British Medical Journal* 3:749–51.

Tyrer, P. (1978) Drug treatment of psychiatric patients in general practice. *British Medical Journal* 2:1008–010.

Wells, F.O. (1973) Prescribing barbiturates: drug substitution in general practice. *Journal of the Royal College of General Practitioners* 23:164–67.

Wheatley, D. (1972) Evaluation of psychotropic drugs in general practice. *Proceedings of the Royal Society of Medicine* 65:317–20.

Williams, P. (1980) Recent trends in the prescribing of psychotropic drugs. *Health Trends* 12:6–7.

——, Murray, J., and Clare, A. (1982) A longitudinal study of psychotropic drug prescription. *Psychological Medicine* 12:201–06.

Wing, J.K., Cooper, J.E., and Sartorius, N. (1974) *The Measurement and Classification of Psychiatric Symptoms*. London: Cambridge University Press.

Winokur, A., Rickels, K., Greenblatt, D.J., Snyder, P., and Schatz, N.J. (1980) Withdrawal reaction from long-term, low dosage administration of diazepam. *Archives of General Psychiatry* 37:101–05.

13

Benzodiazepine withdrawal in general practice

David R. Hopkins, Kulwant B.S. Sethi, and John C. Mucklow

Summary A study of benzodiazepine prescribing in a single-handed general practice was carried out over a period of three months. It seemed that the existing pattern of prescribing was indiscriminate and ineffective, and that repeat prescriptions were poorly controlled. A programme of controlled withdrawal was instituted for patients whose consumption of benzodiazepines was felt to be no longer appropriate. Of 103 patients identified who had been taking benzodiazepines for longer than three months, 78 were entered into the programme. On completion, 45 patients (58 per cent) had discontinued benzodiazepines completely, and a further 13 (17 per cent) were taking less than half their original dose. Four patients had failed to reduce consumption at all and two were lost to follow-up. At follow-up between three and five months later, 49 patients (63 per cent) had discontinued benzodiazepines completely and only two had restarted treatment. The median time taken to complete the programme was 3.2 weeks, with 95 per cent of patients completing within six weeks. Withdrawal was generally well tolerated, with a temporary increase in insomnia as the main symptom. Two patients experienced severe symptoms, but both had stopped treatment abruptly.

Introduction

Long-term prescribing of benzodiazepines accounts for a considerable work-load in general practice, and many patients are involved. Balter and colleagues (1974) showed that 8.6 per cent of adults surveyed in the UK had, at some time during the previous year, taken anxiolytics for at least one month continuously, and in 1974 diazepam accounted for 4.3 per cent of all NHS prescriptions (Skegg *et al.* 1977).

Reprinted, with permission, from the *Journal of the Royal College of General Practitioners* 32: 758–62, 1982.

Benzodiazepines can produce psychological and, if given over a prolonged period, physical dependence (Marks 1978). Their hyponotic effects can decrease or disappear over periods as short as two weeks (Kales *et al*. 1974). There is little convincing evidence that benzodiazepines are efficacious in the treatment of anxiety after four months' continuous treatment (Committee on the Review of Medicines 1980), and some patients will then develop a psychological dependence on continual treatment.

For these reasons we felt it was desirable to carry out an audit of benzodiazepine prescribing in general practice, and to try to withdraw treatment. It has already been shown feasible to discontinue or substitute barbiturates in general practice (Wells 1973), and we felt that a similar exercise could be applied to benzodiazepines.

Aims

1. To prevent or cure psychological dependence in patients taking benzodiazepines over prolonged periods by withdrawal of treatment from those for whom the original indications for treatment had become inappropriate.
2. To reduce the amount of repeat prescribing.
3. To reduce prescribing costs.
4. To develop a more critical and rational use of benzodiazepines.
5. To study the effects of withdrawal on sleep and mood.

Methods

The study was carried out in a single-handed urban practice of approximately 2,800 patients. Those included had all been taking benzodiazepines for at least three months and were identified when they requested a repeat prescription, at consultation or from receptionists. Those with acute physical illness or a history of psychosis were excluded, as were patients under hospital supervision for psychiatric illness.

At the first interview (conducted by D.R.H. or K.B.S.S. using a questionnaire) enquiry was made about treatment, the reasons for starting it and continuing it, and sleep pattern. When and who (general practitioner or consultant) started treatment were determined from the records or, if these were not available, from patients' recollection.

Mood was assessed using a series of visual analogue scales rating subjective feelings (Bond and Lader 1974). The dangers of dependence on long-term treatment and the benefits of withdrawal were then explained. Patients satisfying selection criteria were invited to participate, and all those doing so gave their informed consent.

Because benzodiazepines can be potentiated by alcohol and other

Table 1   *Regimen for withdrawing benzodiazepine tranquillisers*

	baseline	stage 1	2	3	4
Nitrazepam	10 mg	7.5 mg	5 mg	2.5 mg	—
	5 mg	2.5 mg	—	—	—
Diazepam	5 mg t.d.s.	5 mg b.d.	5 mg daily	2 mg daily	—
	5 mg b.d.	5 mg daily	2 mg daily	—	—
	5 mg daily	4 mg daily	2 mg daily	—	—
	2 mg t.d.s.	2 mg b.d.	2 mg daily	—	—
Chlordiazepoxide	10 mg t.d.s.	10 mg b.d.	10 mg daily	5 mg daily	—
	10 mg b.d.	10 mg daily	5 mg daily	—	—
	10 mg daily	5 mg daily	—	—	—
Lorazepam	2.5 mg b.d.	2.5 mg daily	1 mg daily	—	—
	2.5 mg daily	1 mg daily	—	—	—
	1 mg daily	0.5 mg daily	—	—	—
Flurazepam	30 mg	15 mg	—	—	—
Temazepam	20 mg	10 mg	—	—	—

cerebral depressants, patients were asked about their alcohol intake. No excessive drinkers (more than six pints of beer or 12 measures of spirits per week) were identified.

Patients were instructed to reduce the dosage and frequency of medication according to a predetermined regimen (*Table 1*) in order to minimize withdrawal symptoms such as poor appetite, nausea, vomiting, trembling, faintness, insomnia and lack of energy (Covi *et al.* 1973). In patients taking medication more than once daily, withdrawal was planned to take four weeks in the first instance. Where medication was taken less frequently or only in response to emotional upset, treatment was stopped abruptly. A check was made on the rate of consumption of tablets by reference to the number of repeat prescriptions obtained recently, and in most cases this accorded with patients' estimates.

Interviews were repeated weekly whenever possible during withdrawal, either at the surgery or at home. A special surgery was arranged for the first

Table 2   *Reasons for exclusion*

unwilling to reduce dosage	6
severe anxiety	7
senile dementia	2
severe psychiatric illness	3*
severe physical illness	3
not contacted after two visits	2
under hospital supervision	1
recent bereavement	1
total	25

* One each of schizophrenia, manic depressive psychosis and endogenous depression.

Table 3 *Benzodiazepines prescribed*

preparation	daily dosage range (mg)	number
Diazepam	2–15	37
Nitrazepam	5–10	26
Chlordiazepoxide	10–30	8
Lorazepam	1–5	3
Flurazepam	30	1
Temazepam	20	1
Diazepam and nitrazepam	—	2
total		78

Table 4 *Duration of treatment prior to study*

months	3–12	13–36	37–60	61–120	>120
patients	8	22	21	17	10
percentage (n = 78)	10	28	27	22	13

few weeks of the study to cope with the additional work. The questions about sleep pattern and mood were repeated at each visit, and any symptoms associated with withdrawal were recorded. We recognized that further supplies of tablets might be obtained from hoarded stocks or from relatives and friends, but that this was impossible to prevent. Interviews were continued until either complete withdrawal for one week had been accomplished or the patient was removed from the study. Indications for removal were intercurrent mental or physical illness, major life events and inability or unwillingness to continue withdrawal.

Patients complaining of increased anxiety or insomnia were encouraged to continue withdrawal, but it proved necessary in some cases to maintain a constant dosage until symptoms were relieved, after which the withdrawal regimen continued. Patients removed from the study continued treatment with the lowest effective dosage. In many cases patients did not adhere closely to the regimen, although this was still used as a guideline. An extra tablet to cope with a stressful situation or the precipitate withdrawal of treatment were amongst the variations noted.

It was recognized that patients might restart treatment after complete withdrawal and all patients were therefore interviewed again (by K.B.S.S.) between three and five months after the end of the study. Patients were questioned about their consumption of benzodiazepines, if any, since the end of the study, and were asked whether they had obtained further supplies from relatives or hoarded stocks. The presence or absence of withdrawal symptoms was again noted, and patients were asked whether their sleep was better or worse than before the study.

Table 5   *Reasons for starting treatment*

	patients	percentage (n = 78)
anxiety	33	42
insomnia	17	22
bereavement*	20	26
hospital admission	7	9
unknown	1	1
total	78	100

* Leading to anxiety (14) or to insomnia (6).

Differences between groups of patients were assessed for statistical significance using the chi-square test with Yates's correction where appropriate.

Results

One hundred and three patients (3.7 per cent of the practice) were identified who had been receiving benzodiazepines for longer than three months. Of all patients over 30 years old, 3.7 per cent of men and 8.2 per cent of women were receiving treatment.

Twenty-five patients were excluded for various reasons (*Table 2*). Of the 78 patients entered into the study, 56 were women. Ages ranged from 30 to 86 years (mean 60.0). *Table 3* shows the preparations prescribed for these patients. The dose and frequency varied widely, and 18 patients took the medication as required rather than regularly. The duration of treatment prior to the study is shown in *Table 4*. Almost two thirds of patients had taken benzodiazepines for more than three years. Treatment had been started by a general practitioner in 79 per cent of cases; the reasons for starting are shown in *Table 5*. In many instances the reason was no longer operative, but 46 patients (59 per cent) had required continued treatment because of recurrent anxiety, and 32 (41 per cent) because of recurrent insomnia. Many patients were receiving other prescribed drugs, analgesics and antihypertensive agents most commonly.

Forty-six patients (59 per cent) were able to stop taking benzodiazepines completely. Another 26 (33 per cent) succeeded in reducing their intake and in 13 of these the final dosage was less than half the original. Two patients were lost to follow-up after the first interview but have requested no further repeat prescriptions. Only four patients proved unable to achieve any dose reduction.

At follow-up between three and five months later, 49 patients (63 per cent) had stopped treatment completely, and 15 (19 per cent) had reduced their intake. Four patients (5 per cent) had not changed their intake and a further eight (10 per cent) were lost to follow-up. Of these, two had left the

Table 6 *Results of withdrawal according to duration of treatment*

| | duration (months) | | | | |
	3–12	*13–36*	*37–60*	*61–120*	*> 120*
complete withdrawal (*n* = 46)	5	17	13	7	4
partial or no withdrawal (*n* = 30)	2	5	7	10	6

practice and the remaining six failed to attend follow-up interviews. Only two patients had started treatment after complete withdrawal.

The time taken to reach the final dosage is shown in the Figure. Ninety-five per cent of patients had either withdrawn completely or reached their final dosage within six weeks. The median time taken was 3.2 weeks.

When patients who were successful in complete withdrawal were compared with those remaining on treatment at the end of the study, it was found that the likelihood of withdrawal was related to duration of previous treatment (*Table 6*), successful withdrawal becoming less likely as duration increased ($x^2 = 7.27$ with two degrees of freedom, $p < 0.05$). There was no relationship between successful withdrawal and either age, sex, who had started treatment (consultant or general practitioner) or the reason for continuing treatment.

The effect of withdrawal on sleep pattern was determined by the main indication for treatment. Patients tended not to complain of disturbed sleep when treatment was taken as an anxiolytic, but insomnia was noticed more readily when it was hypnotics that were being withdrawn. Subjective estimation of duration and quality of sleep is notoriously unreliable, but in general patients noted either difficulty falling asleep or frequent waking. Early waking was rare. In most cases sleep disturbance was transient, lasting up to two weeks. Patients usually persisted with withdrawal after encouragement, but 13 patients were unable to tolerate this disturbance and withdrawal was terminated. In these patients dosage was either increased to the original level or kept at the reduced level, depending on the severity of the disturbance. Withdrawal appeared to have little effect on waking, and indeed several patients noted increased alertness and a sense of well-being on waking once treatment had been withdrawn.

Many patients reported agitation or tension during withdrawal which usually settled within one or two weeks and which often settled with reassurance; another 13 patients were unable to tolerate these symptoms and withdrawal was terminated.

The results of the visual analogue scales were analysed by allocating a score from 0 to 100 for each rating according to its position on the 10 cm

Time taken to reach final dosage or complete withdrawal (n = 76)

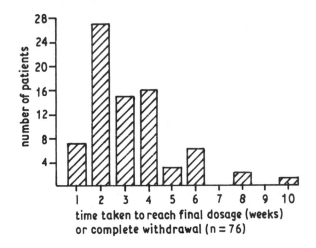

line, a score of 100 corresponding to maximum mental sedation, physical sedation or tranquillisation. Fewer than half of all patients had a fully completed analogue scale at each interview. Many had difficulty in comprehending what was required, and any recordings from these subjects would have been meaningless.

No statistically significant difference was found between ratings of symptoms before and after the study, and no difference was found in the ratings between those who were successful in withdrawal and those who continued treatment after the study. Further statistical analysis of results was thought to be inappropriate because of the lack of a control group and the small numbers studied.

It was difficult to distinguish between true withdrawal effects and those attributable to anxiety or psychological dependence. Most symptoms (*Table 7*) were subjective, their severity was difficult to quantify, and there were far fewer recorded at follow-up. In most cases symptoms were transient and mild, and both the patients who experienced severe reactions had discontinued treatment abruptly.

Discussion

The idea for this study arose when the practice took on a trainee (D.R.H.) for the first time. It was noted that prescribing of benzodiazepines appeared excessive, and patients were often able to obtain repeat prescriptions without a consultation. Most patients were anxious to stop treatment after the risks of going on had been explained, and were co-operative and ready to admit lapses in withdrawal.

Table 7 *Symptoms associated with withdrawal*

| | after withdrawal (n = 76) | | at follow-up (n = 68) | |
	patients	%	patients	%
insomnia	41	54	4	6
trembling	28	37	4	6
lack of energy	28	37	2	3
poor appetite	25	32	0	—
nausea	20	26	0	—
weakness	18	24	2	3
faintness	15	20	0	—
numbness	8	11	0	—
vomiting	3	4	0	—
palpitations	2	3	1	1

We now realize that the indications for initiation of treatment were, in some instances, inappropriate. This criticism applied particularly to bereavement, and the use of psychotropic drugs to suppress a natural grief reaction must be questioned. Patients admitted to hospital may require hyponotics and/or anxiolytics, but several of our patients had been given further supplies following discharge.

We were encouraged that 57 per cent of patients were able to discontinue treatment completely, and this rose to 63 per cent at follow-up several months later. These results suggest that withdrawal is feasible in the majority of patients on long-term treatment. The importance of this study has been highlighted by the recommendation of the Committee on the Review of Medicines (1980) that benzodiazepine therapy be limited to short-term use.

Although our regimen had allowed four weeks for withdrawal of medication, most patients required less time than this. We preferred to err on the side of caution rather than to risk withdrawal reactions. The fact that the only two severe reactions occurred when treatment was stopped abruptly suggests that advice to withdraw treatment slowly is sound (Tyrer 1980). It was found more difficult to withdraw treatment in patients who had been taking it for many years. Our results suggest that this difficulty is not due solely to advancing age, as there was no relation between age and success in withdrawal.

The effect of withdrawal on sleep pattern confirms that patients may suffer a period of rebound insomnia (Kales *et al.* 1974), lasting one or two weeks and being followed by reversion to a normal sleep pattern. Further comments on sleep pattern would be inappropriate, since the measurements of quality and duration of sleep were subjective. Our attempts to assess changes in mood pattern failed to reach any firm conclusions. The small number of patients studied and the lack of a control group made detailed statistical analysis of ratings invalid. Symptoms associated with withdrawal were as difficult to assess as changes in sleep or mood pattern. They may be due to either true physical dependence, psychological dependence or unmasking of a continuing anxiety state by withdrawal. These may be impossible to distinguish, although the occurrence of headache, dysphoria or other symptoms unrelated to the original anxiety state might suggest physical dependence (*Lancet* 1979). The two patients who withdrew treatment abruptly both experienced such symptoms. Others experienced milder symptoms which were probably due to anxiety or psychological dependence.

We feel that a programme of withdrawal similar to this is practicable for any general practitioner to undertake. The time spent will be repaid in the long term by reduction in the work-load of repeat prescriptions. For most patients 10 to 15 minutes would be needed for an initial interview to explain that long-term treatment is risky and ineffective, to achieve the patient's co-operation and to suggest a programme of withdrawal. Subsequent interviews should be at weekly intervals and need last no longer than 5 to 10 minutes to enquire about withdrawal symptoms, to give encouragement and to suggest a new dosage for the following week. Most patients should need no more than six weeks to reach their final dosage. The severity of withdrawal symptoms varies considerably and Tyrer and colleagues (1981) have suggested that this variation may relate to the variable rate at which benzodiazepines and their active metabolites are eliminated. They found propranolol superior to placebo in the alleviation of symptoms during the withdrawal.

Conclusion

Our patients have benefited in several ways from the study. The dangers and cost of unnecessary and ineffective treatment have been eliminated, and other, more effective treatment can be explored (for example simple psychotherapy or relaxation therapy for anxiety states). The study teaches patients that long-term therapy cannot cure long-standing social or emotional problems. The problems we have outlined need never arise if a time limit is placed on the duration of therapy. We continue to use benzodiazepines for acute episodes of insomnia or anxiety as before, but it is explained that no further supplies will be given. We feel that this study is a good example of medical audit, the impetus coming from ourselves. As a result, the prescribing habits of the practice have altered, and improved standards of patient care have resulted.

Acknowledgements

We are grateful to Dr Douglas Garvie for his helpful criticism, and to Mrs Maureen Lowe, who typed the manuscript.

References

Balter, M.B., Levine, J., and Manheimer, D.I. (1974) Cross-national study of the extent of anti-anxiety/sedative drug use. *New England Journal of Medicine* **290**:769–74.

Bond, A. and Lader, M. (1974) The use of analogue scales in rating subjective feelings. *British Journal of Medical Psychology* **47**:211–18.

Committee on the Review of Medicines (1980) Systematic review of the benzodiazepines. *British Medical Journal* **280**:910–12.

Covi, L., Lipman, R.S., Pattison, J.H., *et al.* (1973) Length of treatment with anxiolytic sedatives and response to their sudden withdrawal. *Acta Psychiatrica Scandinavica* **49**:51–64.

Kales, A., Bixler, E.O., Tan, T-L., *et al.* (1974) Chronic hypnotic-drug use; ineffectiveness, drug-withdrawal insomnia and dependence. *Journal of the American Medical Association* **227**:513–17.

Lancet (1979) Withdrawal symptoms with benzodiazepines. Editorial 1:196.

Marks, J. (1978) *The Benzodiazepines: Use, Overuse, Misuse, Abuse*, Lancaster: MTP Press.

Skegg, D.C.G., Doll, R., and Perry, J. (1977) Use of medicines in general practice. *British Medical Journal* 1:1561–563.

Tyrer, P. (1980) Dependence on benzodiazepines. *British Journal of Psychiatry* **137**:576–77.

Tyrer, P., Rutherford, D., and Huggett, T. (1981) Benzodiazepine withdrawal symptoms and propranolol. *Lancet* 1:520–22.

Wells, F.O. (1973) Prescribing barbiturates: drug substitution in general practice. *Journal of the Royal College of General Practitioners* **23**:164–67.

14

Self-help groups as an alternative to benzodiazepine use

E.M. Ettorre

Abstract This paper focuses on the social context of benzodiazepine groups with special reference to self-help groups. It outlines and discusses five areas of interest. These are: (1) a brief review of the self-help literature; (2) general observations on 'self-help concepts'; (3) the social implications of self-help groups and psychotropics with special reference to minor tranquillisers; (4) a case study of TRANX; and (5) future research directions. The aim of this paper is to illustrate how benzodiazepine self-help groups can be a viable alternative to benzodiazepine use, and to highlight some of the key issues which emerge from this area of study.

Introduction

The aim of this paper is to examine the nature, purpose, and context of benzodiazepine self-help groups and to illustrate how these groups can be a viable alternative to benzodiazepine use. This paper attempts to break new ground and should help to form the basis for future evaluative and theoretical work related to the social context of benzodiazepine use, an emergent area of social policy. As the editors suggest in the Introduction, public concern about the extent of tranquilliser prescribing abated in the late 1970s, while the 1980s have seen a new concern with physical dependence on benzodiazepines. In 1984, the Advisory Council on the Misuse of Drugs (1984) noted that while, on the one hand, benzodiazepines may be prescribed on a short-term basis without harmful effects, the long-term prescribing of benzodiazepines, particularly to women, has generated considerable social concern.

One way of analysing the social context of the benzodiazepine problem is to examine the linking of the 'concept', self-help, with the 'practice' withdrawal from benzodiazepines. In Britain this is a relatively new social phenomenon, although there is an increasing number of groups accompanied by insightful literature (RELEASE 1982; SCODA 1984; MIND 1984; Trickett 1984; TRANX 1984). This paper aims to focus on some key issues which have become socially visible with the development of these new initiatives, and five areas of sociological interest are discussed. These are: (1) a brief review of self-help literature; (2) general observations on 'self-help' concepts; (3) the social implications of self-help groups and psychotropics with special reference to minor tranquillisers; (4) a case study of TRANX (Tranquilliser Recovery and New Existence); and (5) future research directions. Although this paper is primarily sociological in orientation, it is hoped that it will be of interest to both practitioners and researchers working in the field.

A brief review of self-help literature

It has been suggested that since the 1950s there has been a rapid increase in the number and variety of self-help groups such as Alcoholics Anonymous, Mencap, Gamblers Anonymous, etc. (Robinson 1978), and that this represents one of the more striking developments in the provision of social care (Richardson and Goodman 1983). While the increased politicization of self-help which is associated with the civil rights movement, the women's movement, etc. emerged as a new social force from the 1950s to the 1970s (Pancoast, Parker, and Froland 1983), a growing number of scholars, researchers, and academics began to define the nature, purpose, and function of self-help groups, or simply to answer the question, 'why self-help?'

For the purpose of understanding future discussions in this paper, it is useful at this stage to classify how self-help researchers have organized their work and, more specifically, how they have defined the social context of self-help. There are two major approaches within self-help research: the *interpretive* approach and the *analytical* one. The former approach is explicitly descriptive and those writing within it focus on the effects self-help organizations have on members, the dynamics of groups, and the processes involved with the inculcation of self-help values in specific supportive contexts. The analytical approach is broad in focus and researchers aim to demonstrate how the notion of self-help links with broad social issues such as the crisis in productivity, professional social work versus social welfare, and mutual aid versus social change.

Self-help researchers within the *interpretive* approach have also been concerned with establishing typologies of the variety of self-help groups and/or defining the activities or dynamics which distinguish self-help groups from other types of social organizations. For example, Sagarin (1969), in the context of deviance management, outlined a two-fold typology based on (1) groups which focus on self-reform (i.e. giving up deviant behaviour) and conforming to social norms, and (2) those which want to reform some aspect of society or aim to change social norms. Katz and Bender (1976), while distinguishing generally between inner focused groups (e.g. providing direct service to members) and outer focused groups (e.g. geared to activities such as education and fund-raising), construct a specific typology based on a group's 'primary focus' which includes self-fulfilment or personal growth; social advocacy; alternative living patterns; outcast havens and 'mixed types'.

Another typology outlined by Levy (1976) suggests that groups could be divided acording to their aims and members. There are groups which aim to manage a 'problem' behaviour; those who share a common situation and want to alleviate their stress; those whose members are labelled as 'deviant'; and those groups who share the aim of personal growth, self-actualization, and enhanced effectiveness in living and loving.

In the now-classic review of self-help literature, Killilea (1976) catalogued twenty 'categories of interpretation' of self-help, while outlining seven characteristics which researchers have emphasized:

(1)　common experience of members;
(2)　mutual help and support;
(3)　the helper principle;
(4)　differential association;
(5)　collective willpower and belief;
(6)　the importance of information; and
(7)　constructive action towards shared goals.

Within the interpretive approach, researchers also construct 'processual' frameworks which help to develop insights into the actual dynamics or day-to-day activities of self-help groups. Authors providing accounts in Lieberman and Borman's (1979) *Self-help Groups for Coping with Crisis*, look at how groups are started and structured, their participants' aims and expectations, and how these groups work. The main research theme is to bring out how groups effect a change in their members. In a similar yet more detailed account, Robinson and Henry (1977), covering over 150 self-help groups in Britain, look at important processual aspects of self-help activity such as how groups are organized, group aims, how people become members, how people 'settle' in, 'what self-help groups do when they are doing self-help', etc. In another British study, Richardson and Goodman (1983) offer a full, descriptive account of self-help activities and focus on four well-established groups. Their findings suggest a wide diversity among these groups regarding their nature and the experience of their members.

Within the *analytical* approach, Gartner and Riessman (1977) outline the dynamics of self-help groups generally and attempt to link the notion of self-help with broader issues such as the focus on the member group or the participants' social backgrounds, the 'consumers as producers' (e.g. those consuming the service produce the service), and ultimately the subordination of a professionally dominant mode of care to one dependent on the experience of 'ex-sufferers'.

Ferrand-Bechmann (1983) offers a model which incorporates self-help groups on a 'voluntary action' (e.g. beyond 'government' or state action) spectrum ranging from various types of self-help activities to informal helping systems that prevail among families, neighbours, and friends. Also, this author presents a model for analysing the relationship between each of these types of informed care and professional social work, and highlights important aspects of the relationship between voluntary action and the welfare state in France.

All research on self-help, whether within an interpretive or analytical approach, is important in providing a clear understanding of self-help group dynamics and activities. It is appropriate at this stage in the discussion to look at key concepts which researchers have developed. Ultimately, this will help to build a framework for understanding self-help groups as an alternative to tranquilliser use, a major aim of this paper.

General observations on self-help concepts

Self-help researchers use over-reaching concepts such as 'mutual aid', 'coping with crisis', 'mutual support for modern problems', 'the self-help process', and 'support systems' to describe organizations which value self-reliance as well as reciprocity in their members. These concepts have close links with two significant sociological concepts: *illness as help-seeking behaviour* and *the norm of reciprocity*.

Mechanic's (1982) analysis of illness as help-seeking behaviour within a medical care network suggests that treatment personnel have often encouraged their patients to assume a dependent stance relative to the professional and have failed to support the patients' ability to struggle for mastery over his or her problems. The end result is often dependence and helplessness. On the other hand, the self-help way to health implies a different form of help-seeking behaviour. Members or potential members seek understanding based on common experience, which produces the necessary common bond of mutual interest and common desire to do something about the problem (Henry and Robinson 1979). While 'doing something' is not about becoming helpless or dependent on one or more professionals within the medical care system, it is about collectively helping oneself in a reciprocal network of relationships.

The process of self-help creates, therefore, a specific organizational structure which demands reciprocity or sharing of problems among members. In a real sense, reciprocity becomes a norm of any self-help group and this norm contributes to the stability of the group. In effect, reciprocity means that each member has rights and duties, and it entails a mutual dependence (Gouldner 1960). Collective help-seeking and reciprocity appear to be the two main types of behaviour which distinguish individuals in self-help groups from those seeking help through the traditional medical care system.

The process of self-help has been described as a 'response to the decline of natural support systems such as the church, the neighbourhood, and the family' (Robinson 1980). It can also be seen as a response to inadequacies in the medical care system, or reflective of the fact that more and better services are needed. While Gartner and Riessman (1977) suggest that the emergence of the self-help movement has arisen out of the needs of modern society, self-help is not a new discovery. Pancoast, Parker, and Froland (1983) report that two distinct historical models have emerged: *the clinical model* and *the structural model*. Within the former model, self-help is a means by which individuals and small groups may deal with their own problems, struggling to survive in a world for which they are not ideally designed. On the other hand, self-help within the structural model is seen as a natural and healthy way for communities to organize themselves both for internal social satisfaction and against loss of control and awareness. While discussions in this paper focus more on the clinical model of self-help and less on the structural one (because of the limitation of length), it is important to be aware of the differences between these two models. Furthermore, the structural notion of self-help can, and indeed does, imply a certain amount of community action in which 'the first step may be to counter the prevailing ideology and show how people do have real interests in common, by raising the appropriate demands' and levels of awareness (Binns 1977). In this light, self-help groups may be seen as critical components of primary care and prime vehicles for social change.

Change is also an important element within the clinical model of self-help. For example, the main reason for the focus on individuals and their problems is to bring about change. The need for change is explicit and effected by those specific functions which self-help groups undertake. Richardson and Goodman (1983) offer a clear account of the five basic functions to which effective self-help groups are devoted. They include: (1) emotional support (such as helping people who feel lonely, confused, isolated); it may be offered in a crisis or over a longer period; (2) information and advice (which helps people to cope better, and may concern methods of self-care or services provided by other organizations); (3) direct services (which help individuals to cope with particular problems and provide back-up services such as babysitting, holiday play schemes); (4) social activities (which are aimed at bringing people together); and (5) pressure group activities (which are aimed at making people aware of their group or changing the services provided).

While all five functions are important for 'effective' self-help groups, variations among groups do occur. Also, the above authors demonstrate how diversity within the spectrum is usual practice. While the above discussions have outlined features which distinguish the two approaches used by self-help researchers, as well as key concepts related to the emergence of self-help groups, the following discussions will focus on the relevance of these specific ideas to benzodiazepine self-help groups.

The social implications of self-help groups and psychotropics with special reference to minor tranquillisers

Self-help groups have a particular role to play in the management of benzodiazepine withdrawal. Whatever techniques are used, sympathetic support is needed to sustain individuals over the withdrawal period and self-help groups are a valuable resource in this respect. While benzodiazepines were believed to be more effective and safer than barbiturates in alleviating anxiety and stress, and furthermore in dealing with the extent of clinical anxiety in society, they tended to be prescribed on a long-term basis (OHE 1984) and often caused problems for those wanting to come off.

Obtaining prescriptions for benzodiazepines is more likely to involve the mediation of the 'treater' (a medical practitioner) on behalf of the 'treated' (the patient) than participation in the 'black market', and the process of becoming addicted to benzodiazepines is different from becoming addicted to other psychotropic drugs, such as alcohol or heroin. The route to addiction for either alcohol or heroin is usually through self-prescription. Subsequently the establishment of self-help groups such as Alcoholics Anonymous or Narcotics Anonymous, the most publicly known groups for those 'talking out of alcoholism' (Robinson 1979) or coming off heroin respectively, implies a less critical response to the medical profession than does the creation of benzodiazepine self-help groups.

That benzodiazepines have been related to psychological and physical dependence (Lader 1978, 1981, 1983), and that there is a lack of firm evidence of efficacy which might support the long-term use of benzodiazepines in insomnia and anxiety (Committee on the Review of Medicines 1980) give a critical focus to the prescribing practices of the medical profession vis-à-vis benzodiazepines. In particular, benzodiazepine self-help groups appear to have a more critical social stance than other psychotropic drug-related self-help groups, although it has been argued that all self-help groups generally arise 'because of the uncorrected failures in the larger system' (Gartner and Riessman 1977). However, Robinson (1979) contends that a 'separate but compatible view of self-help groups and the professions' is evident in the overall AA philosophy; but this view is not shared by all AA groups. On the other hand, a critical view of the medical profession is implicit with the growth of benzodiazepine self-help groups, and these groups give support, advice, and information about an 'iatrogenic' condition. For example, the very real lack of information that has existed about minor tranquillisers has been a major concern for MIND (the National Association for Mental Health). In their recently published guide to setting up self-help groups for benzodiazepine users, they outlined some of the key issues which concerned participants in the National Tranquilliser Study Day, held in November 1983:

> 'They (minor tranquillisers) were brought on to the market as the new "sugar pills" that are safe and non-addictive and many GPs still believe them to be harmless. The participants called for information to be made available on the optimum way to use the drug, its side effects and its withdrawal effects. More information needs to be given to patients being prescribed these drugs as well as the general public.'
>
> (MIND 1984)

For minor tranquilliser users, self-help groups are important in helping them see that withdrawal symptoms are not unique to themselves and that other members, who are perhaps feeling better, have been in a similar position. Presenting her life story, the coordinator of one of these groups conveys the feeling that she 'has been there' and that 'she is not unique in her experience'. She says:

> 'Once we are off these pills all our lost confidence ultimately returns and we can cope so much better with everything than we used to do on our "crutches". If there are problems of whatever nature, pressurisation (sic) of a job, unhappy marriage, whatever, these problems need to be solved. No pill will solve these problems and anyone who's ... (been) prescribed (tranquillisers) for reasons of anxiety will tell you that they are far more anxious on these pills than they ever were before they were prescribed them.'
>
> (Jerome 1984)

With nearly 30 million benzodiazepine prescriptions in 1981 (OHE 1984) at a cost to the NHS of almost £30 million a year (Lacey 1984), the use of benzodiazepines should be considered a social issue worthy of critical attention. It should be considered a matter of community care, which Abrams (1978) defines as 'that end of the continuum of social care functions at which the commitment of a society as a whole to social care is most directly tested and most critically enacted'. Although self-help groups within this nexus of community care can be seen as an alternative to benzodiazepine use, their organizational activities can be understood as a complement, not as an alternative, to the statutory system of health care.

While on the one hand self-help may be seen as a basic and perhaps critical 'component of primary health care' (Robinson 1980), self-help groups do provide, as the Report of the Wolfenden Committee (1978) suggests, a service which is different from what is provided by the NHS. As alternative groups, self-help organizations may be viewed as pressure groups seeking changes in NHS prescribing practices, pioneers of new services, providers of additional services to the NHS, or indeed the sole provider of services. In whatever way they are viewed, self-help groups are organizationally different from the NHS as well as being cornerstones of primary health care and thus motivated by the goal of public health. Their unique social position is evidenced by their 'complementarity' to the statutory health system and the reinforcement role they play in relation to the informal network of support provided by family, friends, and neighbours. However visible these groups become, they focus critical attention on the need to examine a variety of broad social issues such as possible failures within the health care system; the aggressive marketing strategies of the pharmaceutical industry; conflicts between two modes of social organization (the communal and the bureaucratic) in relieving anxiety and stress; and the social impracticabilities which exist between the value of public health within a political democracy and the pursuit of social welfare in a market economy. Although this discussion has not attempted to delve into these broad social issues, it has not only provided the basic foundation for an understanding of the social implications of self-help groups with special reference to minor tranquillisers, but also outlines the framework necessary for doing a case study of one of these groups, TRANX.

A case study of TRANX

Given that benzodiazepine self-help groups appear to have a more critical stance than other self-help groups concerned with psychotropic drug use, an examination of one of the most visible self-help groups working in the area of minor tranquillisers should be illuminating.

In December 1983, a national tranquilliser advisory council, TRANX, obtained £53,000 state funding for two years from the Department of Health and Social Security. Pioneered by the coordinator and founder, a benzodiazepine user for seventeen years, TRANX is guided by an advisory panel consisting of several consultant psychiatrists and local general practitioners. A 24-hour support network among the group's 40 core members has been organized and the TRANX phonelines, staffed by 12 volunteers, receive an average of 300 calls for help per week. Advice and information to minor tranquilliser users, their families, and their friends are a crucial part of this service. Groups for those suffering from withdrawal effects are held two evenings per week and these groups enable members to gain mutual aid and reciprocal understanding for their problems in a collective context. For example, one member recalls:

'My first TRANX meeting was terrifying because it confirmed that the symptoms are again experienced by most people in withdrawal but it also served to strengthen my determination to get off.'

(TRANX 1984)

Along with the paid coordinator and secretary, the twelve voluntary workers who act as the telephone support team give advice and information to other members in the groups, as well as to those seeking help by visiting the agency. One member of the 'team' said that her experience with TRANX was like being born again. After withdrawing from her pills, she said:

'Thank you all my friends at TRANX for my second chance in life, for without all of you this would not have been possible.'

(TRANX 1984)

Besides running support groups, organizing a phoneline, and acting as an advisory body, TRANX produces information and advice leaflets as well as a quarterly newsletter. TRANX also liaises with local GPs whose patients may want to come off tranquillisers, as well as receiving enquiries from many areas in Britain, although most come from the Greater London area. Referrals are from the media, friends and relatives of prospective clients, GPs, local hospitals, a local alcohol advice agency, and the local social services.

Although the majority of TRANX clients are women over thirty years of age, there are both male and female clients who include all age groups, both those employed and unemployed, and local and non-local residents.

By the end of 1984 (a year after opening), TRANX had received 1,500 enquiries and 130 clients had successfully withdrawn from tranquillisers through the groups or the phonelines, and/or letters (TRANX 1984). ('Success' for TRANX members means they are 'completely off' their medication.)

Given that TRANX is a relatively young organization with a less than perfect record-keeping system, it cannot yet know an effective way of working with its large number and variety of clients, and a proper scientific evaluation is not yet possible. A two-hour interview with TRANX's coordinator, half-hour discussions each with the full-time administrator and three volunteers, attendance at two group meetings, an investigation of TRANX's files on 'ongoing' and 'new' clients, and a perusal of *all* TRANX literature in October 1984 on the research site, revealed that TRANX reflects in a particular way Richardson and Goodman's (1983) five basic functions of effective self-help groups. These are: (1) emotional support to those coming off and wanting to come off; (2) information and advice on withdrawal; (3) follow-up groups and back-up services for those coming off; (4) social activities such as jumble sales and sports competitions; and (5) pressure group activities such as writing to members of parliament and local health authorities. While collective help-seeking about the 'nature' of tranquilliser withdrawal is an objective goal of TRANX, reciprocity linked with mutual dependence is a group norm.

The above-mentioned information-gathering exercise focused on TRANX's social benefits and revealed that it fulfils key criteria for an effective self-help group, while maintaining the norm of reciprocity and upholding the goal of mutual dependence. In April 1985 a further information-gathering exercise, which focused on TRANX's organizational limitations, was carried out and emphasis was placed on obtaining information related to potential 'problem areas'. Four specific areas which may need further evaluation emerged: (1) the self-identity of the user; (2) the method of receiving enquiries and helping clients; (3) client variations; and (4) accepting 'media referrals'.

First, those approaching TRANX, unlike those using street drugs and approaching helping agencies (Dorn and South 1985; Jamieson, Glanz, and MacGregor 1984) receive little, if any, benefit from being part of a subculture and having an alternative self-identity. Often benzodiazepine users feel very isolated and live within restricted social networks (Gabe and Thorogood in this volume; Ettorre, forthcoming). Although TRANX offers users 'a second chance', members withdrawn from benzodiazepines may find themselves without pills in a restrictive environment (e.g. lack of social support) similar to the one in which they lived while on pills.

Second, the great majority of individuals withdrawn from pills with TRANX's help were withdrawn through phone contacts or letters (N=104), while the number for those in groups was 35. The former, most successful, methods of helping members tend to neglect those 'help seekers' who would benefit from a face to face assessment of their needs on an individual basis, or through individual counselling. Additionally, it is still early days to see clearly the different benefits received by those withdrawn by phone or letter, and those withdrawn in groups.

Third, there could be major organizational drawbacks for an agency whose members have different social backgrounds, different personalities, and different needs, as well as using different dosages and type of drugs. For example, TRANX's suggested methods of reducing daily dosages not only vary according to the type of benzodiazepine being taken (e.g. Valium, Serenid-D, Ativan, etc.) and the usual daily dose prescribed, but also according to the 'perceived' needs of members who want to come off. Some members may not be fully motivated to come off their prescribed dosages, since a prolonged period of withdrawal is often recommended by TRANX. In this way, it may be difficult to keep members motivated for long periods of time and some clients, lacking the required motivation, may postpone or continue to postpone the process.

Fourth, TRANX receives a substantial number of 'media referrals' (i.e. individuals who hear about TRANX from local newspaper articles, television shows, etc.). For 'media referral' members, unlike those seen and assessed on the premises, it is difficult to know what the outcome will be, what their motivation entails, and most importantly, from the agency's point of view, how suitable they are as members. By allowing 'media referrals', TRANX may be accepting members whose motivation to come off stems from a 'moral panic' rather than a sincere desire to get well. There is also a danger that the organization is perpetuating the less than accurate media images of the 'junkie housewife' as well as feeding into 'sensationalist' images which do not match the experience of users.

Since TRANX is in the early stages of its development, the limitations and drawbacks presented in this case study are perhaps to be expected in a self-help group which has thus far only two paid workers and a relatively small telephone support team. While the above discussion has outlined specific areas which may need more research, further discussion is needed on how research can be developed in the overall area of benzodiazepine self-help groups.

Future research directions

The discussions in this paper have suggested how self-help groups can be a viable alternative to benzodiazepine use, while providing a sociological framework in which 'self-help' concepts can be understood. Future research could examine two types of self-help groups: one for those coming off legal drugs (i.e. alcohol or benzodiazepines) and one for those coming off illegal drugs (i.e. heroin), and offer comparisons between the groups' self-image of members, the process of coming off, variations in help-seeking behaviour, and the creation of alternative identities. Research on links between benzodiazepine self-help groups and other agencies in both the statutory and non-statutory sector would perhaps point out gaps within the helping network, and the level of coordination or presence of 'complementarity' within the system of social care. Research in this area could also assess whether or not the development of inter-agency links with GPs, health authorities, educational authorities, social services, etc. is a viable way of tapping local community resources or, alternatively, of generating public awareness of tranquilliser issues. Comparison of benzodiazepine self-help groups with other 'campaigning groups' such as CURB (Campaign on the Use and Restriction of Barbiturates) or the women's movement could, on a national level, help those working in the area to translate the WHO goal, 'Health for all by the year 2,000' (Declaration of Alma Ata 1978), into effective political action. In addition, naturalistic or natural history studies to assess the social and public health consequences of benzodiazepine use (Cooperstock and Parnell 1982) would be useful in providing a close examination of the processes involved prior to becoming a member of a particular self-help group.

A study currently being planned by the author will look at helping agencies and the management of help-seeking behaviour vis-à-vis withdrawal from minor tranquillisers. This study will trace the progress over time of patients/clients who require help in coming off tranquillisers from GPs and self-help groups, and will compare both types with regard to their overall treatment/service philosophy; their attitude toward withdrawal; patient/client biography; doctor-patient relationship or client self-help group interaction; and overall service cost. It is hoped that this study would provide data on the similarities or differences in the management of withdrawal by respective agencies, and elucidate why some forms of help may be more successful than others.

Finally, research in this area relates implicitly to the increased level of clinical anxiety in society (OHE 1982). What are the reasons for increasing social anxiety and how can practitioners faced with growing numbers of depressed and anxious patients provide a service consistent with changing social needs? If theory-building in this area is to be effective and related to social policy, both treater and treated need to know some of the contradictions and social tensions which exist in our present system of social care.

Acknowledgements

I would like to thank Jon Gabe, Paul Williams, Professor Malcolm Lader, and Professor Griffith Edwards for helpful comments on earlier drafts of this paper.

References

Abrams, P. (1978) Community care: some research problems and priorities. In J. Barnes and N. Connelly (eds) *Social Care Research*: 78–103. London: Bedford Square Press.

Advisory Council on the Misuse of Drugs (1984) *Report on Prevention.* London: HMSO.

Binns, I. (1977) What are we trying to achieve through community action? In J. Cowley, A. Kaye, M. Mayo, and M. Thompson (eds) *Community or Class Struggle?*: 108–11. London: Stage 1.

Committee on the Review of Medicines (1980) Systematic review of the benzodiazepines. *British Medical Journal* 29 March: 910–12.

Cooperstock, R. and Parnell, P. (1982) Research on psychotropic drug use: a review of findings and methods. *Social Science and Medicine* 16:1179–196.

Declaration of Alma Ata (1978) *Report of the International Conference on Primary Health Care* WHO/UNICEF/ICPHC/ALA: October.

Dorn, N. and South, N. (1985) *Helping Drug Users*. Aldershot: Gower Press.

Ettorre, B. (forthcoming) Psychotropics, passivity and the pharmaceutical industry. In A. Hensman and R. Lewis (eds) *The Illicit Drug Business*. London: Pluto Press.

Ferrand-Bechmann, D. (1983) Voluntary action in the welfare state: two examples. In D.L. Pancoast, P. Parker, and C. Froland (eds) *Rediscovering Self-help: Its Role in Social Care*: 183–201. Beverly Hills: Sage Publications.

Gabe, J. and Thorogood, N. (1986) Tranquillisers as a resource (this volume).

Gartner, A. and Riessman, F. (1977) *Self-help in the Human Services*. San Francisco: Jossey-Bass.

Gouldner, A. (1960) The norm of reciprocity. *American Sociological Review* 25 (2): 161–78.

Henry, S. and Robinson, D. (1979) The self-help way to health. In P. Atkinson, R. Dingwall, and A. Murcott (eds) *Prospects for the National Health*: 184–211. London: Croom Helm.

Jamieson, A., Glanz, A., and MacGregor, S. (1984) *Dealing with Drug Misuse: Crisis Intervention in the City*. London: Tavistock Publications.

Jerome, J. (1984) *The founding of TRANX*. Unpublished paper presented to Department of Social Administration seminar, London School of Economics, November.

Katz, A.H. and Bender, E.I. (eds) (1976) *The Strength in Us: Self-help Groups in the Modern World*. New York: Franklin Watts.

Killilea, M. (1976) Mutual help organisations: Interpretations in the literature. In G. Caplan and M. Killilea (eds) *Support Systems and Mutual Help: Multidisciplinary Explorations*: 37–93. New York: Grune & Stratton.

Lacey, R. (1984) Prescriptions – what price official secrecy? *Open Mind* 9:13.

Lader, M. (1978) Benzodiazepines – the opium of the masses? *Neuroscience* 3:159–65.

Lader, M. (1981) Epidemic in the making: benzodiazepine dependence. In G. Tognoni, C. Bellantuono, and M. Lader (eds) *Epidemiological Impact of Psychotropic Drugs*: 313–24. Amsterdam: Elsevier/North Holland Biomedical Press.

Lader, M. (1983) Dependence on benzodiazepines. *Journal of Clinical Psychiatry* 44 (4):121–27.

Levy, L. (1976) Self-help groups: types and psychological processes. *Journal of Applied Behavioural Science* 12:310–22.

Lieberman, M.A. and Borman, L.D. (eds) (1979) *Self-help Groups for Coping with Crisis*. San Francisco: Jossey-Bass.

Mechanic, D. (1982) The epidemiology of illness behavior and its relationship to physical and psychological distress. In D. Mechanic (ed.) *Symptoms, Illness Behavior and Help-seeking*: 1–24. New York: Prodist.

MIND (National Association of Mental Health) (1984) *Come Off It*. London: MIND.

OHE (1982) Medicines and the quality of life. *OHE Briefing* 19.

OHE (1984) *Compendium of Health Statistics* (5th edn). London: OHE.

Pancoast, D.L., Parker, P., and Froland, C. (eds) (1983) *Rediscovering Self-help: Its Role in Social Care*. Beverly Hills: Sage Publications.

Release (1982) *Trouble with Tranquillisers*. London: Release.

Report of the Wolfenden Committee (1978) *The Future of Voluntary Organisations*. London: Croom Helm.

Richardson, A. and Goodman, M. (1983) *Self-help and Social Care: Mutual Aid Organisations in Practice*. London: Policy Studies Institute.

Robinson, D. (1978) Self-help groups. *British Journal of Hospital Medicine* September: 106–10.

Robinson, D. (1979) *Talking Out of Alcoholism: The Self-help Process of Alcoholics Anonymous*. London: Croom Helm.

Robinson, D. (1980) The self-help component of primary health care. *Social Science and Medicine* 14A:415–21.

Robinson, D. and Henry, S. (1977) *Self-help and Health: Mutual Aid for Modern Problems*. London: Martin Robertson.

Sagarin, E. (1969) *Odd Man in Societies of Deviants in America*. Chicago: Quadrangle Books.

SCODA (1984) Standing conference on drug abuse. *Report of the National Study Day on Tranquillisers*. London: SCODA.

TRANX, (1984) *First Annual Report*. Harrow, Middlesex: TRANX.

Trickett, S.A. (1984) *Coming Off Tranquillisers*. Newcastle upon Tyne: SAT Publishing.

© *1986 E.M. Ettorre*

## PART 5

The meaning of tranquilliser use

15

Introduction

In a recent review of research on psychotropic drugs Cooperstock and Parnell (1982) identified what they felt to be an important gap: namely, a lack of studies considering the characteristics of psychotropic drug use from the point of view of those involved – the users, their families, and doctors. Such studies, they argued, would draw attention to the processual, developmental nature of drug usage and start to provide a basis for understanding *how* the association between psychotropic drugs and various causal variables came about.

In this section the reader is introduced to the work of those who have begun to fill this gap. The papers which follow all have one thing in common – a desire to elucidate the *meaning* of psychotropic drug use. Meaning in this context refers to the interpretation a person gives to an object or event in his or her life. Such meanings arise out of interaction with others and are subject to development and change over time (Blumer 1969:2).

For present purposes we can distinguish two levels of meaning: the symbolic and the social. *Symbolic* analysis focuses attention on the underlying or hidden meaning of an object or event, and the way in which it 'stands for something else' (Firth 1973:26). Such symbolism is not immediately apparent but is perceptible to the analyst on reflection (Gusfield and Michalowicz 1984). *Social* meanings are those which are taken at face value as immediately apparent to actor and analyst alike. Those focusing on this level are concerned with the way in which meanings are used to achieve practical results. The emphasis is thus on the rational and instrumental aspects of everyday life (Gusfield and Michalowicz 1984:418-19).

In the first paper in this section Helman illustrates both these levels of meaning. He describes how a group of long-term benzodiazepine users account for their drug use, their feelings about the drug, and its effects on themselves and their families before identifying the underlying symbolic role which the drug plays in their everyday lives. Drawing on ideas from structural anthropology he suggests that benzodiazepines have three symbolic meanings for his sample: they are perceived of and used as a tonic, fuel, or food.

In the second paper Cooperstock and Lennard concern themselves with the level of social meanings and offer an analysis of the ways in which tranquillisers are used by long-term takers of the drug to manage a variety of role conflicts. Their approach, like those of the remaining authors in this section, is sociological in that they are concerned to place the meaning expressed by their respondents within the context of their everyday lives as members of particular social groups. In their paper the focus is primarily on the *gender*-specific aspects of the roles their respondents are called upon to play.

In the third paper Gabe and Thorogood treat benzodiazepines as one of a number of 'resources' which are differentially available to members of particular social groups – in this case, white and black working-class women – as they go about the business of managing their everyday lives. Using this approach involves considering the social meanings of benzodiazepine use within a broader context and provides a basis for explaining why the white women in the sample were more likely to be the long-term users of the drug.

In the last paper of the section Gabe and Lipshitz-Phillips relate their analysis of the social meaning of tranquilliser use to the debate about whether tranquillisers are a means of social control. Drawing on data for middle- and working-class women patients *and* their doctors they describe the ways in which different categories of benzodiazepine user and their doctors looked upon the causes, nature, and consequences of benzo-diazepine use; the relationship between tranquilliser use and gender and class stereotypes; and the extent to which the level of drug prescribing is influenced by the pharmaceutical industry, the inadequacies in doctors' training, and their conditions of work.

References

Blumer, H. (1969) *Symbolic Interactionism*. Englewood Cliffs: Prentice-Hall.

Cooperstock, R. and Parnell, P. (1982) Research on psychotropic drug use: a review of findings and methods. *Social Science and Medicine* 16(12): 1179–196.

Firth, R. (1973) *Symbols: Public and Private*. New York: Cornell University Press.

Gusfield, J.R. and Michalowicz, J. (1984) Secular symbolism: studies of ritual ceremony and the symbolic order in modern life. *Annual Review of Sociology* 10: 417–35.

16

'Tonic', 'fuel', and 'food': social and symbolic aspects of the long-term use of psychotropic drugs

Cecil G. Helman

Abstract This paper examines some of the many dimensions of meaning that psychotropic drugs can have for those that use them on a long-term basis. It aims to shed light on the problem of psychological dependence on these drugs, and the different forms this dependence can take. To put this study in context, some of the recent literature on psychotropic drug use is reviewed, before reporting the findings of the pilot-study. From this data a classification of chronic users into three different 'types' – called 'Tonic', 'Fuel', and 'Food' – has been developed, each of which embodies a different perspective on psychotropic drugs, their symbolic meanings, and modes of usage. It is hoped this classification will be useful to clinicians and others working in this field.

The growth of psychotropic drug prescribing

Psychotropic drugs have become a familiar feature of modern life, especially in the industrialised world. The prescribing – and ingestion – of these 'chemical comforters'[1] or 'pills for personal problems'[2] has become a widespread and socially acceptable habit. Society, in Warburton's view[3], is in danger of becoming a 'pharmacotopia', where 'chemical coping'[4] becomes a predominant way of dealing with the problems of everyday life.

Several studies have shown the progressive rise in the prescribing of psychotropics, particularly in the past 20 years. In Britain, for example,

Reprinted, with permission, from *Social Science and Medicine* 15B: 521-33. 1981.

from 1965 to 1970, prescriptions for tranquillisers increased by 59 per cent and non-barbiturate hypnotics by 145 per cent[5]. In 1972 45.3 million prescriptions for psychotropics were issued by National Health Service general practitioners in England alone (17.7 per cent of the total number of prescriptions), at a cost of £23.8 million[6]; of the more than 46 million psychotropic prescriptions issued the following year, 13.6 million were for benzodiazepines[7]. Dunlop[8] estimated that every tenth night of sleep in England was induced by a hypnotic drug, and that in any 1 year 19 per cent of British women and 7 per cent of men were prescribed a tranquilliser, while Tyrer[9] estimates that more patients in Britain take tranquillisers regularly for over a month than in any other Western country. In Canada, Sellers[10] estimates that 1 in 10 Canadians receive a prescription for a benzodiazepine each year, and more than 30 per cent of hospitalized patients are given these. In the United States, an estimated 250 million prescriptions for psychotropics are issued annually[11]; the most commonly prescribed drugs in the U.S.A. are the benzodiazepines[12], and in 1973 it was estimated that prescriptions for one of these, diazepam (Valium), was increasing at the rate of 7 million annually[13]. Valium is now reported to be the most widely prescribed drug in the world[14]. In Britain, three of the benzodiazepines, introduced in the early 1960s, have accounted for the majority of the increased prescribing; diazepam (Valium), nitrazepam (Mogadon) and chlordiazepoxide (Librium)[15].

Many reasons have been advanced to explain this increase in prescribing. Blame has been laid at several doors, including that of: *doctors*, and particularly the 'mix of influences' on them such as advertising and societal expectations[16], rushed consultation times and increased workload[17], increased delegation of repeat prescribing to receptionists[18], alleged limited ability to deal with emotional problems of patients in a non-pharmacological way[19], their need to exercise moral authority over patients[20], and give a visible token of this relationship[21], and their acquired 'habits' of prescribing[22]; the *patients*, and their demands for anti-anxiety and sleeping pills[23], and expectations of these drugs[24], their belief in the 'chemical road to success'[25], their 'fashions' of drug ingestion[26], lowered tolerance to emotional distress[27] and need for a token of the doctor's interest in them[28]; the *pharmaceutical industry*, and the impact of its advertising on the medical profession[29], and on the public[30] in promoting the necessity for, and efficacy of, 'pills for personal problems'; and *socio-cultural factors*, including the competitiveness of modern life[31], effects of social and demographic change[32], free availability of health care under the National Health Service in Britain[33], 'stress' of daily life, especially role stresses in women[34], a lowered threshold of physical and psychological pain[35], excessive faith in science and technology in dealing with personal problems[36], the 'medicalisation' of everyday life[37], and cultural beliefs about sleep and its necessity for health[38].

Most authors on the subject agree that there are dangers in this increased prescribing. The benzodiazepines, in particular, are considered to be over-used or mis-used[39], especially the hypnotics[40]. Although some of them are marketed as minor tranquillisers, and others as 'sleeping tablets', their effects are similar, and there is little to choose between them[41]. Numerous of their side-effects have been reported[42], both physical and psychological[43]. In particular, there is a tendency to cause psychological dependence on them[44], and this can occur at virtually any dose[45], and after only a short exposure[46].

This paper is primarily an enquiry into the nature of this psychological dependence, and the many dimensions of meaning these drugs have for those who use them on a long-term basis.

Psychological dependence on drugs

Lader[47] has provided a useful definition of psychological dependence, as:

'the need the patient experiences for the psychological effects of a drug. This need can be of two types. The patient may crave the drug-produced symptoms or changes in mood – a feeling of euphoria or a lessening of tension, for example. Or the patient may take the drug to stave off the symptoms of withdrawal.'

This dependence is sometimes, though not always, associated with drug tolerance: i.e. 'the need to increase the dosage of a drug in order to maintain its therapeutic effect'[48]. True physical dependence, or addiction, is more likely to be associated with tolerance, and with severe physical and psychological withdrawal symptoms[49]. However, as Claridge[50] points out, the distinction between psychological and physical dependence may be more theoretical than real. Physical addiction, for example to narcotics, is just one end of a continuum of drug-taking, with more socially acceptable 'chemical comforters' such as alcohol, tobacco, coffee, and 'tonics' at the other end[51] – a similar point to that made by Peele[52]. Peele sees addiction as an extension of ordinary behaviour, 'a pathological habit' or compulsion; while Stepney[53] sees 'drug-based habits' such as drug dependence and addiction as having a 'family resemblance' to other forms of repetitive and engrossing behaviour with similar psychological functions. These non-pharmacological habits include food-based habits (e.g. overeating, tea drinking); oral-manipulative habits such as smoking, nail-biting, thumb-sucking; social habits and rituals, including gambling and games; thrill-seeking habits, and certain hobbies. In practice these tend to overlap, but they all share the characteristics of escapism, instantaneous gratification, development of some degree of tolerance, and symptoms of withdrawal.

Both personality and socio-cultural factors are as important as the pharmacology of the drug, in both psychological dependence and addiction[54]. Several studies have shown the importance of the socio-cultural matrix of drug users, even if they are physically addicted. Peele[55] quotes the radical drop in the number of U.S. soldiers addicted to heroin, once they returned from Vietnam to the context of civilian life. Jackson[56] reports a case from St Louis in the 1960s where the life-style and behaviour of heroin addicts remained unchanged when the supply of heroin dried up, and was replaced by methamphetamine – whose pharmacological action is opposite to that of heroin. The effect of any drug is influenced by a variety of non-pharmacological factors, including the colour and appearance of the drug itself[57], the standing of the prescriber, the personality of the person taking it, and the setting in which it is taken. As Claridge puts it:

> 'The subject's .. attitude towards and knowledge of drugs, what he has been told about the particular drug he is taking, and the setting in which it is given, will all contribute to the total drug effect.'[58]

There has been speculation as to the attributes of personalities most likely to become psychologically dependent on or addicted to drugs, though no clear picture has emerged. Among the cluster of personality traits isolated are: over-anxiety, emotional dependency and immaturity, and hypo-chondriasis[59]; a painful consciousness of life, with low self-esteem, a sense of inadequacy, and poor personal relationships[60]; and a tendency to depression with anxiety[61].

The importance of both personality and socio-cultural factors is clearly seen in the case of *placebos*, or pharmacologically-inactive preparations. These can cause a wide variety of physical and psychological changes[62], including side-effects such as drowsiness[63], as well as psychological dependence on them[64]. In Britain there is a long history of self-medication with placebos such as 'bitters' and 'tonics'[65], as well as 'nerve tonics' and 'elixirs of life'[66].

Symbolism of drug prescribing and ingestion

In Joyce's view[67] there is a strong symbolic, or placebo element in virtually all drugs prescribed by doctors – even if they are pharmacologically active preparations. He estimates that nearly 1 in 5 of all prescriptions written by general practitioners in Britain are for their symbolic functions; that there are about 500,000 people in the United Kingdom who each year are 'symbol-dependent' patients; and that any drug given for more than 2 years has a large symbolic component. Psychological dependence on this symbolic function is particularly important in the case of psychotropics, all of whom can be regarded as drugs of dependence[68]. According to Tyrer[69], dependence is more likely when fixed dosage regimes are followed for long periods. Parish[70] has shown in his Birmingham study (1971), that 14.9 per cent of patients surveyed had taken psychotropic drugs continuously for one year or more, and 4.9 per cent for 5 years or more. Yet Williams[71] quotes studies showing that most hypnotics lose their sleep-promoting properties within 3–14 days of continuous use by the patient, and that there was little convincing evidence that benzodiazepines were efficacious in the treatment of anxiety after 4 months' continuous treatment; i.e. with long-term use, the pharmcological element in the effect of these drugs declines, to be replaced by a largely symbolic element – particularly if the drug has been used in a fixed, regular, 'habit-type' regimen[72].

The prescribing and ingestion of drugs is imbedded in a matrix of cultural values and assumptions. Unlike in some non-Western societies (and in hospital medicine, here in the West) where healing frequently takes place in a public setting, drug treatment in general practice has two distinct phases (a) the *public* domain, or act of prescribing, and (b) the *private* domain of drug ingestion, self-medication, and compliance with the doctor's instructions. Both domains have strong symbolic elements.

Pellegrino[73] sees three interacting levels of symbolism: that of the act of chemical ingestion itself; its enhancement by the fact of illness; and the potent investiture of this symbolism by the doctor's act of prescribing. Both prescription and drug can be viewed as what Turner[74] calls 'multi-vocal' symbols; i.e. representing many things at the same time. In the case of the *prescribing* act, the prescription has both 'manifest' and 'latent' functions; this has been described by several authors, including Lennard and Cooperstock[75], Smith[76], Balint[77], and Pfefferbaum[78]. Among 'manifest' functions of the prescription, Smith mentions: a method of therapy, of communication, of medical control, and of clinical trial. He lists 27 possible latent functions of the prescription[79], including: as symbols of the doctor's power, and the power of technology, the legitimation of long-term illness, an indication of the doctor's concern, and a way of terminating the consultation. Balint has also described latent functions of the prescription, in particular the placebo function of the consultation itself, where the doctor himself becomes a form of 'drug'. Hall[80] also focuses on this relationship and sees prescribing as a form of 'social exchange'.

After being issued a prescription, the patient enters the private domain of drug *ingestion*, equivalent to a form of self-medication. In a middle-class Western setting, this is the domain of privacy, autonomy and choice. Here, as Stimson[81] has shown, the patient 'has the potential for considerable autonomy' in deciding whether, or how, to comply with the doctor's instructions. He estimates 'non-compliance' in this domain at about 30 per cent and notes that patients make decisions whether to take prescribed drugs or not, based on their lay theories of how the drugs work, their effectiveness and dangers, and their own previous experience of them. Joyce[82] has noted that an individual's experiences with a drug, for example a psychotropic, have cumulative effects, so that people who have had one favourable outcome from the drug will probably experience a similar outcome on subsequent occasions, and this is particularly important in the development of psychological dependence.

This study deals with the symbolic significance of psychotropic drugs to a group of long-term users of these preparations; in particular, the part played by these drugs in their daily lives and social relationships.

Research setting and methods

The survey was essentially a pilot-study, designed to collect both qualitative and quantitative data and to formulate concepts which would then be evaluated in a second, larger survey. It was carried out in Edgware and Stanmore, Middlesex, two adjacent middle-class suburbs on the outskirts of London. 50 patients were interviewed, each of whom had been receiving repeat prescriptions for one of the benzodiazepines[83] for at least 6 months prior to the date of the interview. They were randomly selected from among all patients who satisfied these criteria, and who attended their National Health Service general practitioners on selected days during a 6-month period in 1979. They were interviewed with their permission, and that of their GP's. It was stressed that their comments would remain anonymous, and would not affect their treatment in any way. The interviews were semi-structured and open-ended, and conducted in an informal atmosphere. Replies and comments were entered on a standardised questionnaire. One aspect of the methodology requires comment: the patients interviewed knew I was a doctor (though not their own), as well as a social anthropologist, and this may have influenced their replies – though the extent of this influence is impossible to assess. Given this, some of the replies may provide interesting data on what Lader calls 'drug-seeking behaviour'[84]; i.e. the steps taken by the psychologically-dependent patient to ensure supplies of the appropriate drug, in this case by the form of self-description given by patient to doctor. Stimson and Webb[85] have noted how patients select and order the information they give to the doctor, in order to influence the outcome of the consultation, and this may also have an effect on the collection of data in a social science setting.

The patient sample are shown in *Table 1*: only 9 were in full-time employment at the time of the survey, the other 41 described themselves as 'retired' or 'housewife'[86]. The average age of the sample was over 60 years. In this survey, as in others, women predominated. Women in Britain are

Table 1 *The patient sample*

age (years)	sex m no.	%	f no.	%	total no.	%	marital status	no.	%	children no.	no.	%
20–39	—	—	4	(8)	4	(8)	married	33	(66)	0	11	(22)
40–59	3	(6)	6	(12)	9	(18)	widowed	10	(20)	1	16	(32)
60+	7	(14)	30	(60)	37	(74)	single	5	(10)	2	16	(32)
total	10	(20)	40	(80)	50	(100)	divorced	2	(4)	3	5	(10)
										4	2	(4)

prescribed psychotropics twice as frequently as men; e.g. in Parish's study[87] the female:male ratio for all psychotropics was 2.14:1, that of tranquillisers was 2.1:1, and non-barbiturate hypnotics 1.8:1. In addition, psychotropic drugs were prescribed more for patients 45 years of age or more, and especially elderly bereaved widows[88].

The questionnaire dealt with the perceived effects of psychotropic drugs on the individual, and on their social relationships and self-image; the social context of psychotropic drug use; and patients' attitudes to 'drugs' in general.

The effects of psychotropic drugs on the individual

The sample were asked why they thought they had been prescribed the psychotropic drug, why they had continued to take it, what effects they noticed on themselves after taking it, and what they would do if it was withdrawn or unobtainable. The original reason for it being prescribed seemed less important than why it was being taken now; e.g. one patient, apparently prescribed Librium after a bereavement 8 years previously was still getting repeat prescriptions for them in order 'to help me unwind'. Another, prescribed Mogadon 5 years ago in hospital for 'insomnia' after an eye operation, was still taking it regularly for the same symptom.

The stated reason for taking the drug now, i.e. the current 'problem' perceived by the patients as requiring psychotropic medication – as well as the perceived effects of the drug on them after ingestion – is shown in *Tables 2* and *3*.

Almost half the sample were taking their drug for 'insomnia', and 19 for symptoms of 'tension', 'anxiety', or physical symptoms associated with these states such as 'a tight stomach', 'a bumping heart'. The point at which patients define sleeping problems and subjective emotional states as being 'abnormal', and thus constituting an 'illness' depends, as Kleinman[89] has noted, on personal, social, and cultural factors; and these factors may in turn shape both the perception of symptoms, and how they are described to

Table 2   *Why the drug is currently being taken (n–50)*

	no.	%
insomnia, 'sleeplessness'	23	(46)
'nerves', tension, anxiety	19	(38)
depression, 'feeling low'	5	(10)
'a nervous breakdown'	3	(6)

others. The part played by ethno-religious variables in defining behaviour and subjective states as 'illness' has been noted by Guttmacher and Elinson[90], and others. Cultural beliefs about the nature of sleep, what constitutes 'normal' sleep, as well as whether 'bad thoughts or memories' occurring at night are 'normal', all have an important influence. Dunnell and Carwright[91] found that 29 per cent of a patient population thought that doctors could 'cure' sleeplessness, while 63 per cent believed they could be helped medically with this symptom. In the U.S.A., Solomon *et al.*[92] estimated that one third of Americans over 18 years of age perceive themselves as having had 'trouble sleeping' within a given year, but only 2 per cent would define it as 'insomnia'. In this sample, 'thinking' and 'memories' occurring during the time culturally defined as 'sleeping time', were classified as an abnormal state requiring treatment: e.g.

> 'It's a nice feeling – a block in my head and I can't think beyond it into my miserable thoughts. Something stops me thinking and then allows me to drift into sleep.'

> '(Without it) I'd lie awake, thinking about this or the other. I would lie awake from 4 to 7 o'clock and be thinking, worrying.'

The effect of insomnia on one's personality the following day was also mentioned, e.g.

> 'I fall into a deep natural sleep. I get a good long night's sleep, and wake up feeling normal.'

> 'If I get no sleep at all, I'm not well in the morning. I don't feel myself. Don't want to do anything, can't be bothered, fed up with myself.'

In both these cases there is a subjective concept of what 'being normal' or 'being oneself' is like; part of this definition depends on the patient's

Table 3   *Perceived effects of the drug on the individual after ingestion (n–50)*

	no.	%
no perceived effect	20	(40)
improvement in mental state	17	(34)
fall asleep	13	(26)

interpretation of their own physical and emotional symptoms, and part on the interpretation of others. The possible origin of this self-concept will be discussed later on.

Patients did not differentiate between hypnotics and tranquillisers; all tablets taken at night – even tranquillisers such as Valium or Ativan – were defined as 'sleeping tablets'. It has been noted[93] that emotional states – in this case 'insomnia' –tend to be named after the presumed actions of the drugs available to treat them. The prescription of a drug to be taken at bedtime may therefore help define the problem as 'a sleeping problem'; i.e. one of sleep-deficiency, rather than as a symptom of emotional unease. Similarly, tranquillisers ingested during the day help define the problem as 'nerves' or 'tension'.

34 patients did perceive some improvement in their mental state after ingestion of the drug; e.g.

'If I get het up, it calms me. I feel calmer. I don't think it's imagination. It keeps me on the level.'

'If I'm in a panic I take it – I can feel the panic subsiding. I can sit still for longer.'

The large number of patients (40 per cent) in *Table 3* who noticed no subjective change after ingesting the drug may reflect the development of tolerance, but they may also serve to confirm Joyce's contention of the symbolic-placebo aspect of drugs taken for a long period. *Thirteen* of these patients cast doubt on whether the drug actually had any pharmacological effect on them, and speculated that it's effect was 'probably psychological', e.g.

'It's probably psychological – I imagine that it's helping. I've got something behind me that will help – it's security.'

'I feel a little more confident. I don't know if it's that or me. Whether it was auto-suggestion or me – it calmed me. You become so reliant on them you feel it's doing you good – even if it isn't.'

'I don't know if it makes me relax or not. Having taken it my mind says, "I'm going to relax soon". It's probably psychological.'

'I take 1 at night. It doesn't work any more. It's like a kind of prop – otherwise I think I won't fall asleep. I kid myself that I feel better with Valium.'

These answers suggest that Joyce's estimation of 2 years before a drug becomes largely symbolic in effect, may be an over-estimation. Seeing the drug's effect as 'probably psychological' may be a way of diminishing its effects and regaining a sense of autonomy; the patient's own mind, rather than the ingested chemical, becomes the therapeutic ally in improving his mental state.

Table 4   *Patients' strategies if drug were withdrawn or unobtainable (n–50)*

	no.	%
taken another 'drug'	18	(36)
done without and coped well	14	(28)
don't know	8	(16)
continued with symptoms as before	5	(10)
suffered a 'breakdown'	3	(6)
seen a psychologist	1	(2)
gone on a 'nature cure'	1	(2)

The theme of the drug being 'a prop', 'a security', 'a helper' recurred several times; in some cases, especially elderly widows, the drug was viewed as almost anthropomorphic in nature; a 'someone' rather than a 'something': e.g.

'I'd be terrified at night all alone – if I didn't have something to fall back upon.'

'I take one at night – it's if you're alone, you see.'

In this sense, a socially-isolated individual's relationship with their drug may have symbolic components which are unrelated to its pharmacology.

Side-effects from the drugs were reported by 10 patients, and included nightmares, depression, and impotence – though they continued asking for repeat prescriptions. 39 patients reported no side-effects, and one was unsure. Emotional side-effects from the drugs, e.g. depression, were seen as different in quality from the identical symptoms occurring without therapy, and did not seem to require treatment.

One aspect of the survey dealt with patient's beliefs about what they would do – or would have done – if their drug was unobtainable or withdrawn, or had never been invented. The results are shown in *Table 4*.

The 18 patients who would have turned to another 'drug' – either self-prescribed or from a doctor – reveal the widespread popular belief in 'chemical comforters'. The self-prescribed drugs here included 'Aspirin', 'Aspro', 'Paracetamol', 'Panadol', 'Veganin' and 'Metatone'. Significantly, all except the last one are analgesics and easily available at any pharmacy. The question arises whether patients are linking physical with psychological 'pain'. Peele[94] sees addiction as 'a pain-relieving experience', whatever the source of the pain, and notes that 'a painful consciousness of life characterizes the outlooks and personalities of addicts'. My hypothesis is that, in addition to their easy availability, analgesics may be used for emotional distress because of the experience of these drugs as having relieved physical pain. Jefferys' study of self-medication on a working-class estate[95], also showed the widespread use of 'Aspirins' for 'nerves', 'sleeplessness', and other mental disorders, particularly by women. Her study showed that self-medication was twice as common as the ingestion of prescribed drugs, though often the two were taken together. Patients' use of self-medication may be a way of expressing their autonomy *vis-à-vis* the medical profession, but the continued demand for prescribed psycho-tropics in addition seems to confirm the views of Balint, Pellegrino and others that the act of prescribing itself has important symbolic components. Self-medication for emotional problems has a long genealogy in Britain; opiates and alcohol have been used for centuries, by both men and women. Gin, known as 'mother's ruin', was commonly used by women in the 18th and 19th centuries, as was laudanum[96]. Several of these medications were pharmacologically inactive: 'paregoric', a common domestic remedy, allegedly a tincture of opium, was found to contain no opium in an inquiry in 1880[97]. In 1912 the British Medical Association investigated dozens of patent 'nerve tonics', 'restoratives' and 'elixirs of life', and found that hardly any contained any active ingredients[98]. In 1968, 23.5 million prescriptions for 'tonics, iron and vitamins' were dispensed, all of which have a largely placebo effect[99]. In 1975 these 'bitters' and 'tonics' cost the N.H.S. £497,000[100]. The belief in 'chemical comforters' is a widespread cultural assumption, and this belief is often unrelated to the pharmacology of the ingested chemical.

Those patients in the sample who would not have turned to 'drugs', reported a continuum of likely outcomes, from 'coping' to 'breakdown'; e.g.

'It wouldn't really worry me – I would cope.'

'I would just have gone on trembling.'

'I would have been in a mental home for the rest of my life.'

Are psychotropics 'drugs'?

While self-medication is common, the preparations taken are not regarded as 'drugs'. This word has a negative connotation, and most patients are against their use. They were asked about their general attitude to 'drugs' (*Table 5*) and whether what they had been prescribed, and were taking, was 'a drug' (*Table 6*); if it was a drug, what type it was; and if not, what they thought it was.

Most of the sample were against 'drug-taking' and 'drugs', presumably associating the latter with narcotic abuse. However, 41 patients admitted that their medication was in fact 'a drug'; they qualified their moral disapproval by pointing out that they were an unfortunate but necessary evil, and – for them – there did not seem to be any other alternative; e.g.

Table 5 *General attitude to 'drugs' (n–50)*

	no.	%
against	34	(68)
in favour	15	(30)
don't know	1	(2)

Table 6 *Whether the prescribed medication is 'a drug' or not (n–50)*

is a drug	41	(84)
is not a drug	8	(16)
don't know	1	(2)

'It drugs you off to sleep. They do people a lot of harm. If only there was something else in place of drugs.'

'I don't like to take them, but I just have to.'

'I'm against it basically. If you can do without it you're lucky.'

'I don't like it – but I'm grateful it's there.'

In some cases, the responsibility for the patient being on drugs was put solely on the doctor: e.g.

'It's necessary if the doctor prescribed it. If the doctor prescribes it, I *must* need it.'

'If it's necessary then you take them – if it's treatment by a doctor.'

'I'm not against drugs – I take whatever I'm given to swallow.'

The moral disapproval of 'drugs' in general, was based on two lay uses of the word 'drug'; i.e. something over which one has no control, and which involves a loss of personal autonomy and choice; and something which greatly alters the level of consciousness, to a degree where one can no longer function in daily life; e.g.

'It's not a drug – if you took more of it, it might become a drug.'

'It doesn't drug me – I keep on the go.'

Jones[101] has pointed out that patients differentiate between 'medicine' as something that makes them better, while 'drug' has more sinister implications. In his study, over 80 per cent of patients agreed that heroin was a drug, but only half classified morphine, sleeping tablets and tranquillisers as drugs, while only one third saw aspirin as a drug. The sinister implications in the word 'drug' are particularly those of loss of autonomy, choice, and self-control. Although many of the patients in my sample were psychologically dependent on psychotropics, how they conceptualised this dependence left some room for their own sense of autonomy and self-control, and to do this they tended to diminish the chemical power of 'their drug', as opposed to the 'hard' variety; e.g.

'It's a little bit of help – not a powerful drug.'

'It's soft, sweet – it's different – it's softer (than other drugs).'

'It's just a calmer, a help – I can cut it off when I want to.'

'It's not a drug – merely a thing for sleeping.'

'It's sort of – just a medium drug – a mild sleeping one.'

'It's a harmless one.'

The social context of psychotropic drug use

Stimson and Webb[102] have noted the importance of friendship and family networks in exchanging ideas and information about drugs, both prescribed and non-prescribed. Blum[103] has mentioned the importance of family attitudes in learning about drugs, and their expected effects. The setting in which any drug is ingested can have an important influence on its effect[104]. The patients in this sample were part of social networks that knew of their taking the drug, in general approved of it, and were often taking the same drug themselves. The survey dealt only with knowledge of the *same* drug used by others; presumably a larger number were using other psychotropic drugs as well. The sample were questioned about who knew they were taking, say Valium, and whom they themselves knew to be taking that same drug. Their social networks included friends, relatives, spouses, neighbours, or workmates[105]; the results are shown in *Tables 7* and *8*.

The fact of taking the same prescribed drugs can create a bond between people; similar to what Turner terms 'a community of suffering'; e.g.

'All my friends are on Valium.'

'All the widows are taking something.'

'Nearly everyone I know (is taking Valium).'

In 7 cases, both spouses were taking the same psychotropic drug; an impression was gained that some of these relationships might be termed 'chemical marriages' – where the marriage is only maintained by frequent ingestion of a psychotropic drug by both partners. Knowledge of psychotropic drugs is widely shared within a family, though not always: e.g.

'I'm ashamed to tell anyone that I'm taking a bit of drug.'

In some cases the family may provide the cue for the patient to take the drug; e.g.

'If I'm tensed up – my husband will say "Take a Librium".'

As Claridge[106] has noted, the perception of how others are reacting to oneself can influence the effect of a drug once it has been ingested. Psychotropic drug use by the patients also took place in an atmosphere of tolerance or neutrality. Only 9 patients reported some disapproval by others of their taking the drug, 10 reported approval, 29 said that those who knew did not care either way, and 2 were not sure. The majority of these patients' social contacts, then, did not regard long-term usage of psychotropic drugs as markedly 'abnormal' or morally undesirable, and so to a large extent saw them as socially harmless. This atmosphere also makes possible 'fashions in drug-taking and the exchanging and sharing of drugs within a social network; patients who have accumulated a large store of drugs may act as what Hindmarch[107] calls 'over-the-fence physicians' to family, friends and neighbours. In this survey, only 12 per cent of the patients admitted to this, but in Warburton's study[108], 68 per cent of young adults interviewed admitted receiving psychotropics from friends or relatives. A large number of drugs prescribed regularly are never or seldom ingested, and tend to be stored at home[109], while one survey showed that 27 per cent of British homes had some psychoactive drug in them[110]. Not only is information about psychotropics shared within a

Table 7   *Knowledge of another person taking the same drug (n–50)*

	no.	%
yes	36	(72)
no	14	(28)

Table 8   *Patient known by others to be taking the drug (n–50)*

	no.	%
yes	44	(88)
no	6	(12)

social network, but the drugs themselves may be shared; in that case, there is a reversal of roles and the 'patient' now becomes the 'prescriber'.

Social relationships, self-image, and psychotropic drug use

An important aspect of psychotropic drug use is the role these drugs are believed to play in maintaining, or improving, relationships with others – particularly within the family. Both aspects of Lader's definition of psychological dependence[111] are relevant here: firstly, the believed positive effects of the drug in maintaining or improving existing relationships and secondly, the fear of what would happen if the drug were withdrawn, or unobtainable. The sample were asked the supposed effects of the drug on their relationships, and what they imagined would happen if the drugs were not available. The results are shown in *Table 9*.

Table 9 *Believed effects of drug, or its withdrawal, on sample's social relationships (n–50)*

| | | effect of drug on relationships | | | |
		no effect	good effect	bad effect	total & (%)
effect of withdrawal of	no effect	19	2	—	21(42)
drug on relationships	good effect	—	—	—	—
	bad effect	15	10	1	26(52)
	don't know	2	1	—	3(6)
	total & (%)	36(72)	13(26)	1(2)	50(100)

These results reveal that, for some patients at least, the drug – or its withdrawal – had a definite impact on their social relationships. This impact was an indirect one – the result of changes in the patient's own emotional state, which would then have an effect on other people; i.e. for some patients the drug was taken as much for the benefit of others, as for their own benefit.

Thirteen of the patients saw some good effect on their relationships from the drug, while none saw any good effect resulting from its withdrawal. A total of 26 patients saw some bad effect arising from its withdrawal, usually as a result of a change in their own emotional state. Significantly, 15 patients – who noticed no effect of the drug on their relationships, did feel that these relationships would suffer if the drug were withdrawn; i.e. without it they would be in a form of 'psychotropic-deficiency state'. They could only be returned to normal social functioning, and a sense of completeness, if the drug were obtainable again – much like the diabetic who can only function normally with the aid of injected insulin. The relationship between this sense of social inadequacy and 'incompleteness' without the drug, and the fact that a large proportion of those on long-term psychotropic therapy are elderly widows[112] who are, in a sense, socially 'incomplete' – needs to be explored in further research projects.

A total of 19 patients in the sample perceived *no* effects, either positive or negative, of the drug on their social lives. In this group, presumably, the perceived site of the drug's effect was on the patient themself, and was taken for their benefit rather than for the benefit of others.

Those patients who saw the drug as necessary for the maintenance of their social relationships, tended to view the drug as helping them conform to an idealised, normative model of behaviour. This model was essentially a static one, and the only element within it that could be changed was the patient's emotional reaction to their life situation; e.g.

'If I could send the 4 children away I might learn to cope (without the drug) – otherwise it would be impossible.'

These patients' self-images included a wide variety of negative personality attributes that could only be minimised or cancelled out by, in a sense, 'titrating' the drug against them. Without the drug's aid the patient is 'incomplete', the negative personality traits predominate, and he or she cannot conform to the idealised model of 'normal' behaviour. Aspects of behaviour in relation to others – particularly family members – that were believed by patients to be linked to psychotropic drug ingestion, are shown in *Table 10*.

In the above cases, the psychotropic drug can be conceptualised as a 'fuel' without which the patient's social persona would not function. This concept of the personality requiring the aid of technology – in this case a psychotropic drug – in order to function adequately, is similar to the 'human beings as machines' metaphor, which Lennard and Cooperstock[113] see as becoming increasingly pervasive in the modern world.

Learnt aspects of psychotropic drug use

Blum[114] has pointed out the 'learning model' aspect of drug use, whereby people acquire knowledge as to what drugs to use, and when, and what sorts of responses are to be expected. Parish[115] has suggested that in prescribing psychotropic drugs for personal problems, doctors are communicating a model of how to deal with these problems – not by confronting them, but by ingestion of the drug; a point illustrated in *Table 10*. Trethowan[116], a psychiatrist, points out that this strategy is a 'non-solution'; anxiety can be biologically purposive, and merely suppressing it chemically may undermine the patient's motivation to confront and deal with the anxiety-provoking situation. In addition, patients can acquire a taste for what Watts[117] calls 'this artificial tranquility' – for a life

Table 10   *The normative model: aspects of behaviour in relation to others affected by psychotropic drugs or their withdrawal*

---

1. *being 'normal'*

e.g. 'Now I feel normal all the time. I don't go off the handle so easily. I'm not so excited, angry, irritable.'

'Without it I couldn't lead a normal life.'

'[Without it] I'd not be doing the normal things I should have done.'

2. *being 'oneself'*

e.g. 'If I don't have it (Mogadon) I don't feel myself. I don't want to do anything'.

'[With it] It's nice – I feel just myself.'

3. *self-control*

e.g. 'If people can't control their emotions, then they need them – like some women.'

'[Without them] I might not be responsible for what I'd do. I could not cope.'

4. *even-tempered*

e.g. '[Without it] it'd make me uptight, irritable, snappy.'

'[Without it] I'd be nervy, impatient with other people.'

5. *good to live with*

e.g. '[Without it] I'd be nasty, jumpy, not nice to live with.'

'[Without it] I'd be difficult to live with – nasty tempered.'

'[Without it] I'd be less patient with the family.'

'[Without it[I'd be miserable – take it out on the family.'

6. *nurturing (to family)*

e.g. '[Without it] I couldn't help those I love.'

7. *non-complaining*

e.g. '[Without it] I'd be all groans and moans.'

8. *sociable*

e.g. '[Without it] I wouldn't want to see people.'

'[With it] I'm friendly – I can associate with people.'

'[Without it] I'm morose – don't want to talk – withdrawn.'

'If I'm calmer, I feel more confident, especially with strangers. I feel confident on Valium.'

9. *assertive*

e.g. '[With it] I'm more assertive – I get the feeling I don't care – to hell with everybody!'

---

theoretically free of interpersonal problems, 'bad thoughts' and 'bad memories'. Patients on long-term psychotropic treatment can also learn emotional dependency on the doctor – what Pfefferbaum terms the 'negative placebo effect'[118] – as well as a new self-image; i.e. a sense of personal unworthiness and 'incompleteness', that can only be corrected by the addition of the drug which 'completes' them. Six patients in this survey referred to this learnt aspect of psychotropic drug use: e.g.

'If it had never been invented – I wouldn't have had the experience of relying on them.'

'[Without the sleeping tablet] I'd have probably banked on getting catnaps during the day – if one's never heard of a thing, one doesn't miss it.'

'If I didn't know of it – there would have been nothing I could do about it – I would think "I'm a miserable so-and-so and I'm stuck with it!" '

'[If it had not been prescribed] I would never have known about it – you would have to rely on yourself.'

Table 11   *A classification of long-term psychotropic drug users*

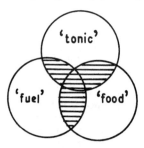

A classification of psychotropic drug users

Although this pilot-study was based on a small and not necessarily representative sample, it is possible to see that long-term users of psychotropic drugs are not a homogeneous group. They differ from one another not only in age, sex, background, and other demographic variables – but also in terms of their attitudes towards the drugs and their usage, as well as the *symbolic* role these drugs appear to play in their daily lives and relationships. This role, as reported by the sample, may be an aspect of their 'drug-seeking behaviour', but is still of crucial importance in psychological dependence.

The hypothesis is that long-term users of psychotropics can be classified into three main groups – called 'Tonic', 'Food', and 'Fuel' – and that each of these groupings represents a different conceptualisation of psychotropic drugs and their use. These three 'types' are *not* discrete groups, but rather clusters of attributes which overlap to some extent, so that no one individual would usually have *all* the attributes of his particular group. This is shown schematically in *Table 11*.

These groups are based on patients' stated beliefs about, and expectations of, their psychotropic drug. However – in further research projects – they need to be related to patients' actual health behaviour, as independently observed, as well as to a variety of demographic variables including age, sex, marital status and ethnicity, and also trends in the consumption of tobacco, alcohol and other 'chemical comforters'. From this survey, though, the classification is based on the following criteria:

1. The degree of perceived *control* by the patient over the drug – under what circumstances, in what manner, and how frequently it should be ingested. On this basis, patients can be placed on a continuum of perceived control; i.e.

Minimum control . . . . Maximum control
    ('Food')   ('Fuel')   ('Tonic')

2. The perceived *site of action* of the drug – whether primarily on the patient, their social relationships, or on both; i.e.

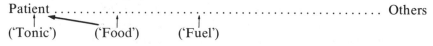

Patient . . . . Others
('Tonic')   ('Food')   ('Fuel')

⇂ = perceived site of maximum effect.

3. Beliefs about the nature of the *effects* of the drug –or its withdrawal – on the patient's subjective emotional state, and social relationships.

4. Beliefs about the nature of 'drugs' in general, and their own prescribed drug in particular.

5. 'Habit' aspects of daily life (cf. Stepney (53)); i.e. whether the patient is subject to other fixed daily rituals or habits, whether pharmacological or not.

The three hypothetical types of chronic users are described below, with examples.

'Tonic'

Patients classified as 'Tonic' (17 patients) in this sample, express maximum control over the drug, its dosage, and when it is to be used ('I can cut it off when I want to', 'I am sufficiently strong willed to overcome it.'). They use the drugs more as a form of *self-medication* when required, rather than on a regular basis. Using the drug in this flexible way they represent what Stimson[119] calls 'the patient as decision making individual', and have a sense of autonomy and choice in relation to how the drug should be used. Despite their less frequent use, they still continued to be prescribed regular supplies of psychotropics by their general practitioners. They placed the site of action of the drug on themselves, rather than on their relationships; these relationships were not affected either by the drug, or its withdrawal (see *Table 9*). They were more likely to describe the drug's effects as 'probably psychological', and to diminish the drug's pharmacological power ('it's a small help', 'it's not addictive – it serves a purpose', 'it's only a mild form'). They tended to be more anti-drug than other groups ('It's a vice – there's too much drug-taking around', 'It's awful', 'It's not a good thing.'). They tended to stress the value of autonomy, choice, and self-control. Five of the men in the sample fell in this group. The use of the drug was episodic, and usually for a short period only; during that time it was used as a temporary 'tonic', 'stimulant' or 'a thing for sleeping'. The subjective emotional states classified here as 'illness' and therefore requiring treatment, were temporary feelings of anxiety or tension, or a sense of 'feeling low' – what Pellegrino[120] would term 'loss of soul' – i.e. 'of vitality, pep, spirit'. These latter symptoms were frequently treated by patent 'Nerve Tonics', 'Restoratives', and 'Elixirs of Life'[121] before psychotropic drugs became easily available.

'Mr A is a Company Director. He is aged 56, is married and has 2 children. He has been on Valium for 3 years for "tension" and following a "mild coronary". He describes himself as "just a mild taker", and stresses that he takes Valium "only when necessary" when he needs to relax a bit and get some sleep. His wife was also taking Valium. He felt that without the drug he "wouldn't really worry" and he could cope well with his everyday life, though it would "take longer to fall asleep". Neither Valium, nor its withdrawal, would have any effect – he said – on his relationships with others. He was against "drugs" in general, though felt that some people needed them: "If people can't control their emotions, they need them – like some women".'

'Fuel'

Twenty-two of the patients could be fitted into this grouping, 5 of them men. They expressed a variable degree of control over their medication, a few speculating that its effect was only 'a habit' and 'probably psychological'. Nevertheless, the drug played an important and constant part in their daily lives; its maximum effect being on their relationships with others (*Tables 9* and *10*). These relationships were affected indirectly by the effect of the drug, or its withdrawal, on the patients' subjective emotional state. The drug can be conceptualised as a 'fuel', without which the patient's personality would not disintegrate but would just not *function* in conformity with familial and social expectations (*Table 10*). This 'functional' definition of 'normality' or 'health' has been noted in other studies; e.g. Blaxter and Paterson[122] studied health beliefs and behaviour of working-class women in Aberdeen; in many cases 'health' was defined in a functional sense – the ability to 'carry on' with work and social obligations, despite feeling subjectively 'ill'. In the 'fuel' group, the drug was seen as an often essential constituent of the patients' relationships, and its ingestion a way of maintaining or improving these relationships. This may also apply, as Balint has suggested, to the maintenance of their relationship with the doctor. Using the drug as a 'fuel' in order to function socially, also has other aspects: e.g. sharing responsibility with the drug for social successes (and failures); and being able to function socially, but still claim some of the benefits of the 'sick role'. The group's beliefs about the desirability of 'drugs' varied from 'I'm against them – but everyone needs a little bit of help' to 'If they do you good – take 'em'. In general drugs were viewed as 'a help' – a necessary element in the smooth running of social relationships and families. An impression gained was that this group was not as 'habit-prone' as the 'Food' group, though the drugs played as important a symbolic role in the lives of both groups; e.g.

> 'Mrs B is a housewife, aged 70, with a grown-up daughter. She has been taking Mogadon "for years" for "insomnia and pain in the back". She takes 1 at night to fall asleep – "it smoothes me down – then I don't know anymore. I feel better in the mornings." It does not have any bad effects on her, but "if I have it with milk it makes me dream." She is worried about what would happen if the drug were not there – "I should just go on worrying about not sleeping" –and the effects of the lack of sleep on the following day – "If I get no sleep at all, I'm not well in the morning. I don't feel myself. Don't want to do anything, can't be bothered, fed up with myself." Without the drug she gets "bad-tempered" with her husband – very "snappy" with him, and "all groans and moans". With the drug she is "nice and calm" in relation to him. Both he and her daughter know of her taking the drug; he very much approves, though her daughter is against it. Without the drug she would have had to have "gone on a nature cure". She is not keen on taking the drug – "I don't like it – but I'm grateful it's there." A friend of her's is also taking Mogadon.'

'Food'

This group contained 11 patients, all of them female and a higher proportion of elderly patients than the first two groups. They express least control over the drug, and its ingestion – and over their life generally; ('I take whatever I'm given to swallow.'). This psychological dependence is as much on the medical profession, as on the prescribed drug. The drug is perceived as acting equally on both the patient's emotional state *and* their relationships; without it, both would disintegrate ('I would end up in a nerve hospital'. 'I would have been in a mental home for the rest of my life.'). The drug is a 'food', in that without it the patient would not 'survive' as a sane independent person; both personality and relationships would disintegrate if the drug were withdrawn ('If I don't get enough sleep I feel desperate – I'd be so exhausted I shall become stupid – unable to concentrate – forgetful – I'd lose control – I'd be irritable', 'I'd go all haywire – worry about the least little thing', 'I wouldn't want to see people – I'd feel stressed'.). Their ingestion of drugs is at fixed times, and with an inflexible dosage – the opposite of the flexible and episodic use of these drugs by the 'Tonic' group. As this group is mostly elderly patients, especially elderly widows (see Parish[87]) who are socially 'incomplete', it can be hypothesised that they perceive the drug as something that 'completes' them, and enables them to survive – as 'a prop', 'a helper', 'a security'. In addition, elderly people tend to be more 'habit-prone' – i.e. to have more fixed daily habits and rituals; also, many of them are already the recipients of what might be termed 'medically-induced habits', i.e. the regular daily ingestion of such prescribed drugs as digitalis, diuretics, thyroid drugs, anti-diabetic drugs, pain-killers and so on. The question arises whether a person who is already socially isolated, 'habit-prone' by age, as well as taking other drugs on a fixed daily basis, is not particularly vulnerable to becoming psychologically dependent on psychotropics and on their symbolic meanings.

Patients in this group, perhaps because of the curative effects of the other medicines they were taking, tended to be more 'pro-drug' than the other 2 groups (e.g. 'They're very good – it calms a person down', 'They help', 'Drugs help people'). They did not try to play down the effect of the drug on them.

If my hypothesis is correct, and psychotropic drugs in this group have become a symbolic form of 'food' – necessary for the patient's very survival (in a psychological sense) – then part of their symbolic power arises from what Pellegrino[123] terms the 'benediction' of the medical profession. This is reinforced every time the drug is prescribed – as is the link with the doctor, and with other members of the 'community of suffering'.

Not all members of this group, though, are elderly or single; e.g.

'Mrs C is a 52-year old housewife, with 4 children, married to a bank manager. Both she and her husband are taking Dalmane for "insomnia". She has been on hypnotics for many years now, even though they give her "a bad taste in the mouth" and make her "tired all the time". She feels she *cannot* cope without them: "If I could send the 4 children away I might learn to cope – otherwise it would be impossible." Without it, she would have "a breakdown" – "I have an uncontrollable fear of a breakdown." The drug helps her relationships "because I sleep"; *without* it, they would suffer – i.e. "I'm irritable with the family. I can't cope, I don't want to cope. I can't keep still", and added "I think I'm unbearable to live with anyway." Her husband, children and friends all knew she was on Dalmane, but "got used to it". She thought that drugs were a good thing "if they are necessary" and if the person's state was "very bad". She thought Dalmane was "a tranquilliser – but I sincerely hope it's not a barbiturate." If it had never been invented "I probably would have had to get on with it".'

Conclusions

The social and symbolic meaings of psychotropic drugs to a group of long-term users of these preparations, in 2 London suburbs, were examined in this pilot-study[124]. The emphasis in the study was on qualitative, rather than large-scale statistical data, in order to formulate concepts which would then be evaluated in subsequent and larger projects. The study reveals that psychotropic drugs can have many dimensions of meaning for those that use them: they can become incorporated into patients' self-images, and become an integral part of their social relationships. This helps explain the nature of their psychological dependence on these drugs. Also, chronic users of psychotropics are not a homogeneous group; they perceive – and use – psychotropics in a variety of ways, and this has important clinical implications. Doctors who regularly issue these drugs to patients by 'repeat prescriptions' or 'refills' – without assessing how the drugs are perceived, or used, can do more harm than good; as well as their side-effects, and tendency to cause psychological dependence, they are often accumulated for exchanging with others, as well as for suicide attempts[125]. To show that these drugs can be perceived and used in different ways, rather than as a single category of consumption, I have described three models of psychotropic drug use – as 'Tonic', 'Fuel', and 'Food'[126] – with some examples. To a large extent, *all* 'chemical comforters' – from coffee, alcohol, tobacco and 'vitamins' to more powerful psychotropic drugs – can be fitted into this classification.

Further study is needed to assess the predictive value of this classification in identifying patients most 'at risk' of becoming psychologically dependent on prescribed drugs, and also to relate these categories to tobacco and alcohol use, and to a larger number of social variables.

Acknowledgements

I wish to acknowledge the help of Drs B.H.J. Briggs, J.A. Cree, D.S. Myers, and M.M. Sundle in the project, as well as Dr Murray Last, Anthropology Department, University College London; and useful comments on the data from Dr Ruth Cooperstock, and also Dr Conrad Harris, Department of General Practice, St Mary's Hospital Medical School, London.

References

1   Claridge G. *Drugs and Human Behaviour*, p. 231. Allen Lane, London, 1970.
2   Trethowan W.H. Pills for Personal Problems. *British Medical Journal* 3, 749–51, 1975.
3   Warburton D.M. Poisoned people: internal pollution. *Journal of Biosocial Science* 10, 309–19, 1978.
4   Pellegrino E.D. Prescribing and Drug Ingestion: Symbols and Substances. *Drug Intelligence and Clinical Pharmacy* 10, 624–30, 1976.
5   Parish P.A. The prescribing of psychotropic drugs in general practice. *Journal of the Royal College of General Practitioners* 21, Suppl.4, p. 10, 1971.
6   Trethowan W.H. *op. cit.*, p. 749, 1975.
7   Tyrer P. Drugs for anxiety. *Prescribers' Journal* 16, No. 1, pp. 1–8, 1976.
8   Dunlop D.M. The use and abuse of psychotropic drugs. *Proceedings of the Royal Society of Medicine* 63, 1279–282, 1970.
9   Tyrer P. Drug treatment of psychiatric patients in general practice. *British Medical Journal* 2, 1008–010, 1978.
10   Sellers E.M. Clinical pharmacology and therapeutics of benzodiazepines. *Canadian Medical Association Journal* 118, 1533–538, 1978.
11   Warburton D.M. *op. cit.*, p. 311, 1978, quoting Pekanen, J. The Tranquillizer War. *New Republic* July 19, 17, 1975.
12   Hall R.C.W. and Kirkpatrick, B. The Benzodiazepines. *American Family Physician* 17, 131–34.
13   *Lancet*. Benzodiazepines: use, overuse, misuse, abuse? Editorial, 1, 1101–102, 1973.
14   Lennard H.L. and Cooperstock R. The Social Context and Functions of Tranquillizer Prescribing. In *Prescribing Practice and Drug Usage*. (Edited by Mapes, R.), pp. 73–82, Croom Helm, London, 1980.
15   Parish P.A. *op. cit.*, p. 67, 1971. Librium was introduced in 1960, Valium in 1963, Mogadon in 1965. In 1970, in England alone, 4.8 million prescriptions for Librium were dispensed, 4.3 million for Valium and 2.5 million for Mogadon. p. 5. From 1965 to 1970, prescribing of Librium and Valium increased by 110 per cent.
16   Segal H.J. The Social Risks and Benefits of Prescription Writing. In *Prescribing Practice and Drug Usage*. (Edited by Mapes, R.), pp. 19–36, Croom Helm, London, 1980.
17   Warburton D.M. *op. cit.*, p. 316, 1978.
18   Dajda R. Who prescribes? The Illusion of Power Sharing in the Surgery. In Mapes, R. *op. cit.*, pp. 147–56, 1980.
19   Melville A. Reducing Whose Anxiety? A Study of the Relationship Between Repeat Prescribing of Minor Tranquillizers and Doctors' Attitudes. In Mapes, R. *op. cit.*, pp. 100–18, 1980.
20   Hall D. Prescribing as Social Exchange. In Mapes, R. *op. cit.*, pp. 39–57, 1980.
21   Hall D. *op. cit.*
22   Parish P.A. *op. cit.*, p. 63, 1971.
23   Hindmarch I. Too many pills in the cupboard. *New Society* 55, 142–43, 1981.

24 Trethowan W.H. *op. cit.*, p. 751, 1975.
25 Warburton D.M. *op. cit.*, p. 314, 1978.
26 Parish P.A. *op. cit.*, p. 51, 1971.
27 Teeling-Smith G. Psychotropic drugs and society.*Journal of the Royal College of General Practitioners* **23**, Suppl.2, 58–62, 1973.
28 Balint M. *The Doctor, his Patient and the Illness.* 2nd edn. Pitman Medical, London, 1974.
29 Parish P.A. *op. cit.*, p. 67, 1971, and Hall, D. *op. cit.*, p. 45, 1980.
30 Warburton D.M. *op. cit.*, p. 314, 1978.
31 Warburton D.M. *op. cit.*, p. 314, 1978.
32 Mapes R. Sociological parameters of increased prescribing rate. In *Prescribing Practice and Drug Usage.* (Edited by Mapes, R.), pp. 33–6, Croom Helm, London, 1980.
33 Mapes R. *op. cit.*, pp. 33–4, 1980.
34 Cooperstock R. and Lennard H.L. Some social meanings of tranquillizer use. *Sociology of Health and Illness* **1**, 331–47, 1979.
35 Pellegrino E.D. *op. cit.*, p. 628, 1976.
36 Lennard H.L. and Cooperstock R. *op. cit.*, pp. 73–4, 1980.
37 Hall D. *op. cit.*, pp. 49–50, 1980.
38 Dunnell K. and Cartwright A. *Medicine Takers, Prescribers and Hoarders.* Routledge and Kegan Paul, London, 1972.
39 *Lancet. op. cit.*, 1973.
40 Solomon F., White C.C., Parron D.L. and Mendelson W.B. Sleeping pills, insomnia and medical practice.*New England Journal of Medicine* **300**, 803–08, 1979.
41 Smith A. and Rawlins M.D. Benzodiazepines. *British Medical Journal* **2**, 447, 1977.
42 Hall R.C.W. and Kirkpatrick B. *op. cit.*, 1978.
43 Sellers E.M. *op. cit.*, 1978.
44 See References 41, 42, 43.
45 Sellers E.M. *op. cit.*, p. 1536, 1978.
46 Smith A. and Rawlins M.D. *op. cit.*, 1977. Even in normal volunteers, two weeks' treatment with a benzodiazepine produces 'rebound' anxiety when the drug is withdrawn, which may last for several days.
47 Lader M. Spectres of tolerance and dependence.*MIMS Magazine*, 15 Aug, pp. 31–5, 1979.
48 Lader M. *op. cit.*, pp. 31–2, 1979.
49 Peele S. Addiction: The Analgesic Experience. *Human Nature* **1**, No. 9, 61–7, 1978.
50 Claridge G. *op. cit.*, p. 225, 1970.
51 Claridge G. *op. cit.*, p. 231, 1970. 'Medically recognized addiction is only the pathological end-part of a continuum of drug-taking that involves us all. Even the most upright of citizens have their chemical comforters, most of which are psychologically harmless when taken in small quantities.'
52 Peele S. *op. cit.*, p. 67, 1978.
53 Stepney R. Men of Habit. *World Medicine*, 19 May, pp. 39–41, 1979.
54 Claridge G. *op. cit.*, pp. 224–26, 1970; and Peele S. *op. cit.*, pp. 61–7, 1979.
55 Peele S. *op. cit.*, pp. 62–3, 1979.

56 Jackson B. Deviance as Success: The Double Inversion of Stigmatised Roles. In *The Reversible World: Symbolic Inversion in Art and Society*. (Edited by Babcock, B.A.), pp. 258–71. Cornell University Press, Ithaca & London, 1978.

57 Keir J. The psychological effects of drug presentation. *MIMS Magazine*, 15 Oct, pp. 41–7, 1979.

58 Claridge G. *op. cit.*, p. 25, 1970.

59 Lader M. *op. cit.*, p. 32, 1979.

60 Peele S. *op. cit.*, p. 62, 1978.

61 Warburton D.M. *op. cit.*, pp. 312–13, 1978.

62 Claridge G. *op. cit.*, pp. 24–50, 1970.

63 *Lancet*. Drug or placebo? Editorial, 1, pp. 122–23, 1972.

64 *Lancet. op. cit.,* p. 123, 1972.

65 Dunnell K. and Cartwright A. *op. cit.*, p. 110, 1972. They are commonly used for 'general health', 'preventive reasons' and 'tiredness'.

66 British Medical Association. *More Secret Remedies: What They Cost and What They Contain*, pp. 44–70. British Medical Association, London, 1912. e.g. 'Phospherine', 'Guy's Tonic', 'Invigoroids', 'Vita Ore', 'Dr Lecoy's Vigoroids'.

67 Joyce C.R.B. Quantitative Estimates of Dependence on the Symbolic Function of Drugs. In *Scientific Basis of Drug Dependence*. (Edited by Steinberg, H.), pp. 271–19. Churchill, London, 1969.

68 Parish P.A. *op. cit.*, p. 31, 1971.

69 Tyrer P. *op. cit.*, p. 1009, 1978.

70 Parish P.A. *op. cit.*, pp. 29–30, 1971.

71 Williams P. Areas of concern in the prescription of psychotropic drugs. *MIMS Magazine*, 1 Jan, pp. 37–43, 1981.

72 See Reference 69.

73 Pellegrino E.D. *op. cit.*, p. 624, 1976.

74 Turner V. *The Ritual Process*, p. 48. Penguin Books, London, 1969.

75 Lennard H.L. and Cooperstock R. *op. cit.*, pp. 78–80. In Mapes, R. 1980.

76 Smith M.C. The Relationship Between Pharmacy and Medicine. In Mapes, R. *op. cit.*, pp. 157–200, 1980.

77 Balint M. *op. cit.*, 1974.

78 Pfefferbaum A. Psychotherapy and Psychopharmacology. In *Psychopharmacology*. (Edited by Barchas, J.D. *et al.*), pp. 481–92. Oxford University Press, New York, 1977.

79 Smith M.C. In Mapes, R. *op. cit.*, pp. 165–67, 1980.

80 See Reference 20.

81 Stimson G.V. Obeying Doctor's Orders: A view from the other side. *Social Science and Medicine*, 8, pp. 97–104, 1974.

82 Joyce C.R.B. *op. cit.*, pp. 271–72, 1969.

83 The number of patients using the benzodiazepines, and names of the drugs were: diazepam ('Valium') – 26; nitrazepam ('Mogadon') – 14; flurazepam ('Dalmane') – 5; chlordiazepoxide ('Librium') – 3; lorazepam ('Ativan') – 1; & oxazepam ('Serenid D') – 1.

84 Lader M. *op. cit.*, p. 33, 1979.

85 Stimson G. and Webb B. *Going to See the Doctor*, pp. 37–40, 48–56. Routledge and Kegan Paul, London, 1975.

86   25 'Retired', 16 'Housewife'. Occupations of male patients, and husbands of female patients ranged from Accountant, Dentist, Bank Manager, Engineer, Businessman, to Machinist, Taxi-driver and Laboratory Technician. All were house-owners.

87   Parish P.A. *op. cit.*, pp. 16–21, 1971.

88   Parish P.A. *op. cit.*, p. 33, 1971.

89   Kleinman A. *Patients and Healers in the Context of Culture*, pp. 72–80. California University Press, Berkeley, 1980.

90   Guttmacher S. and Elinson J. Ethno-Religious variations in perceptions of illness. *Social Science and Medicine* 5, pp. 117–25, 1971.

91   Dunnell K. and Cartwright A. *op. cit.*, 1972.

92   Solomon F., White C.C., Parron D.L. and Mendelson W.B. *op. cit.*, p. 803, 1979.

93   *Lancet. op. cit.*, p. 1102, 1973.

94   Peele S. *op. cit.*, pp. 61–7, 1978.

95   Jefferys M., Brotherston J.H.F. and Cartwright A. Consumption of medicines on a working-class housing estate. *British Journal of Preventive and Social Medicine* 14, pp. 64–76, 1960.

96   Jarrett D. *England in the Age of Hogarth*. Hart-Davis MacGibbon, London, 1974.

97   Public Health Administration: The Report of the Local Government Board. *The Practitioner* 25, p. 390, 1880.

98   See Reference 66.

99   Dunnell K. and Cartwright A. *op. cit.*, p. 110, 1972.

100 *Department of Health and Social Security Circular* No. ECL 106/69 Serial No. 1/78. 1978. Sent in March, 1978, to all general practitioners in Britain.

101 Jones D.R. Drugs and prescribing: what the patient thinks. *Journal of the Royal College of General Practitioners* 29, 417–19, 1979.

102 Stimson G.V. and Webb B. *op. cit.*, pp. 86–7, 1975.

103 Blum R.H. Social and epidemiological aspects of psychopharmacology. In *Psychopharmacology: Dimensions and Perspectives*. (Edited by Joyce C.R.B.), pp. 243–82. Tavistock Publications, London, 1968.

104 Claridge G. *op. cit.*, pp. 123–46, 1970.

105 The numbers of patients known by various members of their social networks to be taking the drug were: Spouse 31; Relative 19; Friend 15; Neighbour 3; and No-one 6. Most patients were known by more than 1 person to be taking the drug.

106 Claridge G. *op. cit.*, p. 131, 1970.

107 Hindmarch I. *op. cit.*, p. 142, 1981.

108 Warburton D.M. *op. cit.*, p. 312, 1978.

109 Hindmarch I. *op. cit.* In a study in Leeds, 80 pills per house were found, an average of 25.9 pills per person.

110 Dunnell K. and Cartwright A. *op. cit.*, 1972.

111 See Reference 47.

112 Parish P.A. *op. cit.*, pp. 33 & 44, 1971.

113 Lennard H.L. and Cooperstock R. In Mapes, R. *op. cit.*, p. 75, 1980.

114 Blum R.H. In Joyce, C.R.B. *op. cit.*, pp. 271–74, 1968.

115 Parish P.A. *op. cit.*, p. 49, 1973. Quotes Lennard on this.

116   Trethowan W.H. *op. cit.*, p. 750, 1975.

117   Watts C.A.H. The Use of Sedatives and Minor Tranquillizers. *Journal of the Royal College of General Practitioners* **23**, Suppl. 2, pp. 30–3, 1973.

118   Pfefferbaum A. In Barchas, J.D. *et al., op. cit.,* p. 488, 1977.

119   Stimson G.V. *op. cit.*, p. 103, 1974. Also, Dunnell K. and Cartwright A. *op. cit.*, p. 58, 1972: 'People's attitudes towards medical care may contribute to the effects of a drug. Self-reliant people, who felt "a person understands his own health better than most doctors do", had lower expectations about doctors' ability to cure or relieve various conditions. They had less faith in doctors.' These independent people were more likely to self-medicate.

120   Pellegrino E.D. *op. cit.*, p. 625, 1976.

121   See Reference 66. As an example, 'Gordon's Vital Sexualine Restorative's' claim was: 'Permanently Cures – "Neurasthenia, Nervous Breakdown, Brain Fag, Depression, Loss of Energy, Sleeplessness, Nervous Headache, Melancholia, Trembling, Poverty of Nerve Force, Nervous Prostration, General Weakness, Loss of Strength, Exhausted Vitality, Premature Decay, Brain Wreckage, Neuralgia, Nerve Tire, etc." '

122   Blaxter M. and Paterson E. *Attitudes to Health and Use of Health Services of Two Generations of Women in Social Classes 4 and 5*. Report to DHSS/SSRC Joint Working Party on Transmitted Deprivation, 1980.

123   Pellegrino E.D. *op. cit.*, p. 628, 1976.

124   A short description of this data, directed to general practitioners and without any theoretical elaboration or conceptual models, has been published as: Helman C.G. Patients' Perceptions of Psychotropic Drugs. *Journal of the Royal College of General Practitioners* **31**, pp. 107–12, 1981.

125   Drug overdoses can, in a sense, be seen as having aspects of all three groups, though the perceived qualities of the drug are negative, rather than positive; these aspects are: autonomy, choice, self-medication and the powerful effects of the drug on personality and relationships.

126   The metaphor of 'Food' was first suggested by a patient who said of her diazepam (Valium): 'But it's just like taking a biscuit with tea.'

17

Some social meanings of tranquilliser use

Ruth Cooperstock and Henry L. Lennard

Abstract With approximately 20 per cent of all prescriptions written for psychotropic drugs, a large proportion of which are tranquillisers, it becomes necessary to examine the consequences of such use and the functions served by these drugs in social as well as pharmacological terms. This paper reports data from an exploratory study of the social and behavioural effects of use based on group interviews with current and former tranquilliser users. It adopts a natural history approach. The informants reflected the age and sex distribution of tranquilliser users generally, predominantly female and middle-aged. The thematic material dealt largely with a variety of role conflicts. Discussion focussed on these conflicts and the individual's ability to perform expected roles or adapt to them. Among females the roles included those of wife, mother, and houseworker, while males primarily discussed tranquilliser use as a means of controlling somatic symptoms in order to perform their occupational role. The function of tranquillisers in maintaining the individual in a dependent patient role was also discussed by a number of informants. This study demonstrates the inadequacy of the biomedical model of disease in explaining continued tranquilliser use.

Over the past fifteen years minor tranquillisers, particularly the benzo-diazepines, have become a part of the armamentarium of physicians as well as an accepted component of the lives of large segments of our population. Social critics and sociologists (1, 2, 3) have described the ways in which these drugs, termed anti-anxiety agents, have become identified as solutions to 'problems of living'. Consistent with this analysis, the preparations acting on the central nervous system, of which the benzodiazepines comprise an increasing part, are those most likely to be prescribed for long term use.(4)

Reprinted, with permission, from *Sociology of Health and Illness* 1: 331–47. 1979.

In an extensive study of prescribed drug use in Oxfordshire,(5) psychotropics accounted for almost one-fifth of all prescriptions, with almost 10 per cent of the males and 21 per cent of the females receiving at least one psychotropic prescription during the year. One Canadian investigation found 13.7 per cent of all adults reporting use of minor tranquillisers within the past 12 months (6) while another found 8.8 per cent of a community sample claiming use of a sedative/hypnotic in the past 48 hours.(7) Over a recent 19 month period in Saskatchewan it was found that one in every seven over age 19 received a prescription for diazepam alone (the generic term for Valium).(8) In all of these studies it is clear that prescribing is not random within populations. Women consistently receive twice the proportion of prescriptions for tranquillisers as do men.(9) Additionally women in the middle and late years are at highest risk; Skegg *et al.* (5) in Oxfordshire report 33 per cent of women aged 45–59 received at least one psychotropic prescription in a year, while 12.9 per cent of these women received at least five such prescriptions over the year and among women 75 and over 20.2 per cent received this number. It has been well established that those using psychotropic drugs also report numerous somatic disorders. While morbidity is generally somewhat higher among women this can not account for the disproportionate prescribing to them.

Prescriptions in general serve important symbolic functions for both physician and patient,(10, 11) but prescriptions for psychotropic drugs must be viewed as a special case. The acceptance of these agents for long term use cannot be viewed as simply the result of vigorous promotion by the pharmaceutical industry. Rather this acceptance has coincided with changes in the nature of 'illness' as presented to physicians today, with chronic and ill-defined illnesses taking precedence, with the enormous growth of the pharmaceutical industry, and the grateful utilization by the medical profession of the new and often life-saving drugs produced in the past 25 years. Ironically, some of the very factors that altered the nature of presenting complaints have reinforced and strengthened the physicians' belief in the bio-medical model of illness. Engel(12) has described this belief system as the dominant model of disease today, assuming disease to be fully accounted for by 'deviation from the norm of measurable biological variables'. He further points out that this 'leaves no room within its framework for the social, psychological and behavioural dimensions of illness'. Given this belief system, the prescription of a tranquillising drug is often the outcome of a negotiation whereby problems and distress arising in a variety of life situations are defined as psychological 'symptoms' of disease. This negotiation results in the labelling and definition of the problem as a medical one, requiring health care resources and, frequently, continued medication. Needless to say, the biomedical model also finds the locus of illness in the individual, thus requiring individual treatment.

Engel(1977: 196) proposes a 'biopsychosocial' model of illness in which the physician must 'weigh the relative contributions of social and psychological factors as well as of biological factors implicated in the patient's dysphoria and dysfunction as well as in his decision to accept or not accept patienthood and with it the responsibility to cooperate in his own health care.' Expanded in this way the problem, for example, of patient 'compliance' with drug regimes could never again be viewed as simple patient unwillingness to accept the greater knowledge of the physician regarding the appropriate treatment of one's bodily systems. Thus the very notion of compliance would be altered to one of therapeutic cooperation or alliance.

What consequences ensue from use of these drugs? What functions do they serve for the individual, or for the families and intimates of users? When sizable segments of a population ingest any drug, particularly one acting on the central nervous system and mood, it becomes necessary to examine the ways in which human interaction may be altered, and the range of functions served by the drugs. This paper reports data from a study of the social and behavioural consequences and meaning of tranquilliser use conducted in Toronto in the spring of 1977. It will not deal with the physical effects of use reported: effects on motor skills, perception, cognition, mood; but rather with those functions, both negative and positive, relating to the use of tranquillisers as a means of maintaining a given social role as expressed by the informants. Numerous drugs in use today do effect mood, and hence would have an effect on relationships, self-image, and so forth, the steroids being an obvious example, but none other merit such close attention as the tranquillisers because of the extent of their use and because of their wide and increasing range of indications.

Studies of the effects of tranquillisers have tended to be either clinical,(13, 14) pharmacological,(15, 16) or based on surveys utilizing prestructured questions.(17) No previous work has focussed on the perceptions of the drug's effects as viewed by the user. The decision was made to bring together groups of individuals to discuss, as freely as possible, the meaning they attribute to their use. Both authors were present at each group and the discussions, which were tape recorded, lasted approximately two hours. They were later transcribed. The approach selected was most akin to a natural history study of a population, with the clear intention of permitting and encouraging spontaneity, group interaction and discussion, and minimal participation on the part of the investigators. An attempt was made to create a non-judgemental atmosphere in the group. By opening discussion with a short statement of their interest in 'any aspect of the drug that you were aware of, physical, emotional, social – it's effect on your work, relationships, etc.' it quickly became clear to the informants that the investigators' interests extended beyond the purely physiological. The informants all responded to a newspaper announcement asking for volunteers who would be interested in discussing the consequences of their use. Only those whose primary drug was a benzodiazepine (in all cases diazepam, chlordiazepoxide or Librax) were included.

The data are based on 14 group interviews with 68 participants and an additional 24 lengthy letters from individuals who could not participate in the groups but wanted to offer their experience. The groups ranged in size from two to eight people. Consistent with general tranquilliser consumption figures, the volunteers were predominantly female (76 per cent), their mean age was 46 with a range from 23 to 74 years. Because of the exploratory nature of this study, the investigators chose to attract a population of articulate individuals and this is reflected in the high educational attainment of the group.[1] Seventy-six per cent had either university or post-secondary technical training. Sixty-six per cent were married, 14 per cent single, and the remaining 20 per cent were separated, divorced or widowed. The majority were in the labour force (58 per cent), 25 per cent described themselves as housewives, 14 per cent were either retired, disabled or not working, and two per cent were students. Of those working outside the home, the majority were in professional or managerial occupations.

Both the high educational and occupational attainment of the population as well as the method of acquiring volunteers prevent direct application of the findings to the Canadian population as a whole. The informants did, however, match tranquilliser users on such characteristics as sex and age. It must be emphasized that this method of sample selection was deliberately chosen because of the richness of the data it was hoped to gather from articulate individuals and because, in this exploratory study, the authors saw greater heuristic value emerging from this method than from more traditional sampling design.

In each group, following the few opening remarks already mentioned, the investigators suggested that the members of the group take turns giving a short history of their drug use, including the reasons for starting, the name of the drug, the amount, typical dosage, and the length of time they used the drug (66 were still using either regularly or intermittently). Three individuals did not receive their tranquillisers from a physician, although all had used this source initially. Only one person had used the drug for less than a month, eight per cent had used it from one month to a year, 24 per cent from one year to four years, and 67 per cent had used tranquillisers anywhere from 4 to 18 years. Thus this is clearly a population of long term users, although their use patterns were close to the usual recommended daily dose. The mean daily dose of diazepam, for example, was 16.2 mgs.

Although many modes of analysis were possible, the investigators studied the data thematically and found the material on initial and continuing use most understandable in terms of the problems of social roles expressed.[2] The initial reasons for use varied widely with 53 per cent citing a somatic problem,[3] although a high proportion of these commented on a social stress as related to the disorder, 30 per cent attributing use to social stresses only and 19 per cent to internal tensions.[4] Continued use, however, was most often discussed in terms of 'permitting' them to maintain themselves in a role or roles which they found difficult or intolerable without the drug.

As might be expected of a predominantly female population, the most common roles discussed related to the traditional ones of wife, mother, houseworker. As will be shown, these were typically discussed in relation to conflict over ability to perform the role or adaptation to its demands. Among males discussion tended to relate to conflict regarding work performance, or more typically, the need to contain somatic symptoms in order to perform an occupational role. Difficulties adapting to the role of the newly separated or widowed were also discussed. Another conflict discussed by more than a few informants revolved around that of the patient role itself.

Some mention should be made of the sex composition of the groups and the impact of this on the discussions. Five of the groups were composed of all females and nine groups contained one or more males. The groups were organized solely on the basis of convenience. Striking differences existed in the two types of groups, despite the fact that one of the investigators was male. Conforming to traditional roles and consistent with other studies,(18) the men tended to be less emotionally expressive than the women, a consequence of which appeared to be greater emphasis on reports of somatic problems and side-effects of the drugs. Again, as shown in other work,(19) the mixed groups, even those with only one male member, tended to follow the lead of the male and focus less on problems of role strains and interpersonal relations than did the all female groups who typically moved rapidly into discussion of social strains. Lacking all male groups it is impossible to know how these would have evolved.

What follows will deal with the ways many of the informants saw tranquillising drugs as helping to maintain them in the traditional female role of wife and homemaker. In a recent symposium on Valium(20) the chairman, attempting to demonstrate the usefulness of the benzo-diazepines, stated,

'We hear much about the adverse effects of the drugs and their costs, while we hear little in terms of how many divorces Valium may prevent.'

The chairman here has clearly identified an important function of these drugs as expressed by our informants, i.e. to sustain strained social systems. Significantly, these strains within family groups were discussed and resulted in drug use by female rather than male informants. The chairman's remark was consistent with the culturally accepted view that it is the role of the wife to control the tensions created by a difficult marriage, and implicit in his comment is that drug use is justified in order to accomplish this. Valium is an aid in the maintenance of a nurturing, caring role, as seen in the following quote:

> 'In the summertime I virtually live on them because we have a boat. And I can't sleep on the boat. My husband doesn't swim and I am up like this (indicating tension) all the time. . . . It's the only way I can get to be nice the next day to all those people we have floating around this boat all the time, preparing meals for them.'

There were clear expressions of anger and resentment directed at their spouse by a number of women, at the same time as they saw no alternative to continued occupancy of the traditional wife, houseworker role. This anger may well reflect the greater sense of powerlessness felt by women than men.(21) For example, a woman with four teenagers said:

> 'I take it to protect the family from my irritability because the kids are kids. I don't think it's fair for me to start yelling at them because their normal activity is bothering me. My husband says I overreact. . . . I'm an emotional person, more so than my husband who's an engineer and very calm and logical – he thinks. . . . But I suppose I overreact, but because I overreact is no reason for the family to suffer from my irritability. . . . So I take the Valium to keep me calm. . . . . Peace and calm. That's what my husband wants because frankly the kids get on his nerves, too. But he will not take anything. . . . He blows his top. . . . When I blow my top I am told to settle down. When he does it, it's perfectly alright. . . . He's the slow volcano kind, but when he loses it, oh boy. He can blow but I can't. And this I have resented over the years, but I've accepted it. I'm biding my time. One of these days I'm going to leave the whole kit and kaboodle and walk out on him. Then maybe I won't need any more Valium.'

Other women spoke about adjusting their dose in relation to family stresses; one said, 'I need more on the weekends when my family is home.'

Ginsberg(22) has found that tranquilliser use may be particularly prevalent among women in role conflict. The following quotes exemplify just such conflicts:

> 'Now I am in a situation which I cannot get out of. There is no way I will drop my responsibilities to my husband who is a very fine man, or my children. My husband's and my interests have gone different ways. The communication has diminished, but he's still a very good husband, and

he's an excellent father to the children. . . . I can't leave them and because I can't leave them I'm sticking to the Valium. That's my escape.

I would like to be off in Australia somewhere, writing. You know, do only my work. But having to stop the writing to get the supper on, it irritates me. And there are so many irritations during the day. But I cannot change the situation because of my family.'

This informant was the only woman expressing this type of conflict who worked at all, and significantly, her writing was done at home and earned her no income. The women quoted above were all middle class, well-educated and had worked prior to marriage or childrearing and at the time of drug use were all economically dependent on their husbands. Again, a sense of powerlessness pervades these quotes. Bahr(23), reviewing the literature, points out that a wife's power in the family relationship tends to increase when she is employed.

Oakley(24) identifies the features of the housewife's role as being: (1) exclusively filled by women; (2) identified with economic dependence; (3) maintaining a status as non-work; and (4) holding priority over other roles. The following quote is an example of a family in which the husband rigidly adheres to the view of the roles' priority over all others and the wife, while attempting to fulfil the role, is nonetheless incapable of accepting or finding gratification from it:

'But the problem started with marriage, where I have a North European background with its stoicism. And I married a husband who was very open and outgoing and for instance would sit down to dinner. . . . and say, "Am I supposed to eat this shit?" And I didn't know how to react to it. I cried a lot, and he was very verbal in his criticisms. . . . And then I went for two years without pregnancy so I was treated for infertility, after which I had nine pregnancies and four live children in four and a half years. I was alternately feeling suicidal and yet feeling responsible to these four lovely little kids. . . . And I am constantly in conflict, because I'd like to get a job. And I'm conflicted with the thought that I should be home with my kids. . . . And I'm into so many things because I am trying to compensate. You know at home there's nothing. There's my kids. . . . You know if you tried to talk to him at this point (and said) "Guess what I did. Guess what I accomplished. Guess what happened today". He says, "I don't want to listen. You clean up the kitchen and then I'll listen." And this is terribly frustrating.'

Another woman explained women's utilization of physicians' services by the fact that wives are not expected to make demands on their husbands. She said:

'And the first thing a man will say to you when you're not feeling well, at least a husband, . . . is "why don't you go to the doctor?" Like, don't bother me that you are feeling sick, go see the doctor. So women do go running off.'

Tranquillisers are also used to help individuals adapt to conflicts generated by intolerable behaviour in a spouse, in the following an alcoholic husband.

' "I started getting sick with stomach pains and I think I just couldn't cope at home anymore. I lived with an active alcoholic. . . . I guess in 1969 it wasn't fashionable that you talk about your problems, especially when you have an alcohol problem. And I do have two children." Subsequently it was found that the informant required major surgery. She continues: "I was in terrible shape after the operation because I knew the problem still existed at home and I was concerned about my children. The doctor gave me tranquillisers afterwards to cope and stop shaking because I just started shaking whenever something came up. . . . When I found I got better (from the effects of the operation) and I learned about alcoholism and about my problem I looked for help myself. I joined Al-Anon (a group for the families of alcoholics) and I stopped taking the tranquillisers." '

Many women reported initial tranquilliser use following the birth of children and the physical and emotional strains that frequently occur at this time. One informant described her inability to cope with her maternal role in the following way.

'And then . . . I realized that I'd better get some of this pressure off at some point, I was afraid I was going to kill my kids. I had one of those days and I just felt that something would snap. And I knew then that I needed something to detach myself from the pile-up of stress and pressure at that point. And it did; I felt very detached so that the next day the situation hadn't changed, but I felt very detached and able to cope without feeling so full of stress and tension. It was almost like I wasn't there. Probably a week's vacation away from the situation would have been just as valid a way of coping with the problem. I couldn't do that so I found that Valium did that. . . . And sort of the end of that week some of the pressures had gone down; like some of the problems with the children were sort of going together, as I got more hyper, they got more hyper. We were interacting and the pitch was getting higher and higher. And once I calmed down after the week, they calmed down.'

She discontinued use at the end of the one week period, finding that the drug had been extremely functional for this short term alleviation of a strained situation but that long term help came via attendance at marriage counselling which was initiated soon after ceasing drug use. She says about this:

'I have since discovered that a lot of the problems that I was bearing totally on myself weren't all mine, which I discovered in some very good marital counselling. So that has relieved it considerably.'

Unlike the woman just quoted, other mothers of infants continued use over prolonged periods. These were women who expressed clearly conflicting attitudes regarding their maternal role. In the following example these conflicts were initially triggered by a difficult infant:

'It turned out I couldn't have children so we adopted . . . and with the adoption of the first child I was deliriously happy . . . . And then I adopted a second child very quickly after the first, and she was a holy terror. She screamed from the minute we brought her into the house and she never stopped screaming. I was absolutely going around the bend and I called my G.P. and he prescribed my first tranquillisers . . . maybe they should have given the kid the tranquillisers! I don't know, or a shot of whiskey or something. But I had to learn how to cope with this screaming and I felt very inadequate. I felt I was a lousy mother. I felt I didn't love her as much as I loved the first and there was something wrong with me. . . . I think that was the start for me of really feeling inadequate in the role of mother, and also feeling that basically I didn't really enjoy it that much.'

Another informant suffered two post partum depressions and used tranquillisers for long periods following the birth of both her children. She began psychotherapy while still using tranquillisers and in the course of the therapy recognized her dislike of the role she had previously accepted as houseworker and mother. She said:

'At the end of the therapy sessions I said one of the things I really wanted to do was to go back to work part-time. I had taught student nurses and I really enjoyed that. And I felt that I really needed to do something that gave me a good feeling about myself. And I've never really had that as a mother or housekeeper. Like I'm always kind of wondering whether I'm doing the right thing as a mother, and I really don't know how to keep house, and don't feel very adequate in that situation.'

Following this statement she was asked by another member of the group whether any shift in her drug use occurred when she returned to work, to which she replied: 'I could cut right down and did'. The reports of the effects of work by our informants are consistent with the general findings that employment tends to protect women from the 'sick role'(25, 26) as well as affect drug use.(27)

For the mother of older children, the time demands of the maternal role cause strains in the form of anger and resentment toward the spouse. For example:

> 'Out at the cottage, even ... I have no escape. My husband wants to escape from the kids. ... He takes the sailboat out and disappears for three or four hours.'

The severe strain of mothering two retarded children was the trigger for one informant, who said:

> 'We found that our retarded children caused trouble in what had been a relatively happy marriage.... Most of us are overwhelmed by the physical care and emotional drain connected with caring for a handicapped child. The disappointment combined with the work is impossible for most of us to bear without help.... The hard work combined with the disappointment made me anxious and depressed.'

Almost all the above women described situations of extreme role strain, inability to comply with traditional role expectations, often feeling they lacked the 'right' to express their dissatisfaction and preferences. They see husbands as having other 'escape routes' when marital difficulties or obligations become burdensome. The issues addressed by almost all of these women are structural and some were able to describe structural, as opposed to individual, remedies to their problems.

Tranquilliser use was also initiated as a response to the strain of adapting to a new role, whether related to loss through widowhood or through separation. The following quote illustrates the use of the drug to aid adaptation to sudden loss and the strains involved in an abrupt change from the traditional role of wife to that of separated and economically independent woman:

> 'All of a sudden my husband decided he's going to be on his own. I thought we had a pretty good household. I liked being a mother and housewife and wife. All of a sudden it's all over. My whole life crumbled all of a sudden; and I had to find a job. I can't change that quickly.... Instead of being able to discuss it rationally, his idea is to say nothing, absolutely nothing. ... I asked what is the matter and he couldn't even tell me. This was when I blew it and went to a doctor.'

The following description of use after the death of a spouse illustrates the function of the drug for this informant in easing his pain.

> 'So then my wife passed away.... I was married for 35 years.... So I went to my doctor and said "You know the situation. I need a little something to lean on for a few days".... So he gave me Valium. It was 5 mg. He said, "Now take one after breakfast and one after supper". He gave me enough to do me for a month. In three days I went through what he gave

me for a month. You know what I mean, I was really upset. I couldn't face people, I couldn't do anything. So I was eating them like popcorn.'

This informant, at the time of the group interview, was still using tranquillisers on a regular daily basis, years after his wife's death.

Continuing use of tranquillisers can be viewed as an adaptation to an unsatisfactory role, or as a means of coping with unresolved conflicts, but it also can be seen as a learned habitual mode of reacting to stresses as seen in the following:

'I started taking them when my father died and I tapered off when I got married. I sort of tried to taper off because my husband wasn't too crazy about my taking them. . . . But after we were divorced I was worse than ever.'

Although males occupy two major roles, an occupational one and as husband or head of household, the males in this population tended to speak of their tranquilliser use in relation to only one of these roles – the occupational one. Significantly, sex role research identifies competence as a dominant value in the male self-image.(28) Most typically, male informants discussed the onset of somatic symptoms in relation to work stresses or new strains brought on by a change in jobs, and the continued use of tranquillising drugs as a means of controlling these symptoms. A number accepted that little change in their job status was possible and therefore they saw no means other than drugs to alleviate the sometimes incapacitating symptoms. The most common symptom mentioned by the men was atrial fibrillation, others included dyspnoea, colitis, muscle spasms, and so forth. Only two female informants mentioned occupational stresses as a factor in their drug use.

One informant, a minister, found his symptoms appearing following a change of jobs:

'I changed jobs about 5 years ago from a preaching . . . job to a human relations job. It's competitive stuff. And about six months later I started having some . . . psychosomatic induced dizziness, a sense of you're about to pass out. I fell enough that my colleagues took me off to a cardiac unit. And that went on. I was told there was nothing there but the fact is every day the dizziness was there and it was something to fight against.'

He was placed on Valium to control his symptoms and continued on the drug for a number of years, varying the dose as necessary. While permitting him to carry on in his competitive job, the drug also affected his self-image. In his words:

'When I do take Valium I'm conscious of being very quiet; I'm conscious of being the way I would like to be on my own, without drugs, but conscious of the fact that it's not me. And I really resent that. And I'd like to achieve that part without any tranquillisers.'

A successful businessman summarized the functions served by Valium in his work. The drug, in this case, produced feelings of calm in situations which the informant found he couldn't control and hence produced stresses. He said he uses tranquillisers:

'if I know I am going into a meeting and I know that it's going to be something that has a lot of tension to it. Sometimes I look at the people and their styles in terms of how they are going to go through the meeting. And so I figure rather than put up with the nonsense of getting myself into an emotional twist I take one of these and I'm quite conscious, I'm in control of myself. . . . I find that I react less. . . . I dislike . . . making a decision and then going through this 'if only' phase. I find that very frustrating. I prefer to look at the risks and the offsets, reach a decision and then put the whole damn thing behind us. If I know I'm going to be there with those type of people and we're going to be sitting on a mountain contemplating our navel for a long period of time I'll say "O.K. I don't want to react to what they are saying". I take a diazepam.'

Another male describes his use of tranquillisers as a means of reducing tensions related to his work that arose from his self-inflicted perfectionistic demands:

'I'm overly conscientious, a perfectionist. I wouldn't dare go home thinking I'd made a mistake. I've got to be sure that I'm right. So that adds to my tension. And because my partners are careless that puts more onus on me.'

A major use for tranquillisers today is adjunctive therapy for individuals with a wide array of chronic conditions.(29, 30) They are typically dispensed for two purposes: the first is prophylactic, to protect the person with a chronic illness from excessive stress which might have adverse effects on the course of the illness, and the second is to allay psychosocial reactions to the illness, prognosis, or treatment.

Three of the informants suffered from lupus erythematosus and all described long-term use of tranquillising drugs which they felt maintained them in a dependent patient role. Unlike the previous examples of role strains in relation to traditional roles, the frustration and anger expressed by these informants related to the drug's use as a means of masking emotions and thus preventing the assumption of just such adult roles. One of these informants had spent the morning with a fellow lupus patient and describes the feelings of a person about to be discharged following long-term hospitalization and what she perceived to be the insensitivity of the health care system in recognizing the difficulties encountered in rejecting the 'sick role'.(31)

'And no one can understand what she's so upset about. She's going home. She should be in a high state. And like she said to me she was upset today. I said, "Oh I understand. Now you've got to face the world". She said, "Yes, before I was using my health as a crutch for not doing things. And now I'm going to be better, and I'm going home. But I have no friends, because I pushed them away in the past year. How do I make my life? I have nothing to go home to. I have my parents, I have my brothers and sisters. But I have nothing and no one to go home to. And I'm scared". I agreed with her wholeheartedly. . . . This is a very real problem. And I resent the doctors trying to cover it up with platitudes, "Oh, everything will be OK", which is ridiculous because it won't, or giving them Valium which will put them into a very mellow type of mood. But that's not going to solve the problem one iota, it'll just postpone the problem. But it won't solve it.'

The inability of a chronically ill person to view herself and be viewed as a mature adult is vividly illustrated in the following quote, as is the way in which tranquillisers, in her view, further prevent the adoption of an adult role:

'But I want to go right back where I say they were using drugs to cover up my true feelings, because with as much anger and hate or anything I had in me I never voiced my anger to my husband or to his family or anyone whom it was obviously directed at. And consequently they knew I was upset, which I was with just cause. So they gave me Valium and Serax and everything. But that did not solve the problem at all because they didn't even know I was angry with them. Then one day I blurted it out and they came back and grabbed me and said, "Why didn't you tell us? We kept doing this to you because you never said anything. You left yourself wide open". Which was very true. You see, when you have a chronic disease, many people tend to put you down. One beautiful statement they used to say to me was, "You were so lucky to have your George stick with you". This is a chronic one: you're so lucky he sticks with you. Consequently you have to be better than normal. You can't be the ordinary person who makes mistakes or does things wrong. You have to prove you're superhuman which is impossible. But you keep trying, you see, because you make these demands upon yourself. And when people make you angry, you figure, "Well I'm so lucky that they're still sticking with me". You're down about this low at that point so that you don't criticize. Even if they're out of line you never put them down or you never tell them off because you feel you're lucky to have this relationship, because since you're sick, you shouldn't have anything. Poor kid, but we don't want to cope with it. Consequently, and I'm not alone in this, we keep our true feelings submerged. But the anger is there, the hurt is there. And until you voice this hurt, until you listen to yourself, until you tell someone where they're stepping out of line, until you're honest enough with yourself and with them, it's never going to be corrected. I keep going back; using Valium or Serax or any of these things to hide them or mask them is not going to solve the problem at all.'

It is clear from the above data that in order to understand the functions served by these drugs it is necessary to look beyond the medical model of disease to the structural factors creating the stresses which bring many to the attention of the health care system.

There has been no mention to this point of the image held by these informants of the prescribers of their drugs. A noteworthy finding was that considerably more anger was expressed by women than men toward their physicians. This may relate to a number of factors, including their greater difficulty in asserting themselves in relation to a male physician,(32) their awareness of differential prescribing to men and women as expressed by a number of informants (reflecting recent studies conducted by members of the medical profession (33, 34, 35)), and, at least as demonstrated in these groups, a greater awareness than the males of the structural, rather than individual nature of the problems. Typifying this awareness is the following statement by a female informant:

'I think the thing that upset me most about the way drugs were used with me was that in the early years when I was so obviously unhappy with what was happening in my life the solution to the doctors was so obviously a drug solution. And I had to push everybody I knew, including the doctors, except my psychiatrist who supported me all the way, that the solution for me was going to be really to quite radically change my life and not to make me comfortable with the life I was in.'

Although some informants saw no alternative to their continued use of tranquillisers, others, particularly those who had already discontinued using them, discussed alternative solutions to their problems. These included both individual and structural solutions such as yoga, relaxation exercises, strenuous exercise, consciousness raising, and self-help groups as well as paid full or part-time employment and changes in marital relationships or type of employment.

Summary and conclusion

By utilizing a natural history approach to data gathering regarding the consequences of tranquilliser use it becomes immediately obvious that the biomedical model of disease is inadequate to explain continuing use of these drugs.

Although 53 per cent of the informants claimed their use began in relation to a somatic disorder, the majority recognized that their continuing use related to a variety of role strains. The most common strains and conflicts mentioned by female informants revolved around their traditional roles as wife, mother, houseworker, while males tended to discuss conflicts regarding their work or work performance. Some of those with chronic illnesses tended to discuss their use of tranquillisers as creating greater strains for them in their efforts to 'normalize' their lives. The drug, by masking feeling, prevented the rejection of the undesirable 'sick role' too often imposed by both the nature of their illness and their family members.

The data presented raises a wide variety of questions for the social scientist, the medical profession and for our social institutions and legislators. A number of middle class informants found they ceased use during or after making structural changes in their lives. Are such alternatives open to all members of society? The poor? The elderly? If not, are tranquillisers to be accepted as adequate solutions to social stresses? These are clearly moral and ethical issues that transcend the bounds of the medical profession and demand social, not medical answers.

The data does, however, demand further studies of the physician-patient relationship. Little is known of physicians' own views of their prescribing, particularly how they view continuing use on the part of their patients. Are they seen as necessary for continuous symptomatic relief? As the best of poor alternatives? To what extent are the sorts of social and role strains discussed by the informants known to their primary care physicians?

Although the study did not intend to focus on the chronically ill, enough material was presented to suggest that use of tranquillisers by this large population is again a means of resolving strains. In this situation the strains were incurred by the individual's inability to perform a healthy 'adult' role in the family. How applicable is this model to a range of chronic conditions? How common is this reaction among the chronically ill? Again, in relation to this group, the data raise the question of the desirability of this solution. Clearly, there is a great need for continuing research to answer these questions.

Notes

1 The call for volunteers appeared in the Toronto Globe and Mail, a newspaper with a predominantly middle class readership. The paper also has a national circulation which resulted in calls and letters appearing from many parts of Ontario and Quebec.
2 Other aspects of use, such as side-effects, problems of dependence, etc. are being reported elsewhere.
3 These problems included: degenerative discs, lupus erythematosus, ulcerative colitis, atrial fibrillation, etc.
4 Totals exceed 100 because of multiple coding.

References

1 Lennard, H.L., Epstein, L.J., Bernstein, A., and Ransom, D.C. (1971) *Mystification and Drug Misuse*. San Francisco: Jossey Bass.
2 Stimson, G. (1975) Women in a Doctored World. *New Society* **32** (656):265–7.
3 Illich, I. (1975) *Medical Nemesis: The Expropriation of Health*. London: Calder & Boyars Ltd.
4 Dunnell, K. and Carwright, A. (1972) *Medicine Takers, Prescribers and Hoarders*. London: Routledge & Kegan Paul.
5 Skegg, D.C.G., Doll, R., and Perry, J. (1977) Use of Medicines in General Practice, *British Medical Journal* **1** (6076):1561–563.
6 Smart, R.G. and Goodstadt, M.S. (1976) Alcohol and Drug Use Among Ontario Adults: Report of a Household Survey, 1976. Toronto: Addiction Research Foundation Substudy No. 798.
7 Chaiton, A., Spitzer, W.O., Roberts, R.S., and Delmore, T. (1976) Patterns of Medical Drug Use – A Community Focus. *Canadian Medical Association Journal* **114**(1):33–7.
8 Harding, J. (1978) A Socio-Demographic Profile of People Prescribed Mood-Modifiers in Saskatchewan. Alcoholism Commission of Saskatchewan: Research Division, Final Report, January.
9 Cooperstock, R. (1976) Psychotropic Drug Use Among Women. *Canadian Medical Association Journal* **115**:760–63.
10 Balint, M. (1964) *The Doctor, His Patient and the Illness*. Toronto: Pitman Medical.
11 Bush, P.J. (1977) Psychosocial Aspects of Medical Use. In A.I. Wertheimer and P.J. Bush (eds) *Perspectives on Medicines in Society*. Washington: Drug Intelligence Publications, Inc.
12 Engel, G.L. (1977) The Need for a New Medical Model: A Challenge for Biomedicine. *Science* **196** (4286):129–36.
13 Greenblatt, D.J. and Shader, R.I. (1974) *Benzodiazepines in Clinical Practice*. New York: Raven Press.
14 Preskorn, S.H. and Denner, L.J. (1977) Benzodiazepines and Withdrawal Psychosis. *Journal of the American Medical Association* **237** (1):36–8.
15 Kleinknecht, R.A. and Donaldson, D. (1975) A Review of the Effects of

Diazepam on Cognitive and Psychomotor Performance. *Journal of Nervous and Mental Disease* **161** (6):399–411.

16 Sellers, E.M. (1978) Clinical Pharmacology and Therapeutics of Benzo-diazepines. *Canadian Medical Association Journal* **118**:1533–538.

17 Uhlenhuth, E.H., Balter, M.B., and Lipman, R.S. (1978) Minor Tranquilizers: Clinical Correlates of Use in an Urban Population. *Archives of General Psychiatry* **35**(5):650–55.

18 Phillips, D.L. and Segal, B.E. (1969) Sexual Status and Psychiatric Symptoms. *American Sociological Review* **34**(1):58–72.

19 Ruble, D.N. and Higgins, E.T. (1976) Effects of Group Sex Composition on Self-Presentation and Sex-Typing. *Journal of Social Issues* **32** (3):125–32.

20 Hollister, L.E. (1977) Valium: A Discussion of Current Issues. *Psychosomatics* **18**(1):44–58.

21 Olson, D. (1969) The Measurement of Family Power by Self-Report and Behavioural Methods. *Journal of Marriage and the Family* **31** (3):545–50.

22 Ginsberg, S. (1976) Women, Work and Conflict. In N. Fonda and P. Moss (eds) *Mothers in Employment*. London: Brunel University Management Programme and Thomas Coran Research Unit, University of London.

23 Bahr, S. (1974) Effects on Power and Division of Labor in the Family. In L.W. Hoffman and F.I. Nye (eds) *Working Mothers*. London: Jossey Bass. Quoted in: F. Fransella and K. Frost *On Being a Woman: A Review of Research on How Women See Themselves*. London: Tavistock Publications, 1977.

24 Oakley, A. (1974) *Housewife*. London: Penguin Books.

25 Nathanson, C. (1975) Illness and the Feminine Role: A Theoretical Review. *Social Science and Medicine* **9** (2):57–62.

26 Brown, G.W. and Harris, T. (1978) *Social Origins of Depression*. London: Tavistock Publications.

27 Cooperstock, R. (1979) A Review of Women's Psychotropic Drug Use. *Canadian Psychiatric Association Journal* **24**(1): 29–34.

28 For a review of this see: F. Fransella and K. Frost *On Being a Woman*. London: Tavistock Publications, 1977.

29 Greenblatt, D.J., Shader, R.I., and Koch-Weser, J. (1975) Psychotropic Drug Use in the Boston Area. *Archives of General Psychiatry* **32**(4):518–21.

30 Blackwell, B. (1973) Psychotropic Drugs in Use Today: The Role of Diazepam in Medical Practice. *Journal of the American Medical Association* **225** (13):1637–641.

31 Parsons, T. (1951) *The Social System*. Glencoe, Ill.: The Free Press.

32 Stephenson, S. (in press) The Physician–Patient Relationship. *Canadian Psychiatric Association Journal*.

33 Milliren, J.W. (1977) Some Contingencies Affecting the Utilization of Tranquilizers in Long-Term Care of the Elderly. *Journal of Health and Social Behaviour* **18**(2):206–11.

34 Bass, M. and Paul, D. (1977) The Influence of Sex on Tranquilizer Prescribing. Paper presented at the North American Primary Care Research Group Meeting, March, Williamsburg, Virginia.

35 Dixon, A.S. (1978) Drug Use in Family Practice: A Personal Study. *Canadian Family Physician* **24**:345–53.

18

Tranquillisers as a resource

Jonathan Gabe and Nicki Thorogood

Abstract Social scientific studies of tranquilliser use have played an important part in heightening awareness that their use can best be understood when considered within a social context. From a sociological point of view, however, these studies often suffer from limitations which restrict their descriptive and explanatory power. This paper discusses these limitations before attempting to develop an alternative approach which focuses on the meanings attached to tranquilliser use, and relates these meanings to the ways in which the users of these drugs manage their everyday lives as members of particular social groups. In order to bridge the gap between structure and experience, tranquillisers are conceptualized as *resources* which, along with other material and socio-cultural resources, are both differentially available and variously experienced. Attention is focused first on the availability of these drugs to samples of black and white working-class women, and the meanings which they attribute to these drugs. The different patterns of drug use which are found are then related to these women's varying access to and experience of a range of other resources (namely paid work, social supports, leisure, cigarettes, and religion). This provides a basis for explaining different patterns of tranquilliser use and hopefully illustrates the usefulness of 'resource' as a bridging concept between social structure and everyday life.

Introduction

Social scientists interested in the use of tranquillisers have generally approached the subject in one of two ways. Some have simply set out to describe the prevalence and pattern of tranquilliser use, and relate these patterns to socio-demographic variables, health status, and physician visits.[1] Others have gone beyond description to measure the strength of statistical association between these and other variables and tranquilliser use. Additional possible determinants which have been considered

244

include the occurrence of stressful events, family structure and role responsibilities, the nature of social supports, prescribed drug use by social network members, and attitudes to health, doctors, and their medicines.[2]

Both these approaches are useful in that they place tranquilliser use within a social context. From a sociological point of view, however, each has its limitations. The former approach provides a social map of tranquilliser use without explaining its genesis, while the latter approach, although encouraging the search for explanations, is premised on a number of assumptions which can be seen as sociologically problematic. The first such assumption is that the individual represents the basic methodological unit. The analysis proceeds by categorizing these individuals in terms of particular attributes which are then aggregated in the search for relations of association. As a result the individual is, in effect, treated as if he or she belongs to a single population instead of to distinctive class, race, and gender groupings whose relations are structured unequally in terms of wealth, power, and privilege.[3]

Second, the very attempt by the authors of these studies to identify causal relations between variables presupposes that such variables can be meaningfully extracted from their context and treated as independent of each other. This approach ignores the fact that many of the phenomena which these authors seek to explain are internally related and mutually constitutive. Separating out such phenomena would appear to violate the very relationship one is trying to explain.[4]

Third, these researchers seem to assume that establishing a strong relationship between tranquilliser use and particular variables is in itself a sufficient explanation for patterns of usage, even though such an approach does not explain *how* the association has arisen.[5] In order to answer the latter question attention needs to be focused on the social processes involved in tranquilliser use, which in turn requires an analysis of the everyday lives of members of particular social groups.[6] One objective of this paper is to provide such an analysis.

Fourth, and finally, on the occasions when subjective meaning (for example, attitudes to tranquillisers) has been introduced as a causal variable, it has been treated as if it were simply a psychological property which can be elicited in a straightforward way by using standardized questionnaires. This approach, however, fails to grasp that the assignment of meaning is generally experienced as problematic by individuals, and that such meanings derive from and arise out of social interaction within a particular social and historical context. An understanding of the tranquilliser users' point of view therefore needs an alternative methodology which, although based on theoretical premises, allows these people to define their experiences in their own terms without the researcher prematurely imposing his or her categories of meaning on them.[7]

Tranquilliser use and the management of everyday life

Given the problems identified above we have set out to develop an alternative approach which can be applied to the study of benzodiazepine drugs like Valium and Librium.

We start from the position that tranquilliser use is best explained if one focuses initially on the *meaning* of such drugs to those who use them. We are not the first to consider such a topic. A beginning has already been made by Helman[8] and Cooperstock and Lennard[9] although these authors have either focused on meaning *per se* without exploring the relationship between such meanings and the users' everyday lives as members of particular collectivities, or have treated meaning solely as a function of being a member of a particular group. For us, meaning must be seen in the context of people's everyday lives, for everyday life represents the 'paramount reality'.[10] This reality is shared with others through common sets of meaning and these meanings lend consistency to a person's behaviour.

It is frequently argued that everyday life is experienced as routine and mundane yet, as Brittan[11] has pointed out, there is more to everyday life than this. Routines are not experienced as indivisible but are interrupted by personal and social crises which infringe on the calm of mundane reality. Moreover, following C. Wright Mills,[12] we would argue that these personal troubles, and the routines of everyday life which they interrupt, can only be understood in the context of the historical and structural processes which shape these experiences. For us, this means that everyday life has to be seen as the lived experience of particular class, race, and gender groupings. This notion underpins our approach to tranquilliser use.

Merely recognizing the interplay between everyday life and structure is not enough, however. What is needed, we believe, is a 'middle range' concept which bridges the gap between what have traditionally been described as the micro and macro levels and, in so doing, helps dissolve what is in reality a false dichotomy premised on a philosophical dualism.[13] One such concept is 'resource', a term which has been used by social scientists working in the health field generally[14] and in mental health in particular.[15]

Before discussing the way in which we intend to use the concept it might be helpful to describe briefly how it has traditionally been used in the health field and to summarize the problems which we feel such a conceptualization involves. This description will provide a background against which to judge the worth of our own use of the term.

In the health literature, resource is generally linked with coping and/or stress. Pearlin and Schooler,[16] for example, state that:

'resources refer not to what people do but to what is available to them in developing their coping repertoires.'

Those who make this linkage, however, tend to treat resource as if it were simply a psychological property: a set of personality characteristics (self-esteem, fatalism, mastery, etc.) to be drawn on in countering threats posed by events and objects in their environment.[17] Sometimes the fact that some resources might be social in nature is acknowledged but rarely developed further, unless social is taken to mean social network.[18]

For us the problem with much of this 'resource' literature, as with the 'coping' and 'stress' literature generally, is that it takes the individual divorced from the social context as the unit of analysis and ignores the significance of social structure and power relations.[19] Life is simply reduced to a series of pathogenic events and problems for the individual to cope with or not as the case may be. Moreover, 'failure to cope' becomes labelled maladaptive with associated moral implications.[20] It also encourages victim blaming.[21]

In an attempt to resolve some of these problems we have tried to conceptualize 'resource' sociologically rather than psychologically. We have also substituted the term 'management' for 'coping' since it could be argued that the former incorporates fewer normative connotations than the latter, being more concerned with what people do to get by than with individual motivation and personality. Following Giddens, we suggest that resources are best conceived of as structural properties which are drawn on (along with rules) by knowledgeable actors in the production of interaction.[22] Giddens developed the concept of structural property as part of his theory of 'structuration', a theory which emphasizes the processual nature of patterned social relations. For him, such structural properties are both the medium and the outcome of the reproduction of social practices, and illustrate the mutual dependence of structure and agency.[23] For this reason Giddens rejects the idea of structure as only constraining. In his words: 'If structure is conceived of as merely external to human action it becomes regarded as a sort of autonomous form independent of such action.'[24] It should thus be seen as enabling as well as constraining.[25] Since structure consists of resources and rules can we therefore say that these properties are also both enabling and constraining? We believe it is justified to draw such a conclusion[26] and intend to demonstrate the utility of this double-edged notion of resource when we discuss our data.

Before doing so, however, we wish to mention two further aspects of Giddens' conceptualization of resource which we have found useful. First, he makes clear that resources should not be seen as inert materials possessed by individuals, but as part of a process or set of relations. As he puts it, 'the material existents involved in resources are the content or vehicles of resources'[27] which exist in time and space only as moments of the constitution of patterned social relations.[28] Second, he stresses that resources and power are integrally related although conceptually distinct. Power, he states, is not a resource itself; rather, resources are the vehicles of power, they are the media through which power is exercised routinely in social interaction, and structures of domination reproduced.[29] In talking about domination Giddens is drawing attention to the fact that resources are structured asymmetrically,[30] affecting differentially the capacity of actors individually and collectively to get others to comply with their wants,[31] or to have behaved otherwise themselves.[32]

In the following pages we identify a range of differentially distributed resources available to people in the management of their daily lives, of which tranquillisers are but one. In so doing we will be particularly concerned to establish the extent to which specific resources are experienced as enabling or constraining.[33] The analysis proceeds by discussing each resource in turn for heuristic reasons only. In reality the management of everyday life cannot be explicated in terms of a single resource: the process has to be located within intersecting sets of resources that ultimately express features of the totality.[34]

Introducing the studies

The utility of our conceptualization of resource will be illustrated by drawing on data collected during the course of two linked studies undertaken in the London Borough of Hackney. The first, a DHSS-funded study,[35] was designed specifically to explore the meaning of benzodiazepines to middle-aged white women; the second, which was SSRC funded, was constructed to explore the broader issue of the relationship between the health beliefs, health behaviour, and structural position of West Indian women. This latter study, however, shared with the former a concern about the meaning of benzodiazepines and used a similar methodology.

In this paper we focus on 45 indigenous white women and 15 West Indian-born black women aged between 40 and 60 who were identified as working class.[36] The indigenous white sample was taken from those attending one general practice in Hackney over three months in 1980–81. Patients who fell into the relevant age group were asked by their GP to allow a researcher to look at their medical records and to agree to be interviewed if we asked to see them. Of those asked only one-tenth refused this permission. Once the patients had agreed to participate we scrutinized their records to establish what drugs they had been prescribed over the previous ten years. As our focus was the meaning of benzodiazepines, as distinct from other psychotropic drugs (such as antidepressants or major tranquillisers), we decided to exclude from our sampling frame those women who had recently received prescriptions for these other drugs.

Consequently, we were left with a sample of 45 indigenous women. These women were divided into two basic groups: 'users', of whom there are 32 in the present sample, and 'non-users', of whom there are 13. Of the 'users' half were currently in receipt of a prescription for a benzodiazepine.

The West Indian women, who were approached during 1981 and 1982, were selected in two ways. Approximately half came from the same practice as the indigenous women, while the remainder were taken from a small 'community sample' gathered by contacts suggesting eligible others who might be willing to participate.[37] Women attending the practice were asked to take part by a researcher rather than by their doctor, and this resulted in a higher refusal rate: just over a quarter declined to be interviewed. Moreover, their medical records were not made available, as had been the case with the indigenous women. As we did not have access to the medical records of the women collected in the community sample either, we have been forced to categorize them as 'users' or 'non-users' of benzodiazepines solely on the basis of their *own* recollections about drug use. Using this criterion, nine of the West Indians could be described as 'users' and six as 'non-users'. Of the 'users' just under half said they were taking benzodiazepines currently, a proportion similar to that among the white 'users'.

Once these two groups of women had agreed to participate, we interviewed them in their own homes for up to four hours, using a checklist which had been developed in the light of our theoretical interests and on the basis of pilot interviews with some of the women. The issues explored with both the indigenous and West Indian women were generally the same, as was the approach adopted. With both groups, the 'life history' method was used; that is, we started the interview by asking them about their memories of health and illness in childhood and adolescence, and gradually took them through to the present. Attention was focused on their feelings about, and the use of, drugs in general and benzodiazepines in particular. Attempts were also made to get these women to relate their experiences of health and illness, and drug use, to their social circumstances over time; they were asked specifically about whether they recognized a relationship between their work, housing and family circumstances, and their health. In addition, the West Indian women were asked about issues such as their experience of personal and institutional racism, which it was hypothesized would be of particular relevance to them.

The interviews, all of which were tape-recorded, were subsequently transcribed and content analysed in terms of the thematic categories used in the construction of the checklist and categories suggested by the data.

No claim is being made about the statistical representativeness of these two samples of women. Rather, we are using our case study data to construct theoretically informed propositions which are generalizable only on the grounds of 'logical inference'.[38] Whether these generalizations are considered justified therefore hinges on the plausibility of our theoretical approach and analysis.

Resources for managing everyday life

During our interviews with the women we paid particular attention to those material and socio-cultural resources which *they* said they turned to in managing their everyday lives. Besides benzodiazepines they mentioned paid work, housing, social supports, leisure activities, cigarettes, alcohol, and religion. Of these eight, six are discussed here. For an account of the other two resources (housing and alcohol) see Gabe and Thorogood.[39] Each of these resources was differentially available, accessible, and acceptable to these women according to their structural position. We will consider each resource in turn, focusing first on its availability and second on the way in which it was experienced.

Benzodiazepines

Psychotropic drugs like benzodiazepines comprise one of the most frequently prescribed categories of drug in Britain, as in other industrialized countries.[40] They are also given more to women[41] and to the middle aged and elderly[42] than to other social groups; that is, the availability of benzodiazepines as a resource is structured asymmetrically towards groups like 'middle-aged' women. In our sample of such women, two-thirds reported that they had been given a prescription for Valium or another benzodiazepine at some time in the previous ten years. Of these women just over half said they had used such a drug consistently over a number of years during the decade: they would thus seem to justify the label 'long-term user'. Others stated that they had only taken the drug for a couple of weeks at a time and over a two-year period at most: they can thus be described as 'short-term users'. The remainder of the sample – one-third of the total – were the 'non-users' of benzodiazepines.

The indigenous women were somewhat *more* likely than the West Indians to be categorized as 'long-term users'. Five-eighths of the white 'users' were so labelled compared with one-third of the black 'users'. Moreover, the indigenous women who were categorized as 'long-term users' said that they had taken the drug for a much longer period of time. Whether this was in fact the case is impossible to establish in the absence of evidence about the prescriptions given to both groups. GP records of prescriptions to the indigenous women over the ten years prior to being interviewed, however, support the assessment of the 'long-term users' among them regarding the duration of their use of these drugs. Those who saw themselves as 'long-term users' had received benzodiazepine prescriptions, on average, in seven of the last ten years. There is also support for those indigenous women who saw themselves as 'short-term users': according to the records, they had received prescriptions, on average, in two of the last ten years.

When the women were asked what they felt about taking benzo-diazepines, a range of opinions was expressed. Some stated that they were concerned about the danger of becoming dependent on or addicted to these drugs, and felt that they might be harming their body or mind by ingesting such unnatural substances. Others said they felt these drugs were helpful in that they offered them 'peace of mind', and yet others expressed both views. Overall, one-quarter emphasized only the dangers and one-tenth only the benefits; the remaining two-thirds expressed mixed views.

The majority of users' apparent ambivalence is well captured in the following remarks. One woman, for example, stated:

'I hate the stuff, I detest the stuff. You know you've taken a drug when you've taken Valium. But I can't say I can do without them. I don't want to break right down because I won't be able to pick up the pieces. I'd rather stay the way I am.'

And another 'user' commented:

'When I take Valium my mind goes blank. I don't worry about anything. It will all sort itself out. It just sort of puts my mind at ease.'

Later on, however, she admitted:

'I'm not really one for taking tablets. I think once you get hooked on these Valium you've had it you know. You really are hooked on them.'

West Indian and indigenous 'users' expressed a similar range of feelings about the drugs. Among the two 'user' groups, however, there were substantial differences. 'Short-term users' were less likely than the 'long-term users' to express ambivalent or positive feelings, and were more likely to talk only of the dangers.

When 'non-users' of benzodiazepines were asked what they felt about the drug they seemed less ambivalent than the 'users'. Although they all talked about the dangers of dependence, very few talked about the benefits. This was so for both indigenous and West Indian women.

The 'users' in the sample were also asked what their drug *use* meant to them. These women responded in one of three ways. Some only talked about benzodiazepines as if they were a *lifeline*; that is, something which they needed to take regularly and depended on simply to keep going in the face of chronic, unresolved problems. Others conceived of the drug only as a *standby*, to be kept in reserve and used occasionally to meet some short-lived crisis. And yet others characterized their drug-taking behaviour in terms of both these meanings. Four-fifths of the 'users', however, looked upon their drug taking in only *one* way, with nearly equal numbers referring to them as a lifeline or standby.

The following quotations illustrate these two basic views of benzodiazepine use:

'Well the Valium I've got to take haven't I really because there's no doubt I do need something. I think even you would recognize the fact that you could easily go to pieces without it.'

'Valium does help if you're that desperate but I tend if I can do without it – I do without it as long as I can and I only take it if it's absolutely necessary. I can go three or four weeks without and then I suddenly feel the need. That's why I keep some in my bag just in case I need it.'

While there were no important differences in the meaning which indigenous and West Indian women attributed to their use of benzodiazepines, there was a difference between the 'user' groups. 'Long-term users' were more likely to see the drug only as a lifeline, whereas 'short-term users' were more likely to conceive of it only as a standby. The meaning attributed to drug use was also related to feelings about the drug. Those who talked of the drug only as a lifeline expressed mixed or positive views, with most choosing to voice the former; whereas those who referred to it as a standby expressed mixed or negative views in equal numbers.

In sum, the difference between the indigenous and West Indian women 'users' was that the former seemed to have used benzodiazepines more often and over a longer period. In every other respect they were similar, expressing the same range of sentiments about the drug and the meaning of its use. For the majority of 'users', both black and white, feelings about the drug were mixed. This was so for both long- and short-term 'users', and for those who treated the drug as a lifeline. As a resource they seemed to see benzodiazepines as *both* enabling and constraining. Negative views were most commonly expressed among the 'short-term users' and those who looked upon the drug as a standby. For these women the drug seemed *more* constraining than enabling. The few who expressed positive views were more likely to be 'long-term users' and to have looked upon the drug as a lifeline. These women were the ones who saw the drug as mainly enabling. As for the 'non-users', both indigenous and West Indian, they generally seemed to consider only its constraining effects.

Paid work

At the time of the 1981 Census the registered unemployment rate for women in Hackney was running at 12.5 per cent, compared with 7 per cent for London as a whole.[43] For middle-aged, black, and working-class women in Hackney the unemployment rate was significantly higher than for some other social groups.[44] As a result the chances of these women being in paid work in the borough were less than elsewhere. This reflects the way in which the resource of paid work is unequally distributed on age, race, and class lines according to geographical area.[45]

In our sample of women two-thirds were in paid work and most of these were working full-time. Indigenous and West Indian women were equally likely to have paid jobs, although the former were more likely to work part-time.[46] The indigenous women were also more likely than the West Indians to be doing routine non-manual rather than manual work, and to be employed in a non-manual capacity in a larger number of occupational settings. Indigenous women categorized as non-manual workers included clerks, shop assistants, and telephonists; among the West Indians in this category almost all were nursing auxiliaries.[47] Those indigenous and West Indian women who were in manual jobs were generally either machinists or cleaners. In terms of their drug-taking status, those in paid work were more likely to be 'short-term users' or 'non-users' of benzodiazepines and less likely to be 'long-term users'. Moreover, the 'long-term users' in paid work were more likely to be employed part-time rather than full-time.

When those in paid work were asked what they felt about what they were doing they responded in two ways. Some emphasized only positive aspects of their work while others *also* referred to negative aspects. Foremost among the benefits which paid work offered were financial independence and the self-respect that stemmed from it, companionship and emotional support, and the opportunity to get out of the house and do something that required concentration, thereby taking their minds off their personal problems. Those who also emphasized the negative aspects referred to low pay and resulting money worries, physical exhaustion at the end of the long working day, and lack of mental stimulation. The following comment was made by an indigenous woman who held mixed feelings about her job as a telephonist:

> 'It helps me forget when I'm working because my mind is on the job. . . .
> Just lately though I've felt so tired. I keep thinking, I don't know, am I
> doing the right thing? Should I pack up work again? But I've got that
> little bit of independence, that little bit of extra money.'

'Long-term users' of benzodiazepines generally expressed mixed feelings about the nature of their employment, whereas 'short-term users' and 'non-users' emphasized the advantages. West Indian women, regardless of their 'user' status, expressed the latter view.

Those not in paid employment *all* held mixed views about their situation, whatever their 'user' status. Although it made it easier for them to fulfil their taken-for-granted domestic responsibilities, they felt constrained by the financial restriction, the lack of economic independence, and 'being stuck within four walls'. As one unemployed, white, ex-factory worker put it:

> 'Since I've been made redundant I've been on my own most of the time
> and I'm home all day. I can get the housework done now but I get so
> depressed. I hate being off work and stuck at home with no one to talk
> to.'

In sum, it would seem that the resource of full-time paid work was more
available to West Indian women, and to 'short-term users' and 'non-users'
than to others. The West Indian women in paid work also experienced it as
enabling, whatever their 'user' status, whereas among the white women this
was so primarily for the 'short-term users' and 'non-users'. White 'long-
term users' generally expressed mixed feelings. There were no major
differences in the way unemployment was experienced.

Social supports [48]

In 1981, according to *Social Trends*, 80.3 per cent of women between 45 and
59 years of age living in Britain were married; the remainder were single,
widowed, or divorced.[49] Of the women in this age group who have had
children it is likely that a significant proportion will no longer have these
children living at home with them. The *General Household Survey*, conducted
in 1980, indicated that approximately 70 per cent of women aged 45 or over
had no children living in the household with them.[50] Evidence regarding
West Indians living in Britain suggests that West Indian women are slightly
less likely to be married than indigenous women, but are more likely to have
children living with them and to have a larger number to support.[51] It would
thus appear that male partners and children, as social support resources, are
differentially available and accessible to middle-aged indigenous and West
Indian women. The white women are slightly more likely to have available a
potentially supportive male partner but are less likely to have immediate
access to their children.

In our sample of women approximately two-thirds were married, one-
quarter were separated or divorced, and most of the remainder were single.
Just over half the sample had children living at home with them and the
mean number of children per household was 1.15. Indigenous women were
slightly more likely to be married and less likely to be divorced than the West
Indian women. The former were, however, noticeably less likely to have any
children still living at home and they had, on average, significantly fewer
children per household than the latter. In sum, our sample contained fewer
married women and more divorcees, and more households with children
living at home than previous surveys would lead one to expect. The
differences between the indigenous and West Indian women, however,
parallel those found in other studies.

When we related the household structure of our sample to benzodiazepine use we found that 'non-users' were the most likely to be married and 'long-term users' to be divorced or single. The association between 'non-use' and marriage was, however, only marked among the West Indians. 'Non-users' were also the most likely to have children living at home and this was so whatever their racial group membership.

When the women were asked about their relationship with household members they responded in a variety of ways. Of those who had a male partner some said he was generally supportive and helped them through emotional crises, while others complained of a breakdown of communication and at times blamed their partner for their current poor state of mental health. 'Non-users', whether indigenous or West Indian, were the most likely to refer to their partner as supportive.

As one of them remarked:

'I can get upset very quickly ... and when I do I shout, I really shout, and I bang doors (laughs). My husband says to me "I don't know what you're getting all upset about!" But he overcomes it with me. He's really good you know. He calms me down. He never loses his temper. He does such a lot for me. We sort of work together.'

Those who had had children were far more likely to talk of their daughters as supportive than their sons. This mother–daughter relationship was often perceived as a particularly important source of practical help and emotional strength, and at times may have countered an unsatisfactory relationship with a partner. 'Non-users' were again the most likely to mention this supportive relationship although this did not hold for the majority of West Indian women who, regardless of their 'user' status, said they were close to their daughters. As one West Indian woman put it:

'When I turned 40 and I was pregnant I was really worried. I didn't think I could cope. But, today she's such a helpful one in the family. Oh dear, she's my right hand. She's useful, obedient, everything.'

It would thus appear that social support resources were differentially available and accessible to the women in our sample. 'Long-term users' were less likely than 'non-users' to have access to a partner or children, and to find them supportive. The relationship between children (daughters) as social supports and tranquilliser use, however, did not hold for the West Indians who, regardless of their 'user' status, saw them as supportive.

Leisure

Research on leisure patterns has been biased towards male pastimes and has frequently failed to take gender differences into account.[52] When such differences have been considered it has been found that women participate less than men in many activities, whether based inside or outside the home[53] and that, for middle-aged women, the most popular activities are visiting or entertaining, listening to records, reading books and magazines, needlework and knitting, watching TV, gardening, and bingo.[54] Many of these activities are home-based and most share the characteristic of being easily fitted into short and unpredictable time periods, thus making it possible for them to be combined with domestic work and child care.[55] This blurring of the boundary between work and leisure reduces the likelihood of women experiencing leisure as a mental or physical change or rest.[56] There is also some indication in the literature that working-class women have less opportunities for leisure than middle-class women,[57] and that black women might experience and construct their leisure in a different way from white women.[58] On the few occasions that West Indian-born women's leisure has been considered by researchers it has only been compared with that of West Indian-born males. These comparisons show that such women participate less frequently in recreational activities than the men, and that this difference can be explained primarily in terms of the unequal sexual division of labour within the household; it is the women who have the major responsibility for domestic work, whatever their employment status.[59] The types of recreation mentioned in these studies also suggest that West Indian women are less likely than white women to watch television, and more likely to listen to recorded music and hold house parties. In sum, it would seem that the resource of leisure, like other resources, is distributed and experienced according to gender, age, class, and race.

When the women in our sample were asked whether they had any particular hobbies one-fifth said they had none at all. Among the remainder the most popular pursuits were knitting and sewing, reading, listening to music, television, gardening, and bingo – activities which, as we noted earlier, are common among middle-aged women. Many of our women said they derived a great deal of pleasure from these hobbies and frequently indicated that such activities helped them to relax. The 'long-term users' of benzodiazepines were markedly more likely than the other women to indicate that they did not have a hobby. Often they said they lacked the time and energy for such activities because of their dual role as wage-earner and housewife:

Int. 'What about hobbies? Have you got any hobbies?'
Res. 'Yeah, Lesneys (local toy manufacturers) and housework!'

Those 'long-term users' with hobbies mentioned fewer, on average, than the other 'user' groups and seemed to have less leisure options open to them. This pattern was also found among the West Indian women, whatever their 'user' status. For these women the most common activities by far were listening to music, dressmaking, and reading. Of these, music was the most frequently referred to as a source of pleasure and a means of lifting their spirits:

'I am always able to get rid of my troubles, to put my problems aside . . . by playing some music. I have a lot of different records. I like Country and Western as well. A little bit of reggae, all sorts. And that helps, music helps, music is very soothing. It lifts you.'

The women were also asked whether they had had a holiday in the last year. Just over half said that they had – a proportion similar to the national average for those belonging to the working class.[60] Of these women a number said that such a holiday provided them with a much-needed break. The opportunity to take such a break, however, varied by 'user' group. 'Long-term users' were far less likely to say they had had a holiday than the other women. The pattern was, however, mediated by race. Black women, whatever their 'user' status, rarely mentioned a holiday.

Overall, then, it would seem that the resource of leisure was less available to 'long-term users' and to West Indian women than to others. Those who had access to it, however, found it completely enabling.

Cigarettes

Survey reports indicate that the proportion of women smoking cigarettes regularly has increased significantly over the last four decades (although in recent years there is evidence of a decline[61]) and is now little different to that found among men.[62] Figures for 1980 indicate a prevalence rate of 37 per cent for women and 42 per cent for men.[63] At the same time the average number of cigarettes smoked by women has increased markedly and is now close to male consumption rates.[64] There are also generational and class differences in smoking. Among women, those between 20 and 59[65] and those belonging to the working class have the highest prevalence and consumption rates.[66] In sum, cigarettes as a resource are now distributed primarily along generational and class lines.[67]

When the women in our sample were asked if they smoked currently three-fifths said that they did – a higher proportion than the survey figures would have led one to expect, even for this age group. Smoking for these women was also strongly linked with benzodiazepine 'use'. 'Users' were more likely than 'non-users' to say that they smoked and, among the former, it was the 'long-term users' who were markedly more likely to say that they did so. This pattern was found in both the indigenous and West Indian samples although the latter were less likely to identify themselves as smokers, whatever their 'user' status.[68]

On being asked what they felt about cigarette smoking they responded in a variety of ways. The most frequent reaction was to view cigarettes as a way of 'calming the nerves'. Other common responses, in declining frequency of mention, were that it endangered physical health, invited habituation, was financially costly, and provided a source of pleasure. The positive view of cigarettes as calming and pleasurable was frequently combined with negative references to ill-health and money. Half the sample expressed these mixed sentiments while the remainder emphasized either positive or negative views in broadly similar proportions. Not surprisingly, non-smokers referred only to the negative aspects of smoking while the smokers expressed mixed views or only stressed the advantages. 'Long-term users' of benzodiazepines were the only ones to take a wholeheartedly positive view and relatively rarely stressed the negative aspects alone. The other two 'user' groups, in contrast, expressed either mixed or negative views in equal proportions. Such meanings were not related to the women's racial group membership.

In our sample cigarettes as a resource were therefore unevenly distributed and variously experienced as enabling and/or constraining. 'Long-term users' and indigenous women were the most likely to avail themselves of the resource, and members of the former 'user' group were the only ones to view it as totally enabling. The following comment from a white, long-term benzodiazepine 'user' illustrates this point of view:

> 'I find sometimes that it (smoking) keeps my nerves down a little. On the switchboard things can be a little bit – you can get a little bit agitated, especially if you get very awkward people, and the first thing I go for is a cigarette. I just think "thank God for that" and I seem to unwind. It's the only pleasure I get out of life is a smoke.'

Religion

There is relatively little survey information about religion in Britain. What evidence there is generally relates to religious behaviour – church membership and attendance – and not to religious beliefs. It suggests that there has been a decline in membership and attendance at most of the main Christian churches, but that this has been paralleled by an increase in membership and attendance among the sects.[69] This pattern is particularly marked in large industrial areas.[70] National surveys and small-scale studies indicate that women make up the bulk of the congregations in Christian churches[71] and that their attendance increases with age.[72] This pattern holds for both the indigenous and West Indian populations,[73] although attendance rates for the West Indians appear to be higher.[74] Whether such behaviour indicates that older women and black women are also more likely than others to adhere to religious beliefs in everyday life is not clear. It would seem plausible to suggest that there is some kind of relationship, which in turn lends support to the view that religion as a resource is distributed by gender, race, and age.

The women in our sample were only asked about religion if they mentioned it first themselves. Just under half did so and, of these, almost all said that they held some religious beliefs. Less than one-third of these believers, however, said that they attended church – often a non-conformist one – at all regularly. 'Non-users' of benzodiazepines were slightly more likely to mention religion than the 'users' and to say that they were regular church attenders. Long-term and short-term 'users' were equally likely to mention religion but the 'short-term users' were far more likely to say that they were regular churchgoers. The sample also divided on racial lines. West Indian women were far more likely to talk about their religious beliefs than the indigenous women, whatever their 'user' status. They were also more likely to consider themselves to be regular church attenders. This only held, however, for those who were 'short-term users' or 'non-users' of benzodiazepines.

The women who mentioned religion were then asked what part it played in their daily lives. The majority responded by talking about the importance of prayer and bible reading. Through such activities they said they were able to obtain the peace of mind and inner strength to overcome the difficulties which faced them. 'Non-users' were slightly more likely than 'users' to make such remarks, but there were no differences between long-term and short-term 'users'. This pattern was, however, only found among the West Indian women. Among the indigenous women, only 'long-term users' said they drew on their religious beliefs to lift their spirits.

The following quotation from a West Indian 'non-user' of benzo-diazepines illustrates the significance of religion to West Indian women in helping them get by:

'Praying, now that's special. You got to do that, haven't you, as a telephone link to the master of all. I don't have to go to church to pray – I walk along and say a little prayer. Every day of my life I do that. It does help you get by. God is your friend and your father – he's always there – you know he's there. So if you've got something bothering you and if you don't want anybody to hear, like I don't want him (husband) to hear, I just whisper it to him and he hears, he knows.... He is my best friend, my very best friend.'

Overall, then, it would seem that religion was viewed solely as an enabling resource. This was far more the case for the West Indian women than the indigenous women and, among the West Indian women, for the 'non-users' of benzodiazepines. Within the indigenous sample the 'long-term users' were the only ones to emphasize its relaxing properties.

Discussion

We have had two related aims in writing this paper: to demonstrate the usefulness of Giddens' notion of resource as a bridging concept between social structure and everyday life; and to illuminate the meaning of tranquillisers for indigenous, and West Indian, working-class women within the context of these groups' structured social existence.

The concept of resource is well equipped to fulfil a bridging function because it contains both structural and experiential dimensions. We have demonstrated these dimensions in our analysis, describing how resources for managing everyday life are asymmetrically distributed according to group membership, and variously experienced as enabling and/or constraining. Such ambiguity is unsurprising, given that resources were theorized as containing both elements. However, there were two resources – leisure and religion – that were described only as enabling. Such unambiguous evaluations suggest that the women's relationships with these resources represented particularly significant features of their daily lives.

Our analysis also enables us to throw light on the nature of benzo-diazepine use and its relationship to the availability and experience of other resources for indigenous and West Indian women. We found that indigenous women reported using benzodiazepines more often and over a longer period than their West Indian counterparts and, given the meanings associated with this pattern of use, were more likely to see the drug as enabling.

How can such differences in benzodiazepine use be explained? Part of the answer would seem to lie with the resources that were primarily available to West Indian women. For instance, we found that these women were more likely than white women to have a full-time job and to view such employment as totally enabling. Such findings have been reported elsewhere and have been interpreted as reflecting West Indian women's greater economic need and historical desire for financial independence.[75] This may help explain why the West Indian women found it less necessary than the indigenous women to resort to benzodiazepines on a long-term basis.

We also found that the West Indian women were more likely than the white women to have children living at home and to find their female children particularly supportive. Such a bond between black working-class mothers and their daughters has also been noted before[76] and can be explained in terms of the historical development of the West Indian family structure, which traditionally has forced women to take sole responsibility for the family's well-being.[77] In contemporary Britain this mother–daughter relationship represents a more enabling resource for West Indian women than white women, and provides a further possible reason for the different patterns of use by the two groups.

Finally, we found that the West Indian women were far more likely than the white women to describe themselves as regular churchgoers, and to state that their religious practices helped them to manage their daily lives. These women's willingness to attach such significance to religion is unsurprising, given its historical importance in the West Indies,[78] especially for women.[79] The latter's high church attendance in the Caribbean has been explained in terms of their lack of opportunity, due to informal taboos, to participate in other activities which afford emotional release and the cathartic nature of church services. Similar reasons have been offered for their continuing high attendance in Britain.[80] Church attendance, along with religious practices at home, were also most common among those black women who were 'short-term' or 'non-users' of benzodiazepines. This suggests that religion played a major part in reducing the likelihood of their becoming regular, 'long-term users'.[81]

Overall, it would seem that black women's experience of these resources – paid work, their daughters, and their religion – combined with their distrust of benzodiazepines to reduce the likelihood of their using these drugs to the same degree as their white counterparts. It may also be the case that the racist attitudes and practices of some doctors and ancillary staff[82] reduce the willingness of black women to seek medical advice and drug therapy for their personal problems. The black women in our sample did not indicate that this was the case, however, giving further credence to the view that the availability of resources other than benzodiazepines played a crucial part in explaining the nature of their drug use.

In addition, our analysis provides a basis for commenting on why white women who are long-term benzodiazepine 'users' are constrained to maintain the pattern of drug use that they do. It would seem that these women not only have access to fewer resources than other white women, but that those resources which are available to them are rarely experienced in such a way as to enable them to manage their everyday lives without recourse to tranquillisers. For instance, we found that white 'long-term users' were not only markedly less likely than others to have a full-time job, but that those who were so employed were more likely to express mixed feelings about their situation. It would thus seem that while the absence of paid work may deprive white 'long-term users' of a resource which might make their lives easier, thereby reducing the need for tranquillisers, those 'long-term users' with access to this resource do not experience it in a sufficiently positive way to enable them to change the nature of their tranquilliser use.

We also found that 'long-term use' for white women was associated with being divorced and not having children living at home. Moreover, if these 'long-term users' were living with partners and/or their children, they were less likely than 'non-users' to find these kin supportive. It would thus appear that white 'long-term users' either lack access to potentially supportive social resources, or find that those who are available are unsupportive and a poor substitute for tranquillisers. In such circumstances the existing pattern of drug use is likely to be maintained, a conclusion which is also in line with the findings of other researchers who have explored the relationship between social supports and long-term psychotropic drug use.[83]

It is also clear from our analysis that the white 'long-term users' were markedly more likely than other white women to state either that they lacked all opportunities for leisure or that they had few leisure options open to them. As this resource was only experienced as enabling and as a relaxant, the limited access to it of these long-term users would seem to place them at a considerable disadvantage, and further helps to explain why they continued to use tranquillisers regularly in managing their daily lives.

Overall, then, it appears that three resources – paid work, children and partners, and leisure – had a particularly important influence upon the drug-taking behaviour of white 'long-term users'. These women's access to and relationship with these resources combined with their greater faith in tranquillisers to maintain their existing pattern of drug use.

Finally, our data also points to a relationship between long-term tranquilliser 'use' among indigenous women and another 'psychotropic' resource – cigarettes.[84] We found that white 'long-term users' were more likely than other 'users' both to smoke cigarettes and to describe their experience as enabling. The relationship of these 'long-term users' with cigarettes is, we suggest, in part at least a consequence of their limited access to and negative experience of the other resources we have considered. In the absence of other resources these women have turned to cigarettes to bolster the apparently insufficient relaxing powers of tranquillisers.

In order to test these case study propositions, further studies with larger, representative samples of tranquilliser users need to be conducted. This will make it possible for individual members of particular 'user' groups to be compared in terms of their access to, and experience of, a *range* of resources instead of simply considering their relationship with each resource separately.

References

The fieldwork on which this paper is based was carried out under the supervision of Professor Margot Jefferys at Bedford College. We are grateful for her advice and should also like to thank Professor Michael Shepherd, Mick Bloor, Mike Bury, Monica Briscoe, and Paul Williams for their comments on an earlier draft of this paper. Still earlier versions of the paper were read to the BSA London Medical Sociology Group in 1983 and the Polytechnic of the South Bank postgraduate medical sociology conference in 1985. Thanks are also due to the women who agreed to be interviewed and to the doctors who participated in the study.

1 Parry, H. (1968) Use of psychotropic drugs by US adults. *Public Health Reports* 83 (10):799–810; Balter, M., Levine, J., and Manheimer, D. (1974) Cross-national study of the extent of anti-anxiety/sedative drug use. *New England Journal of Medicine* 290 (14):769–74; Dunnell, K. and Cartwright, A. (1972) *Medicine Takers, Prescribers and Hoarders*. London, Routledge & Kegan Paul; Mellinger, G.D., Balter, M.B., and Uhlenhuth, E.H. (1984) Prevalence and correlates of the long-term regular use of anxiolytics. *Journal of the American Medical Association* 251 (3):375–79.

2 See for example, Linn, L. and Davis, M. (1971) The use of psychotherapeutic drugs by middle-aged women. *Journal of Health and Social Behaviour* 12 (4):331–40; Pflanz, M., Basler, H.-D., and Schwoon, D. (1977) Use of tranquilizing drugs by a middle-aged population in West Germany. *Journal of Health and Social Behaviour* 18 (2):194–205; Murray, J., Dunn, G., Williams, P., and Tarnopolsky, A. (1981) Factors affecting the consumption of psychotropic drugs. *Psychological Medicine* 11 (3):551–60; Radelet, M. (1981) Health beliefs, social networks and tranquilliser use. *Journal of Health and Social Behaviour* 22 (2):165–73; Cafferata, G., Kasper, J., and Bernstein, A. (1983) Family roles, structure and stressors in relation to sex differences in obtaining psychotropic drugs. *Journal of Health and Social Behaviour* 24 (2):132–43; Riska, E., and Klaukka, T. (1984) Use of psychotropic drugs in Finland. *Social Science and Medicine* 19 (9):983–89.

3 For a general discussion of this problem see Davies, C. and Roche, S. (1980) The place of methodology: a critique of Brown and Harris. *Sociological Review* 28 (3):641–56; Graham, H. (1983) Do her answers fit his questions? Women and the survey method. In E. Gamarnikov, D. Morgan, J. Purvis, and D. Taylorson (eds) *The Public and the Private*. London: Heinemann.

4 Harre, R. (1979) *Social Being: A Theory for Social Psychology*. Oxford: Basil Blackwell.

5 This critical point has also been made by Robert Dingwall when considering studies of illness behaviour, and by Roy Wallis and Steve Bruce in their discussion of the explanatory value of multi-variate analysis. See Dingwall, R. (1976) *Aspects of Illness*. London: Martin Robertson; Wallis, R. and Bruce, S. (1982) Accounting for action: defending the common sense heresy. *Sociology* 17 (1):97–111.

6 Raymond Illsley made a similar point when considering the adequacy of existing analysis of the relationship between social structure and health. See Illsley, R. (1980) *Professional or Public Health*. London: Nuffield Provincial Hospital Trust, ch. 2.

7 Cicourel, A. (1964) *Method and Measurement in Sociology*. New York: Free Press; Douglas, J.D. (1971) Understanding everyday life. In J.D. Douglas (ed.) *Understanding Everyday Life*. London: Routledge & Kegan Paul.

8 Helman, C. (1981) Patients' perceptions of psychotropic drugs. *Journal of the Royal College of General Practitioners* 31 (223):107–12; Helman, C. (1981) Tonic, fuel, and food: social and symbolic aspects of the long-term use of psychotropic drugs. *Social Science and Medicine* 15B (4):521–33.

9 Cooperstock, R. and Lennard, H.L. (1979) Some social meanings of tranquilliser use. *Sociology of Health and Illness* 1 (3):331–47.

10 Schutz, A. and Luckmann, T. (1974) *The Structures of the Life-World*. London: Heinemann, p. 3.

11   Brittan, A. (1977) *The Privatised World*. London: Routledge & Kegan Paul.

12   Mills, C.W. (1970) *The Sociological Imagination*. Harmondsworth: Penguin.

13   Giddens, A. (1981) Agency, institution and time-space analysis. In K. Knorr Cetina and A.V. Cicourel (eds) *Advances in Social Theory and Methodology: Towards an Integration of Micro and Macro Sociologies*. London: Routledge & Kegan Paul, p. 162.

14   Croog, S.H., Lipson, A., and Levine, S. (1972) Help patterns in severe illness: the roles of kin network, non-family resources and institutions. *Journal of Marriage and the Family* 34 (1):32–41; Finlayson, A. (1976) Social networks as coping resources. *Social Science and Medicine* 10 (2):97–103; Ben-Sira, Z. (1981) The structure of readjustment of the disabled: an additional perspective on rehabilitation. *Social Science and Medicine* 15A (5):565–81; Bury, M. (1982) Chronic illness as biographical disruption. *Sociology of Health and Illness* 4 (2):167–82; Graham, H. (1984) *Women, Health and the Family*. Brighton: Wheatsheaf Books.

15   Kohn, M. (1972) Class, family and schizophrenia: a reformulation. *Social Forces* 50 (3):295–304; Pearlin, L. and Schooler, C. (1978) The structure of coping. *Journal of Health and Social Behaviour* 19 (1):2–21; Antonovsky, A. (1979) *Health, Stress and Coping*. San Francisco: Jossey-Bass; McCubbin, H.J., Joy, C.B., Cauble, A.E., Comeau, J.K., Patterson, J.M., and Needle, R.H. (1980) Family, stress and coping. *Journal of Marriage and the Family* 42 (4):855–70; Wheaton, B. (1983) Stress, personal coping resources and psychiatric symptoms: an investigation of interactive models. *Journal of Health and Social Behaviour* 24 (3):208–29.

16   Pearlin, L. and Schooler, C. (1978) The structure of coping. *Journal of Health and Social Behaviour* 19 (1):5.

17   This is particularly so of those working in the mental health field.

18   There are two recent exceptions. Antonovsky (1979) and Graham (1984) have both discussed the health consequences of a range of social resources besides social networks. Additional resources considered include income, housing, food, and transport.

19   Gerhardt, U. (1979) Coping and social action. *Sociology of Health and Illness* 1 (2):195–225; Young, A. (1980) Discourse on stress and the reproduction of conventional knowledge. *Social Science and Medicine* 14B (3):133–46; Davies, C. and Roche, S. (1980) The place of methodology: a critique of Brown and Harris. *Sociological Review* 28 (3):641–56.

20   We are grateful to Mike Bury for pointing out the link between coping and morality.

21   Crawford, R. (1977) You are dangerous to your health: the ideology of victim blaming. *International Journal of Health Services* 7 (4):663–80.

22   Giddens, A. (1982) *Profiles and Critiques in Social Theory*. London: Macmillan, p. 38.

23   Giddens, A. (1979) *Central Problems in Social Theory*. London: Macmillan, p. 69.

24   Giddens, A. (1981) Agency, institution and time-space analysis. In K. Knorr Cetina and A.V. Cicourel (eds) *Advances in Social Theory and Methodology*. London: Routledge & Kegan Paul, p. 169.

25   Giddens, A. (1979) *Central Problems in Social Theory*, London: Macmillan, p. 69.

26 This is what Giddens would seem to be implying when he says that: 'To conceptualize structure as rules and resources is to acknowledge that structure is both enabling and constraining' (1981: 171).

27 Giddens (1979:104).

28 Giddens (1982:36).

29 Giddens (1979:91–2).

30 Giddens, A. (1981) *A Contemporary Critique of Historical Materialism*. London: Macmillan, p. 50.

31 Giddens (1979:93).

32 Giddens (1979:88).

33 While all resources are simultaneously enabling *and* constraining in theory, in practice they may be experienced as more one than the other. Recounting such experiences does not, however, put one in a position to specify under what conditions a resource is more one than the other, as to do so would involve dualistic theorizing.

34 Giddens (1979:82).

35 This study was undertaken by one of the present authors and Susan Lipshitz-Phillips, and involved fieldwork in another part of London besides Hackney. Reports of this study can be found in Gabe, J. and Lipshitz-Phillips, S. (1982) Evil necessity? The meaning of benzodiazepine use for women patients from one general practice. *Sociology of Health and Illness* 4 (2):201–09; Gabe, J. and Lipshitz-Phillips, S. (1984) Tranquillisers as social control? *Sociological Review* 32 (3):524–46.

36 The class position of the women was defined by the class position of their household, in turn determined by the highest ranked household member according to primarily economic criteria (such as conditions of employment). It should be noted that routine clerical, sales, and rank and file service work were categorized as working-class occupations on the grounds that the market and work conditions of those in these occupations had more in common with those in other working-class occupations than those in middle-class ones. Foremost among these conditions are rates of pay, promotion prospects, and levels of skill. Support for such a categorization is found in the work of the following: Westergaard, J. and Resler, H. (1976) *Class in a Capitalist Society*. Harmondsworth: Penguin; Garnsey, E. (1978) Women's work and theories of class stratification. *Sociology* 12 (2):223–43; West, J. (1978) Women, sex and class. In A. Kuhn and A.M. Wolpe (eds) *Feminism and Materialism*. London: Routledge & Kegan Paul; Crompton, R. (1979) Trade unionism and the insurance clerk. *Sociology* 13 (3):403–26; Allen, S. (1982) Gender inequality and class formation. In A. Giddens and G. Mackenzie (eds) *Social Class and the Division of Labour*. Cambridge: Cambridge University Press; Crompton, R. and Jones, G. (1984) *White-Collar Proletariat: Deskilling and Gender in Clerical Work*. London: Macmillan Press; Stanworth, M. (1984) Women and class analysis. *Sociology* 18 (2):159–70.

37 Two sampling techniques were employed to see whether the technique chosen affected the responses given (e.g. whether sampling in a doctor's surgery resulted in the researcher being allied with the doctor, regardless of what the researcher said). There was no evidence to suggest that the technique affected the answers given. Moreover, it should be noted that the black 'community

sample' did not differ from the 'general practice' sample in terms of any of the resources discussed in the remainder of the paper.

38   Clyde Mitchell, J. (1983) Case and situation analysis. *Sociological Review* 31 (2):200.

39   Gabe, J. and Thorogood, N. (1986) Prescribed drug use and the management of everyday life: the experiences of black and white working-class women. *Sociological Review*. (In press.)

40   Blackwell, B. (1973) Psychotropic drugs in use today: the role of diazepam in medical practice. *Journal of the American Medical Association* 225 (13):1637–641; Skegg, D., Doll, R., and Perry, J. (1977) The use of medicines in general practice. *British Medical Journal* 1 (6076):1561–563; Williams, P. (1980) Recent trends in the prescribing of psychotropic drugs. *Health Trends* 12 (1):6–7; Mellinger, G. and Balter, M. (1981) Prevalence and patterns of use of psychotherapeutic drugs: results from a 1979 national survey of American adults. In D. Tognoni, C. Bellantuono, and M. Lader (eds) *Epidemiological Impact of Psychotropic Drugs*. Amsterdam: Elsevier/North Holland Biomedical Press; Balter, M., Manheimer, D., Mellinger, G., and Uhlenhuth, E. (1984) A cross-national comparison of anti-anxiety/sedative drug use. *Current Medical Research and Opinion* 8 (suppl.4).

41   Parish, P. (1971) The prescribing of psychotropic drugs in general practice. *Journal of the Royal College of General Practitioners* 21 (92):suppl. no. 4; Lader, M. (1978) Benzodiazepines – opium of the masses? *Neuroscience* 3 (2):159–65; Cooperstock, R. and Parnell, P. (1982) Research on psychotropic drug use: a review of findings and methods. *Social Science and Medicine* 16 (12):1179–196; Cafferata, G. and Kasper, J. (1983) Psychotropic drugs: use, expenditure and sources of payment. *US Department of Health and Human Services*. Data Preview 14, Rockville; Balter, Manheimer, Mellinger, and Uhlenhuth (1984).

42   Parish (1971); Skegg, Doll, and Perry (1977); Cafferata and Kasper (1983).

43   Office of Population Censuses and Surveys (1984) *1981 Census: Key Statistics for Local Authorities*. London: HMSO.

44   Young, M., Young, H., Shuttleworth, E., and Tucker, W. (1981) *Report from Hackney: A Study of an Inner City Area*. London: Policy Studies Institute, No. 593; Harrison, P. (1983) *Inside the Inner City*. Harmondsworth: Pelican.

45   Mackie, L. and Pattullo, P. (1977) *Women at Work*. London: Tavistock Publications; Smith, D. (1977) *Racial Disadvantage in Britain: The PEP Report*. Harmondsworth: Penguin; Bruegel, I. (1979) Women as a reserve army of labour: a note on recent British experience. *Feminist Review* 3:12–23; Barber, A. (1980) Ethnic origin and the labour force. *Employment Gazette* 88:841–48; Friend, A. and Metcalf, A. (1980) *Slump City: The Politics of Mass Unemployment*. London: Pluto Press; Smith, D. (1981) *Unemployment and Racial Minorities*. London: Policy Studies Institute; Showler, B. and Sinfield, A. (1981) Unemployment and the unemployed. In B. Showler and A. Sinfield (eds) *The Workless State*. Oxford: Martin Robertson; Brown, C. (1984) *Black and White Britain: The Third PSI Survey*. London: Heinemann.

46   Nationally it seems that West Indian women are more likely than white women to be employed full-time and less likely to be employed part-time (see Smith (1977); Runnymede Trust/Radical Statistics Group (1980) *Britain's*

Black Population. London: Heinemann; Brown (1984)). Our sample thus replicates the national pattern only for part-time work.

47 This is not surprising given the number of Afro-Caribbean women working for the National Health Service (see Doyal, L., Hunt, G., and Mellor, J. (1981) Your life in their hands: migrant women in the National Health Service. *Critical Social Policy* 1 (2):54–71).

48 In this section we focus on partners and children because our respondents did so when they were asked who they found to be the most socially supportive (outside the workplace). References to friends and neighbours were relatively infrequent.

49 Central Statistical Office (1982) *Social Trends, no. 13, 1983*. London: HMSO, p. 20.

50 Office of Population Censuses and Surveys (1982) *General Household Survey 1980*. London: HMSO.

51 Deakin, N. (1970) *Colour, Citizenship and British Society*. London: Panther; Rex, J. and Tomlinson, S. (1979) *Colonial Immigrants in a British City*. London: Routledge & Kegan Paul; Phizacklea, A. and Miles, R. (1980) *Labour and Racism*. London: Routledge & Kegan Paul; Central Statistical Office (1981) *Social Trends, no. 12, 1982*. London: HMSO, p. 181.

52 Delamont, S. (1980) *The Sociology of Women: An Introduction*. London: George Allen & Unwin, p. 184.

53 Deem, R. (1982a) Women, leisure and inequality. *Leisure Studies* 1 (1):29–46; Deem, R. (1984) Paid work, leisure and non employment: shifting boundaries and gender differences. Paper to the British Sociological Association Conference, Bradford; Central Statistical Office (1981).

54 Central Statistical Office (1981).

55 Deem (1982a:39).

56 Delamont (1980:183); Griffin, C., Hobson, D., MacIntosh, S., and McCabe, T. (1982) Women and leisure. In J. Hargreaves (ed.) *Sport, Culture and Ideology*. London: Routledge & Kegan Paul.

57 Talbot, M. (1979) *Women and Leisure: A State of the Art Review*. London: Social Science Research Council/Sports Council Joint Panel on Sport and Leisure; Talbot, M. (1981) Women and sport – social aspects. *Journal of Biosocial Science* Supplement no. 7:33–47; Deem, R. (1982b) Women's leisure: does it exist? Paper to the British Sociological Association Conference, Manchester.

58 Deem (1982b); Stanley, L. (1980) The problem of women and leisure: an ideological construct and a radical feminist alternative. Paper to the 'Leisure in the 80s' Forum, London; Griffin, Hobson, MacIntosh, and McCabe (1982).

59 Foner, N. (1978) *Jamaica Farewell: Jamaican Migrants in London*. Berkeley: University of California Press; Pearson, D. (1981) *Race, Class and Political Activism: A study of West Indians in Britain*. Farnborough: Gower.

60 Delamont (1980:184); Central Statistical Office (1982:141).

61 Royal College of Physicians of London (1983) *Health or Smoking?* London: Pitman.

62 Cox, H. and Marks, L. (1983) Sales trends and survey findings: a study of smoking in 15 OECD countries. *Health Trends* 15 (2):48–51.

63 Office of Population Censuses and Surveys (1982).

64 Jacobson, B. (1981) *The Ladykillers*. London: Pluto Press.

65 Royal College of Physicians of London (1983:62).

66 Royal College of Physicians of London (1977) *Smoking or Health?* Tunbridge Wells: Pitman Medical; OPCS (1982); Townsend, P. and Davidson, N. (eds) (1982) *Inequalities in Health: The Black Report*. Harmondsworth: Penguin; Royal College of Physicians of London (1983).

67 Smoking data for Great Britain has not been broken down by race. In the United States, however, it seems that black and white women (although not men) have similar prevalence rates. See United States Department of Health, Education and Welfare (1980) *The Health Consequences of Smoking for Women: A Report of the Surgeon General*. Washington, DC.

68 The West Indian women were also asked if they smoked ganja (cannabis). All said they did not, either because it was 'too powerful' or because it was unfeminine, illegal, or irreligious.

69 Central Statistical Office (1980) *Social Trends, no. 11, 1981*. London: HMSO; Delamont (1980:179).

70 Delamont (1980:181).

71 See for example, Butler, D. and Stokes, D. (1970) *Political Change in Britain*. London: Macmillan; Stacey, M., Batstone, E., Bell, C., and Murcott, A. (1975) *Power, Persistence and Change*. London: Routledge & Kegan Paul.

72 Central Statistical Office (1981).

73 Davison, R.B. (1966) *Black British*. London: Oxford University Press for the Institute of Race Relations; Rex, J. and Moore, R. (1967) *Race, Community and Conflict*. London: Oxford University Press for the Institute of Race Relations; Pearson, D.G. (1978) Race, religiosity and political activism: some observations on West Indian participation in Britain. *British Journal of Sociology* 29 (3):340–57; Pearson (1981).

74 Ratcliffe, P. (1981) *Racism and Reaction: A Profile of Handsworth*. London: Routledge & Kegan Paul. It is also the case, however, that West Indian attendance rates are lower in Britain than in the West Indies and are declining. See, for example, Hill, C. (1963) *West Indian Migrants and the London Churches*. London: Oxford University Press for the Institute of Race Relations; Philpott, S.B. (1977) The Montserratians: migration, dependence and the maintenance of island ties in England. In J. Watson (ed.) *Between Two Cultures*. Oxford: Basil Blackwell; Pearson (1981).

75 Foner, N. (1976) Women, work and migration: Jamaicans in London. *New Community* 5 (1–2):85–98; Foner (1978); Phizacklea and Miles (1980); Phizacklea, A. (1982) Migrant women and wage labour: the case of West Indian women in Britain. In J. West (ed.) *Work, Women and the Labour Market*. London: Routledge & Kegan Paul; Stone, K. (1983) Motherhood and waged work: West Indian, Asian and white mothers compared. In A. Phizacklea (ed.) *One Way Ticket: Migration and Female Labour*. London: Routledge & Kegan Paul.

76 Smith, R.T. (1956) *The Negro Family in British Guyana*. London: Routledge & Kegan Paul; Foner (1978).

77 Clarke, E. (1957) *My Mother who Fathered Me*. London: George Allen & Unwin; Smith, M.G. (1962) *West Indian Family Structure*. Seattle: University of Washington Press; Patterson, S. (1965) *Dark Strangers*. Harmondsworth: Penguin; Standing, G. (1981) *Unemployment and Female Labour: A Study of*

Labour Supply in Kingston Jamaica. London: Macmillan. The structure of West Indian families (e.g. the high rate of single-parent families) in Britain has frequently been cited as evidence of the 'pathology' of the black family. We wish to disassociate ourselves from such a position. As our analysis shows, the striking thing about the black family in Britain is its strength and resilience in the face of considerable adversity.

78 Davison (1966:127); Cross, M. (1979) *Urbanization and Urban Growth in the Caribbean*. Cambridge: Cambridge University Press, p. 93; Pearson (1981:124).
79 Foner (1978).
80 Foner (1978).
81 This finding is in line with evidence from the United States that commitment to a religious denomination or sect enhances the ability of both blacks and whites to handle stress and manage their personal problems. See, for example, Najman, J. (1980) Theories of disease causation and the concept of general susceptibility. *Social Science and Medicine* 14A (3):231–37; Baer, H. (1981) Prophets and advisors in black spiritual churches: therapy, palliative or opiate? *Culture, Medicine and Psychiatry* 5:145–70.
82 Brent Community Health Council (1981) *Black People and the Health Service*. London; Torkington, N. (1983) *The Racial Politics of Health: A Liverpool Profile*. Liverpool: Merseyside Area Profile Group.
83 Linn and Davis (1971); Borgman, R. (1973) Medication abuse by middle-aged women. *Social Casework* November:526–32; Murray, J., Williams, P., and Clare, A. (1982) Health and social characteristics of long-term psychotropic drug takers. *Social Science and Medicine* 16 (18):1595–598.
84 To our knowledge no other studies have reported this relationship specifically for long-term tranquilliser users. However, there is some evidence from the United States that tranquilliser users as a whole are more likely to be smokers than non-tranquilliser users, and that women who smoke are more likely to take tranquillisers than those who do not smoke. See Uhlenhuth, E.H., Balter, M.B., and Lipman, R.S. (1978) Minor tranquillisers: clinical correlates of use in an urban population. *Archives of General Psychiatry* 35 (5):650–55; US Department of Health, Education and Welfare (1980).

© *1986 Jonathan Gabe and Nicki Thorogood*

19

Tranquillisers as social control?

Jonathan Gabe and Susan Lipshitz-Phillips

Abstract In this paper we use findings from an empirical study of the meaning of tranquilliser prescribing and use to examine the contention that these drugs are a means of social control, and to assess the explanatory value of the concept of social control when applied to the doctor–patient relationship. We first outline the historical application of the concept to the health field, specify the cultural mechanisms by which social control is said to be achieved and look at the ways in which the mechanisms are thought to operate through the prescribing of the most widely used kind of tranquilliser/hypnotic – benzodiazepines (e.g. Valium, Mogadon). We then draw on our data to see how far they substantiate the arguments which have been developed. In the final section of the paper we suggest some alternative explanations regarding the nature of doctors' power and of patient dependence. We also discuss problems involved in conceptualizing gender and class ideologies, note an inherent tendency towards an over-socialized view of the person and assess the usefulness of functionalist explanations stemming from the application of the social control concept to the doctor–patient relationship.

Social control and the institution of medicine

The concept of social control, which broadly refers to the ways in which social order and stability are maintained, has a long intellectual history.[1] Since the beginning of the twentieth century sociologists, especially in the United States, have described institutions such as the family, the school and the church as performing a social control function. It was not, however, until the 1950s that medicine was seen in this way and then only indirectly via a theory of the sick-role as deviance.[2] In terms of this theory the medical profession, by regulating who should be allowed to deviate temporarily from their usual role obligations and adopt the sick-role, was

Reprinted, with permission, from the *Sociological Review* 32 (3):524–46. 1984.

seen to act as an agent of social control. In the 1960s, it was applied to the mental health field by radical psychiatrists who saw psychiatry as preserving the *status quo* by labelling social non-conformists as 'mad',[3] and, since the mid-1970s, it has been used by other radicals to describe how doctors reinforce the existing sexual,[4] racial[5] and class[6] structures.

A reading of this most recent body of writing suggests that there is a measure of agreement about the way in which the institution of medicine, through the medical profession, exerts social control. Two mechanisms are generally identified: the medicalisation of everyday life and the reinforcement of existing hierarchical social relations.

Doctors, it is said, medicalise everyday life by defining patients' problems which have a social origin in terms of a medical model[7] and an individualised aetiology, thereby reifying the person and their illness and focusing solely on their symptoms.[8] In doing so they encourage patients to be dependent on them and their medicines, discredit lay advice and help, and generally make little attempt to help them to handle their own lives or to become aware of the links between social structure and ill health.[9]

Doctors are said to legitimise and reinforce existing hierarchical social relations by their attitudes and behaviour towards patients. A frequently quoted example of such behaviour is the doctor indicating to a female patient that her symptoms are merely a reflection of her sex's inherently unstable physiology and personality, or of her unwillingness to direct herself to her 'natural' maternal role.[10] Again, it is believed that doctors are more likely to suggest to working-class than to middle-class patients that their symptoms are a consequence of *their* failure to look after themselves adequately.[11] Both mechanisms it is held, minimize the likelihood of people attempting by collective action to change the way in which their society is organised.

Benzodiazepine[12] use as a means of social control

Given the popularity of the concept of social control amongst radicals working in the health field, it is not surprising that this concept has recently been applied to the prescribing and the use of benzodiazepines[13] – one of the most widely prescribed category of drugs in America, Britain and other industrialised countries.[14] In doing so most writers have focused on the first of the two mechanisms discussed above, the medicalisation of everyday life. They argue that benzodiazepines are generally prescribed for socially induced symptoms, that in prescribing them doctors are encouraging patients to deny or ignore social concomitants of distress and that in this way they help to minimise pressure for social change.[15] It has been noted too that benzodiazepines tend to be prescribed more frequently to older people and to women and, on a long-term basis, to members of lower socio-economic groups.[16]

One question which arises is why do doctors rely to the extent that they do on benzodiazepine prescribing? An important answer would seem to be that doctors have traditionally provided sedatives or tranquillisers for patients in distress because they have neither the time nor the training to deal with these patients in other ways.[17] It would seem, however, that in the past the safety of mood-altering drugs was often in question and, to some extent, acted as a brake on prescribing. Benzodiazepines, on the other hand, are believed to be 'safer' and to have fewer adverse effects than earlier sedative drugs; a factor which has been exploited heavily by the drug companies. As a result, doctors have felt free to prescribe them liberally.[18] Patients, in turn, have become dependent on benzodiazepines and, by demanding that the doctor continue to relieve their distress, have helped to maintain the high level of prescribing of these drugs.[19]

Our reading of the literature suggested to us that the concept of social control as applied to medicine in general, and benzodiazepine prescribing in particular, has been useful for medical sociology in that it has brought into relief the influence of structural factors on the doctor–patient relationship which had previously been ignored. To determine how far doctors and patients experience benzodiazepine prescribing and use as social control, we applied the model to data obtained from a small sample of doctors and patients. The data were collected in the course of an exploratory study of the meaning of benzodiazepines to those who prescribed and those who received them.

Background: the empirical study

Our findings are based on in-depth interviews which were conducted by the authors in 1980–81 with fourteen general practitioners and eighty-seven patients from two practices in Inner London. The practices were chosen because they served populations with different socio-demographic characteristics, one being in a mainly working-class neighbourhood and the other in a more middle-class area. There were ten principals and four trainees in our sample of doctors with equal numbers of each in each practice. The average age of the doctors was thirty-five and six of them were women.

Our sample of patients was chosen from that category of patients known to be frequent recipients of benzodiazepine prescriptions, namely, indigenous, white women in the forty to sixty age group.[20] As we wanted to examine the effects of social class, as well as these other structural factors on patients' perceptions and experience of benzodiazepines, we aimed to obtain approximately equal numbers of middle and working-class patients in our sample.[21] In addition, as our focus was the meaning of benzodiazepines, as distinct from that of other psychotropic drugs (such as antidepressants or major tranquillisers), we decided to exclude from our sampling frame patients in the relevant age/sex category who had recently received prescriptions for these other drugs. All indigenous, white women between the ages of forty and sixty, who consulted a GP in one of the two practices in a three-month period were asked by the GP to allow us to look at their medical records and to agree to be interviewed if asked. Only one-tenth of those asked refused this permission. The records of those agreeing to participate were scrutinised and depending on the prescriptions noted they were excluded or included, thus providing us with a sample of eighty-seven women.

These doctors and patients were interviewed with the aid of a checklist by one or other of the authors in the surgery or in the patient's home. An open-ended technique encouraged the interviewees to talk freely and express their feelings, many of which were ambivalent and apparently contradictory. Themes discussed with the doctors included their reasons for prescribing benzodiazepines, the factors which they felt influenced their decision to prescribe, whether or not they offered alternatives to a prescription and what, if anything, they did to reduce patient dependence on these drugs. These interviews usually lasted between half-an-hour and an hour.

With the patients, attention was focused on their feelings about these drugs and about other drugs, the people who took them, their attitude to doctors and their views on the National Health Service (NHS) in general. Patients who were using or had used benzodiazepines were asked about their reasons for taking them, the ways in which they used them and what such usage meant to them. These interviews frequently continued for three hours or longer. All the interviews, both those with doctors and patients, were tape-recorded and transcribed and subsequently analysed both in terms of pre-determined thematic categories and categories suggested by the data.

In this paper we deal with the data from all the doctors but have limited the patient sample to those who were, according to their medical records, either 'high users'[22] or 'non users' of the drug, that is, seventy-four patients in all. Our criteria for determining the frequency of 'use' were the number of years out of the last ten in which patients had received a benzodiazepine prescription and the mean number of prescriptions over this period. If patients had received a benzodiazepine prescription in five or more years and had averaged ten or more prescriptions they were called 'high users'. Thirty-nine fell into this category. 'Non users' were patients who had *not* received a benzodiazepine prescription in the last ten years according to their records. There were thirty-five in this group. A third category, namely, 'intermittent users' were those who had had prescriptions over less than five years and averaged less than ten prescriptions. There were thirteen women in this group. We excluded the latter from the following discussion because we feel the issues with which we are concerned are best explored by focusing on those who exemplify clearly opposing patterns of use.

Two-thirds of the women in our patient sample were defined as working-class, the rest as middle-class.[23] There were proportionately more working-class patients amongst the 'high users' than the 'non users'. Just over two thirds of the 'high users' were working-class compared with just over half the 'non users'.

No claim is being made for the representativeness or typicality of these samples of doctors and patients. Rather we use our case study data to explore the validity of the *theoretical* assumptions which underpin the notion of benzodiazepine prescribing and use as a means of social control and have organised our data accordingly. Following Clyde Mitchell we suggest that 'the validity of the extrapolation depends not on the typicality or representativeness of the case but on the cogency of the theoretical reasoning'.[24]

To what extent then do our data confirm the argument that benzodiazepine use results in the medicalisation of everyday life and the reinforcement of hierarchical social relations? Do they support contentions that doctors prescribe benzodiazepines because of the inadequacy of their training, the conditions of modern medical practice, the impact of drug company advertisements and because they believe they do little harm? Whereas information on all these themes was obtained from doctors, the information obtained from patients referred only to some of them. Wherever possible we draw on both sets of data.

Data from the case study

The medicalisation of everyday life

(a) Individualised aetiology and the use of the medical model
The doctors said they prescribed benzodiazepines to patients presenting with symptoms of anxiety and insomnia. When asked what they felt caused these symptoms the majority offered multi-causal explanations. Most frequently mentioned were interpersonal and domestic problems such as marital strife, child care difficulties and the 'empty nest', the kinds of reasons referred to by nine doctors. Next most frequently listed were physical and/or psychosomatic conditions, such as rheumatism or epilepsy, or a transitionary period such as the menopause. Six doctors put forward such reasons. However, four doctors perceived structural factors – stresses of paid work, poor housing or financial difficulties as the cause of anxiety or insomnia. It would seem then that the majority

of doctors in our sample did not operate with a unicausal model[25] and were unlikely to impose individualised explanations on a patient if they felt that interpersonal or structural factors were relevant to their patient's predicament.

The patients also saw benzodiazepines as being prescribed for anxiety and insomnia. Amongst these patients those who were 'users' were more likely to adopt a multi-causal explanation of benzodiazepine prescribing and use than were the 'non users':[26] just under half the former mentioned interpersonal problems in comparison with one in seven of the 'non users' and a quarter of the 'users' referred to structural factors in comparison with one in nine of the 'non users'. Equal proportions, that is, two-thirds from each group, perceived physical and psychosomatic problems as causing anxiety and insomnia and hence leading to a benzodiazepine prescription. It would seem then that patients were rather more likely than doctors both to perceive a single cause for their symptoms and to suggest physical and psychosomatic factors as the cause.

(b) Patient dependence

Our data suggested that the issue of patient dependence on doctors and their drugs is rather more complex than the social control thesis allows.

The doctors themselves referred to the danger of dependence which, as they emphasised, ran counter to their long-term goal of promoting patient autonomy. All prescribed benzodiazepines in varying degrees but six said they had such doubts about it that they preferred not to prescribe. The remainder expressed mixed feelings and said that while they felt the drug had some value in the acute stage of the crisis there was a danger of patients becoming reliant on them and treating them as 'magic pills'.

Whatever their prescribing patterns or their feelings about them all the doctors emphasised that they did offer alternatives to benzodiazepines and that these at times met their patients' needs. For example, eight said that they used themselves as a therapeutic alternative,[27] five said they recommended certain leisure activities to help their patients relax; and eight said they sometimes referred patients to other members of their primary care team or to allied professionals in other organisations, or corresponded with housing officials on their patients' behalf. Whether these alternatives were more or less likely to make patients dependent on doctors and allied professionals, the doctors at least seemed to be united in their concern to restrict their prescribing of benzodiazepines to crisis situations. Moreover, all seemed to hold the guiding principle that they should help their patients to become autonomous managers of their own lives.

Amongst the patients a majority too expressed mixed feelings about benzodiazepines.[28] More than four-fifths of the 'users' and just over half of the 'non users' said they were fearful of taking them either because of the danger of addiction or because there was a possibility that such unnatural substances would harm their body or mind. At the same time just under four-fifths of benzodiazepine 'users' and just over a fifth of the 'non users' *also* thought they could be helpful. Nevertheless, just under half of the 'users' who saw benzodiazepines as potentially beneficial held what we called a self-help ideology and were concerned not to become too dependent on drugs. This ideology resulted in their trying out various 'fringe' medicines and religions, as well as benzodiazepines, to help them cope with their lives.

When the benzodiazepine 'users' were asked what using these drugs meant to them they responded in different ways. Some seemed to see benzodiazepines as a *life-line*: that is something which they felt they had to take continuously and thus depended on simply to keep going in the face of unresolved problems. Others seemed to view the drug as a *standby* to be kept in reserve and used occasionally to meet some short-lived crisis, and yet others talked as if they had conceived their drug usage in both these senses at some point in time. Three-quarters of the 'users' however seemed to look upon their drug-taking in only *one* way, with slightly more referring to them as a life-line than as a standby. When the 'users' accounts of the meaning of their drug-taking behaviour were related to their feelings about these drugs we found that those who talked about them only as a life-line were far more likely to express mixed feelings whereas those referring to them only as a standby were more likely to express consistently negative feelings about the drugs. Thus, using benzodiazepines as a life-line was directly linked with feelings of ambivalence.

Not surprisingly those who talked of benzodiazepines as a life-line were markedly less likely than other patients to have stopped taking them recently or in the past. In all over half the 'users' said they had stopped taking the drug and most of these claimed to have done so on their own initiative. They said they had been motivated to stop either because they feared they were becoming over-reliant on them or because they were worried by the drug's physical side-effects or, more positively, because they no longer needed them. A minority said they had given up the drug on their doctor's advice.

Despite the differences in the meaning of benzodiazepine use and attitudes to benzodiazepines the patients in general considered that the doctors in both practices were reluctant to prescribe the drug and three-quarters maintained that they only did so after talking the patient's problem through with them and establishing their need for a minor tranquilliser or hypnotic. Further, half the 'users' said that their doctor had either restricted their supply or suggested that they cut down or stop taking the drug and a quarter believed that their doctor shared their doubts about benzodiazepines.

In short, the patients seemed to be aware of the danger of dependency on a drug and, by extension, on the doctor, and the 'users' amongst them seemed to feel that their doctors were equally aware of this danger. At the same time most 'users' felt they had been helped by benzodiazepines, but were aware of other sources of help and of the need to try and help themselves. Indeed a significant number had at some stage stopped using the drug. It would seem, therefore, that these patients were not merely passive recipients of what doctors prescribed but active participants in the process, aware of the dangers of relying on benzodiazepines and trying themselves to alter their behaviour.

The legitimation of existing gender and class relations

We look next at the extent to which the doctors reinforced existing gender and class relations. Did the doctors in our sample see themselves as employing negative stereotypes in their dealings with their patients?

(a) Gender

All but two of the doctors believed that gender was not a factor influencing their decision to prescribe benzodiazepines to a patient. The remaining two admitted that it might play a part but if so, they were not consciously aware of it doing so. However, twelve of the doctors acknowledged that they prescribed more benzodiazepines to women than to men. Nearly all attributed this excess to the stresses women rather than men experience as a result of their social position, for example, having two jobs – one inside and one outside the home. Five felt they prescribed more to women because they attended surgery more frequently than men, largely as a result of difficulties relating to reproduction; only two referred to women's psychological make-up and in particular their allegedly greater emotionality.

The patients in many respects held similar views to those of the doctors. Three-quarters of the thirty-eight women[29] who commented on the sex of the average recipient of a benzodiazepine prescription felt that women were more likely to be recipients than men; and two-thirds thought this was because of the effect on women of their social position in general and the unequal division of labour within the family in particular. Unlike the doctors, however, they were more likely to suggest that gender-specific psychological traits explained why women received more benzodiazepines and were less likely to link prescribing to female physiology. One in three felt that women had lower self-esteem and a tendency to 'worry more' than men and that these traits resulted in their being given these drugs: only a fifth referred to problems concerning reproduction.

'Non users' were as likely as 'users' to recognise gender differences in prescribing. They were, however, less likely than the 'users' to explain the differences in social terms and more likely to refer to psychological factors.

What are we to make of these data? On the one hand, there are grounds for suggesting that both doctors and patients operated with negative stereotypes such as perceiving women as more psychologically or physiologically fragile than men and as limited by their reproductive function. They employed these stereotypes to explain why women received and used more benzodiazepines than men. The proponents of the social control argument would contend that to a considerable extent it is the pattern of differential prescribing which reinforces such negative stereotypes.

On the other hand there is much in our data which would appear to contradict the social control thesis. First, nearly all the doctors maintained that they did not respond to their patients in terms of preconceived ideas about gender differences in illness or psychological make-up. Instead they pointed out that more women than men experiencing anxiety symptoms come to the surgery; consequently they prescribed more benzodiazepines to women. It could be argued, therefore, that it is the women patients who are acting in terms of negative gender stereotypes independently of their doctors.

Second, even if the women patients showed signs of operating in terms of negative gender stereotypes there was no evidence to suggest their experience of the consultation reproduced or enhanced these stereotypes. Although a number of patients amongst both 'users' and 'non users' made a link between gender inequalities and benzodiazepine use in general they seldom made such a link as far as they themselves were concerned. It would thus seem that they were operating with a dual consciousness which acknowledged gender inequalities at an abstract but not at a personal level: a consciousness which the social control thesis does not allow for. This dual consciousness would seem to result from women living their lives in a cultural milieu based upon negative gender stereotypes while rejecting the stereotypes as applying to themselves. If this is so, it becomes difficult to sustain the argument that the experience of the consultation and the receipt of benzodiazepine prescriptions necessarily reproduces women patients' acquiescence in the structure of a male dominated society.

(b) Class

Ten of the fourteen GPs said they felt they were more likely to prescribe benzodiazepines to their working-class patients than to patients of other social classes. They mostly attributed their tendency to do so to three factors: first, working-class patients were more likely than those from other classes to exert pressure for pills; second, they were somewhat less likely to accept 'talk'; third, they perceived their working-class patients' social circumstances as particularly difficult and hence creating greater stress and need for the drugs. Only four attributed their prescribing bias to their own inability to communicate with working-class patients.

The patients were not asked whether they thought benzodiazepine taking was related to class, but were asked about whether they acknowledged the existence of class, to locate themselves in a social class if they felt able to do so, and to say whether they felt health care provision in Britain favoured some social classes more than others. Three-quarters of the patients felt there were class divisions. They seemed to be using the concept to mean collectivities distinguished by the amount of money possessed, the nature of employment and the ownership of property, and identified themselves in class terms. The remainder denied such divisions; they talked in terms of a liberal individualism which envisaged everyone as both individually different from and yet similar to each other. Working-class patients seemed more likely than middle-class patients to accept the existence of class and to criticise inequalities of access to private health care facilities which they felt depended on class differences in material resources. They were less likely than middle-class patients to relate class to differences in the quality of care received within the NHS. 'Users' were less likely than 'non users' to acknowledge class differences but more likely to relate these differences to the quality of NHS care and to criticise what they saw as a class factor in the degree of access to the private health care sector.

As with gender there are several ways of interpreting the data on social class. Again, they could be interpreted as evidence of negative stereotypes which in turn would reinforce social control. For example, the fact that the doctors said that they were prescribing more to working-class patients and justified doing so on the grounds that such patients only wanted pills or were in greater need could be taken to mean that, whether conscious of it or not, they were operating with a notion of the working-class as incapable of resolving their social problems on their own.

A counter interpretation is possible. Our data did not suggest that the doctors held a view of working-class patients as inferior to others. A significant number indicated that, irrespective of social class, they talked to their patients and tried to encourage them to reduce the number of benzodiazepines taken. They were no more likely, they maintained, to acquiesce to working-class than to middle-class patients' requests for pills. It could be argued, then, that doctors' acknowledgement of the fact that they prescribed more frequently to working-class than to middle-class patients reflected a recognition of the social origins of the suffering of working-class patients and the need to try and alleviate this suffering.

Further, the fact that not all the patients denied the existence of class differences in the quality of care in the NHS would suggest, either that the doctors had not sought to impose an egalitarian view of health services on their patients, or that the patients had been able to resist such attempts. It seems that the social control thesis, therefore, does not take sufficient account of the persistence of pre-existing oppositional class consciousness.

Factors which lead to benzodiazepine prescribing and use

Earlier we listed reasons given by proponents of social control theory to explain the widespread use of benzodiazepines. These were the inadequacy of doctors' training, the conditions under which they practice, the influence which drug company advertising has on them and their belief in these drugs' safety. In this section we examine these contentions in the light of our data.

(a) The inadequacy of doctors' training

The doctors in our sample were all aware that there were alternatives to a benzodiazepine prescription and did *not* seem to feel that they lacked the training to pursue these alternatives with their patients. For them benzodiazepines represented just one option; an option which half of them, especially the younger ones and the trainees, said that their medical school and general practice training had made them cautious of choosing. It would seem therefore that medical schools may be changing to meet the criticisms which have been levelled against them and that these changes are being encouraged and reinforced by the development of general practice training schemes.[30] If so, the notion that inadequate professional training in the social aspects of medicine promotes benzodiazepine prescribing would no longer seem so tenable.

The patients for their part, seemed to confirm the latter view. Three-quarters of the 'users' and five-sevenths of the 'non users' of benzodiazepines were wholly complimentary about their doctors and frequently made a point of saying that they liked them because they seemed to be interested in them as people, listened to what they had to say and talked to them, whether or not they prescribed benzodiazepines. Only a few of the patients were totally critical of their doctors' behaviour and most of them were 'non users'.

(b) Conditions of general practice

There was, however, evidence to suggest that organisational factors did affect the prescribing of benzodiazepines, even if this appeared to be the case for only a minority of the doctors. Five of the fourteen said that they felt that running behind time, a full waiting room and administrative interruptions combined to increase the likelihood that they would take the 'easy option'; that is to prescribe benzodiazepines rather than try to reach agreement with the patient about an alternative course of action..The other nine did not mention the impact of organisational factors on their prescribing. As for the patients only a sixth of those who had been critical of their doctor referred to a lack of time to discuss their problems. Nearly all of these patients were 'non users'. It would thus seem that the effect of organisational factors on the consultation was a concern of only a few doctors and hardly any patients.

(c) The impact of drug company advertising
The idea that drug company advertising is affecting doctors' attitudes to benzodiazepines and encouraging them to prescribe them for social problems is indeed a widely held view.[31] However, most of the doctors in our sample maintained that they were not influenced by drug companies, either by their literature or personal visits from their representatives. Indeed, six doctors said they had a policy of not seeing representatives of drug companies at all. Only two claimed that they had changed their prescribing on the basis of what drug representatives had told them. On the advice received they had switched to newer benzodiazepines which were claimed to have a shorter half life and hence the likelihood of more limited side-effects.

It could be argued that in providing this evidence the doctors were seeking to project themselves as independent, judicious prescribers not open to the influence of the drug companies. We feel it is unlikely that they were trying to project themselves in this way, however, as their remarks are consistent with their attitudes about benzodiazepine prescribing. In saying this we are taking the view that the reasons individuals advance for their behaviour should be taken seriously and accepted unless there are grounds for thinking otherwise.[32] This point is important for the argument about social control and is returned to in the discussion.

(d) The lack of side-effects
Finally, it has been argued that doctors favour benzodiazepines because they see them as considerably less likely than many other drugs to cause adverse side-effects. The doctors in our sample did not view benzodiazepines so favourably. All expressed doubts about prescribing the drugs. The most reluctant, six in number, said they always warned patients, and in particular first time users, of the drugs' possible side-effects such as 'dopiness' or slowness of thought or movement. The remaining eight, although more willing to prescribe these drugs, nevertheless expressed worries about them and in general did not attempt to defend their actions by emphasising benzodiazepines' *lack* of side-effects. Only two of them talked about their safety and then specifically in relation to suicide.

The patients too seemed to reject the view of benzodiazepines as safe and free from side-effects. Those who had received benzodiazepine prescriptions said they felt they could be helpful but, at the same time, recognised that they might be harmful to their body or mind and give rise to a hangover or make them 'feel low'. A quarter of the 'users' who were no longer taking the drug said that it was the side-effects which had led them to stop. And both 'users' and 'non users' knew others who had taken the drug and experienced unpleasant side-effects.

It would thus seem that significant numbers of doctors and patients in our study claimed to be well aware of the side-effects of benzodiazepine use and did *not* appear to hold beliefs which encouraged benzodiazepine prescribing and taking. This is perhaps not surprising for, as we have noted elsewhere,[33] there has been considerable publicity about the effects of these drugs in the medical press,[34] the popular press[35] and on radio and television.[36] Such publicity is likely to have heightened the doctors' and patients' sensitivity[37] to the effects of benzodiazepines.

Discussion

We have had two aims in writing this paper: to use our empirical material to evaluate the claim that benzodiazepine prescribing and use represent a form of social control; and to consider the theoretical problems which stem from the use of this concept.

Taking the substantive issue first, there was little to indicate that benzodiazepine prescribing and use necessarily involved the individualisation of social problems or the creation of patient dependence. The data on gender and class was more equivocal; it could be used both to support and to reject the social control thesis. Finally, there was little to substantiate the claim that factors such as the inadequacy of professional training, the conditions of modern medical practice, the influence of drug company advertising and a belief in benzodiazepines' lack of side-effects were promoting benzodiazepines as a form of social control.

As for the theoretical problems stemming from the use of the concept of social control we want to reiterate at this point that we are aware of the contribution which the concept has made to understanding social action and value its emphasis on the effect of structural factors on the doctor–patient relationship. We feel, however, that it has frequently been applied too mechanistically, giving rise to over-generalisations. In the discussion which follows we use our data to highlight these over-generalisations and to provide a basis for suggesting certain theoretical modifications. There are five issues to consider: doctors' power, patients' dependence, gender and class ideology, an over-socialized view of the person, and the limits of functionalism.

Doctors' power

The social control argument would seem to be premised on the assumption that doctors are all powerful, that they manipulate the consultation to maintain their professional dominance and that, by keeping the lid tightly on the interaction, they keep patients in line and get them to accept their lot. The patients, for their part, are seen as the victims of this unequal distribution of power, accept their doctors' definition of their problem, allow them to make decisions on their behalf and accept their instructions about how to conduct themselves with regard to health matters. As Sharrock[38] has pointed out, however, this 'pressure cooker' approach to the interaction involves certain misconceptions.

First, it defines the doctor–patient relationship only in terms of power and ignores the extent of willing co-operation on the part of the patient in the consultation in the hope that the doctor might help resolve his or her problems. It also ignores the fact that the consultation involves a considerable amount of routine medical work with the doctor enquiring into the patient's welfare, establishing symptoms and discussing lines of action with the patient. Second, it fails to explain the necessity for doctors to engage in a continuing struggle for dominance. If doctors are all powerful why is such a struggle necessary? Third, it ignores the fact that patients are often less constrained by their doctors' power than by the constraints which they as patients impose upon themselves in that they come to the consultation accepting if not welcoming the doctors' right to make decisions on their behalf. Regarding this last point we feel that Sharrock is correct to emphasise the role which patients' expectations play in the consultation but do not believe that the institutionalization of professional dominance has been internalized by patients to the extent that he suggests. Patients may appear to accept the doctor's authority during the consultation but this does not mean that they therefore refrain from criticising the medical profession as a whole or from using 'atrocity stories'[39] of past encounters with doctors to redress the balance and present an image of an active rather than passive participant in the consultation.[40] To these three points we would add a fourth. We feel that the 'pressure cooker' approach tends to assume that patients who do not openly contest their doctor's power automatically come out of the consultation having accepted uncritically their doctor's definition of their situation. We found, however, that this was not necessarily the case as far as the patients in our sample were concerned. They seemed to hold a set of reasons for taking benzodiazepines which differed in order of priority from those of their doctors and did not all talk as if they had internalised negative gender and class stereotypes which, it could be argued, had informed their doctor's actions.

To take account of these issues we feel a more sophisticated analysis of the doctor–patient relationship is required; an analysis which moves beyond a discussion of professional dominance and patient subordination and takes as its starting point the fact that this relationship is essentially both dialectical and deferential.[41] It contains potentially contradictory elements of differentiation/opposition and association/co-operation which mean that the relationship is at the same time both stratified (in terms of power) and co-operative (in terms of interchange). These contradictory elements, we suggest, create an inherent tension which threatens the traditional deference which patients normally show to doctors and needs to be managed by the superordinate doctor if this deference is to be maintained. One of the advantages of this model over the 'pressure cooker' model is that it takes account of the problems we have encountered in making sense of our material. It sees the relationship between doctor and patient as about co-operation as well as about power, and it allows for the fact that patients are often deferential because of constraints which they themselves impose and yet are active participants in the consultation, evaluating the interaction from their own point of view. It also represents a conscious attempt to synthesize the two polar positions which have been taken by medical sociologists when discussing the doctor–patient relationship over the last three decades; namely the currently fashionable conflict view[42] and the previously popular notion of reciprocity.[43] Such a synthesis[44] enables us to avoid the current tendency within medical sociology for 'doctor bashing'[45] whilst retaining a critical view of medicine and its practice in modern society.

Patients' dependence

It was noted that doctors are alleged to act as agents of social control because they make patients dependent on them and their medicines, offer a medical solution to social problems, and make little attempt to help patients to help themselves. Yet when we tested this argument against our data we found the situation to be more complex: doctors and patients expressed mixed views about benzodiazepines, doctors often stressed that they encouraged patients to try alternatives to drugs and patients said they tried such alternatives and, if they used benzodiazepines, did not necessarily look upon them as a permanent life-line. In other words, the doctors seemed concerned to prevent their patients becoming dependent on a medical solution to their problems and the patients seemed to dislike this prospect and to try to avoid it, even though they all live in a society in which faith in medicine is said to have increased as it has become more available.[46] What this suggests is that it is possible to prescribe and take benzodiazepines without necessarily creating or experiencing total dependence on them and that to think otherwise is to overstate the argument about patient dependence.[47] The popularity of the latter notion is perhaps in part a result of what Strong[48] has called sociological imperialism: the tendency for sociologists for their own professional purposes to search for, focus on and exaggerate the negative aspects of medical practice. It can also be said to reflect a failure to take seriously the possibility that both doctors and patients differ in the extent to which they think about what they are doing; consequently they vary in their behaviour and the extent to which it can be meaningfully described as controlling. If this is accepted doctors and patients cannot be categorised en masse as the creators and victims of dependency.

Gender and class ideology

The argument that doctors control and oppress, if subtly, their patients through the use of negative gender and class stereotypes is premised on two incorrect assumptions: that all doctors think *and* act continuously in terms of the dominant ideology, and that women and working-class patients passively accept all that doctors tell them regardless of other influences on their consciousness. These assumptions appear to have been challenged by our data. The doctors in our sample differed considerably in their consciousness of the link between benzodiazepine prescribing, gender and class and there was no necessary fit between this consciousness and what they felt actually happened in the consultation. Moreover, a significant number of patients expressed what we chose to call a dual consciousness – in part accepting the dominant ideology and in part opposing it – with different sets of beliefs being appealed to according to the issue under discussion and the extent to which they were personally implicated. This more sophisticated view of consciousness[49] is a more accurate representation of the way in which people think and at the same time undermines the thesis that doctors can, in some simple way, control patients by ideological means. It may well be that some doctors at times express beliefs *and* behave in terms of the dominant set of values, and that some women and working-class patients who are already more accepting of the dominant ideology may find that such an experience reinforces what they already believed. Other patients with more oppositional views are, however, likely to be unaffected by doctors' comments or may find that what they say actually makes them *more* antipathetic to the dominant ideology.

Over-socialised view of the person

The social control thesis also seems to us to fall into the trap of defining human behaviour *only* in social terms and of ignoring any behaviour which falls outside socially organised boundaries. It is this over-socialised view of the person, as Wrong put it,[50] which has resulted in attention only being focused on the social reasons for the prescribing and use of benzodiazepines with no consideration of physical, psychosomatic or psychological factors. To rectify this omission, we feel a more complex model of human behaviour is required which draws on a variety of psychological and psychodynamic theories and takes account of the work of holistic doctors like Balint[51] as well as of sociology. This approach might lead us to consider whether patient dependence, in so far as it exists, is a consequence of psychological need resulting from the level of suffering being experienced, independently of whether the resulting dependence has a controlling effect. It also warns against assuming a direct correspondence between a patient's social structural position and the form of the doctor–patient interaction. Other factors such as the personal attributes of individual patients may also play a crucial role.[52]

The limits of functionalism

Lastly, we would like to consider the problems raised by the concept of social control's functionalist origins.[53] We have shown that the concept of social control, like its functionalist forebears, only relates to the consequences of human behaviour – how such behaviour functions to meet the needs of the existing system – and tells us nothing about why such behaviour took place or about the processes involved. At best it is merely descriptive and at worst it is teleological, treating the consequences of behaviour as their cause.[54] What would seem to be necessary is a model which distinguishes causes from consequences, is grounded in an adequate theory of human agency which takes actors' reasons seriously (and does not treat them as synonymous with society's needs) and places action within a framework of structural constraints. Such a model would not deny social control as a possible consequence of human agency, but would treat it as context dependent and not some thing to be assumed in advance.

Notes

This study was supported by a DHSS grant and was carried out under the direction of Professor Margot Jefferys at Bedford College. We would particularly like to thank Margot Jefferys, Hessie Sachs, Mike Bury and Paul Williams for their comments on earlier drafts of this paper; and the patients and their general practitioners who made this study possible.

1   J. Pitt, Social control: the concept, *International Encyclopaedia of the Social Sciences*, 1968, pp. 381–96.

2   T. Parsons, *The Social System*, Free Press, New York, 1951, pp. 428–79.

3   R.D. Laing, *The Divided Self*, Pelican, Harmondsworth, 1965; T. Szasz, *Manufacture of Madness*, Free Press, New York, 1970; T. Szasz, *The Myth of Mental Illness*, Paladin, St Albans, 1972.

4 See M. Barrett and H. Roberts, Doctors and their patients: the social control of women in general practice, in C. Smart and B. Smart (eds), *Women: Sexuality and Social Control*, Routledge & Kegan Paul, London, 1978; B. Ehrenreich and D. English, The 'sick' woman of the upper classes, in J. Ehrenreich (ed.), *The Cultural Crisis of Modern Medicine*, Monthly Review Press, New York, 1978; M. Howell, Pediatricians and mothers, in J. Ehrenreich (ed.), ibid; D. Scully and P. Bart, A funny thing happened on the way to the orifice: women in gynaecology textbooks, in J. Ehrenreich (ed.), *op. cit.*; L. Doyal, *The Political Economy of Health*, Pluto Press, London, 1979, pp. 215–38.

5 J. Ehrenreich, Introduction, in J. Ehrenreich (ed.), *op. cit.*; Brent Community Health Council, *Black People and the Health Service*, London, 1981; Black Health Workers and Patients Group, Psychiatry and the corporate state, *Race and Class*, vol. 25, no. 2, 1983, pp. 49–64.

6 J. Ehrenreich, *op. cit.*, p. 15; B. Ehrenreich and J. Ehrenreich, Medicine and social control, in J. Ehrenreich (ed.), *op. cit.*; H. Waitzkin and B. Waterman, *The Exploitation of Illness in Capitalist Society*, Bobbs-Merrill, Indianapolis, 1974; H. Waitzkin, Medicine, superstructure and micropolitics, *Social Science and Medicine*, vol. 13a, no. 6, 1979, pp. 601–9.

7 A model which conceptualises disease primarily in terms of a breakdown in underlying physical mechanisms and encourages doctors to search for physical signs in their patients while ignoring possible social and psychological reasons for their distress. G.L. Engel, The need for a new medical model: a challenge for biomedicine, *Science*, vol. 196, no. 4286, 1977, pp. 129–35.

8 B. Ehrenreich and J. Ehrenreich, *op. cit.*, p. 40; H. Waitzkin, *op. cit.*, pp. 605–7; I.K. Zola, Medicine as an institution of social control, in C. Cox and A. Mead (eds), *A Sociology of Medical Practice*, Collier-Macmillan, London, 1975; I.K. Zola, In the name of health and illness: on some socio-political consequences of medical influence, *Social Science and Medicine*, vol. 9, no. 2, 1975, pp. 83–7.

9 J. Ehrenreich, *op. cit.*, pp. 14–15; B. Ehrenreich and J. Ehrenreich, *op. cit.*, p. 54; H. Waitzkin, *op. cit.*, p. 606; I. Illich, *Medical Nemesis*, Calder and Boyars, London, 1975; I. Illich, Medicalization and primary care, *Journal of the Royal College of General Practitioners*, vol. 32, no. 241, 1982, pp. 463–70.

10 M. Barrett and H. Roberts, *op. cit.*, p. 41; D. Scully and P. Bart, *op. cit.*, p. 130; L. Doyal, *op. cit.*, p. 215; A. Oakley, Normal motherhood: an exercise in self control?, in B. Hutter and G. Williams (eds), *Controlling Women: the Normal and the Deviant*, Croom Helm, London, 1981.

11 H. Waitzkin, *op. cit.*, p. 605; V. Navarro, Social class, political power and the State and their implications for medicine, *Social Science and Medicine*, vol. 10, no. 9/10, 1976, pp. 437–57.

12 Benzodiazepines are psychotropic or mood-modifying drugs with a particular chemical structure and pharmacological action and are used therapeutically as anti-anxiety agents and as hypnotics. Drugs belonging to the benzodiazepine 'family' are marketed as the following: Valium, Librium, Mogadon, and Dalmane.

13 I. Waldron, Increased prescribing of valium, librium and other drugs – an example of economic and social factors in the practice of medicine,

International Journal of Health Services, vol. 7, no. 1, 1977, pp. 37–62; P. Conrad, Types of medical social control, *Sociology of Health and Illness*, vol. 1, no. 1, 1979, pp. 1–11; K. Koumjian, The use of valium as a form of social control, *Social Science and Medicine*, vol. 15E, no. 3, 1981, pp. 245–9.

14   B. Blackwell, Psychotropic drugs in use today: the role of diazepam in medical practice, *Journal of the American Medical Association*, vol. 225, no. 13, 1973, pp. 1637–41; M. Balter, J. Levine and D. Manheimer, Cross-national study of the extent of anti-anxiety/sedative drugs use, *New England Journal of Medicine*, vol. 290, no. 14, 1974, pp. 769–74; D. Skegg, R. Doll and J. Perry, The use of medicines in general practice, *British Medical Journal*, vol. 1, 1977, pp. 1561–3; P. Williams, Recent trends in the prescribing of psychotropic drugs, *Health Trends*, vol. 12, no. 1, 1980, pp. 6–7; G. Mellinger and M. Balter, Prevalence and patterns of use of psychotherapeutic drugs: results from a 1979 national survey of American adults, in D. Tognoni *et al.* (eds), *Epidemiological Impact of Psychotropic Drugs*, Elsevier/North Holland Biomedical Press, Amsterdam, 1981; J-R Laporte *et al.*, The utilization of sedative-hypnotic drugs in Spain, in D. Tognoni *et al.* (eds), ibid.

15   I. Waldron, *op. cit.*, p. 43; K. Koumjian, *op. cit.*, p. 246.

16   K. Koumjian, *op. cit.*, p. 247.

17   Ibid., p. 248.

18   Ibid., pp. 247–8.

19   See, for example, I. Waldron, *op. cit.*, p. 41.

20   See G. Cafferata and J. Kasper, Psychotropic drugs: use, expenditure and sources of payment, *United States Department of Health and Human Services*, Data Preview 14, Rockville, 1983; R. Cooperstock and P. Parnell, Research on psychotropic drug use: a review of findings and methods, *Social Science and Medicine*, vol. 16, no. 12, 1982, pp. 1179–96; P. Parish, The prescribing of psychotropic drugs in general practice, *Journal of the Royal College of General Practitioners*, Supplement No. 4, vol. 21, no. 92, 1971; H.J. Parry, Use of psychotropic drugs by U.S. adults, *Public Health Reports*, vol. 83, no. 10, 1968, pp. 799–810.

21   Upper class women were excluded from the study for pragmatic reasons.

22   'User' has been placed in inverted commas because it is realised that there is no necessary relationship between receiving a prescription and using the drug prescribed.

23   The class position of the women was defined by the class position of their household, in turn determined by the highest ranked household members according to primarily economic criteria (such as conditions of employment and ownership of productive property).

24   J. Clyde Mitchell, Case and situation analysis, *Sociological Review*, vol. 31, no. 2, 1983, p. 207.

25   Another recent study of psychotropic drug prescribing and use provides evidence that other GPs also considered that factors besides physical and psychological ones were relevant to the predicament of the women patients to whom they were prescribing drugs like benzodiazepines. See P. Williams, J. Murray, and A. Clare, A longitudinal study of psychotropic drug prescriptions, *Psychological Medicine*, vol. 12, no. 1, 1982, pp. 201–6.

26   The author of another study of long-term psychotropic drug use found that

users expressed a variety of reasons for their having been prescribed such drugs (most of which were minor tranquillisers). J. Murray, Long-term psychotropic drug-taking and the process of withdrawal, *Psychological Medicine*, vol. 11, no. 4, 1981, pp. 853–8.

27 i.e. they believed in giving their patients a 'dose of the doctor'. M. Balint, *The Doctor, his Patient and the Illness*, Tavistock, London, 1957, p. 1.

28 We discuss this ambivalence further in J. Gabe and S. Lipshitz-Phillips, Evil necessity? The meaning of benzodiazepine use for women patients from one general practice, Research Note in *Sociology of Health and Illness*, vol. 4, no. 2, 1982, pp. 201–9. See also J. Murray, *op. cit.*, p. 857; and C. Helman, Tonic, fuel, and food: social and symbolic aspects of the long-term use of psychotropic drugs, *Social Science and Medicine*, vol. 15B, no. 4, 1981, pp. 521–33.

29 The issue of gender stereotyping and benzodiazepine prescribing was raised first of all by some women respondents when the interviewing was well under way. Although it was subsequently incorporated in the interview checklist it meant that it was only discussed systematically with half the sample.

30 For further discussion of this point see J. Gabe and S. Lipshitz-Phillips, Doctors perceptions of benzodiazepine prescribing: an unhappy compromise? Unpublished paper, 1982.

31 See, for example, J. Prather and L. Fidell, Sex differences in the context and style of medical advertisements, *Social Science and Medicine*, vol. 9, no. 1, 1975, pp. 23–6; G. Stimson, Women in a doctored world, *New Society*, vol. 32, 1975, pp. 265–7; I. Waldron, *op. cit.*; S. Chapman, Advertising and psychotropic drugs: the place of myth in ideological reproduction, *Social Science and Medicine*, vol. 13A, no. 6, 1979, pp. 751–64.

32 R. Wallis and S. Bruce, Accounting for action: defending the commonsense heresy, *Sociology*, vol. 17, no. 1, 1982, pp. 97–111; S. Bruce and R. Wallis, Rescuing motives, *British Journal of Sociology*, vol. 34, no. 1, 1983, pp. 61–71.

33 J. Gabe and S. Lipshitz-Phillips, *op. cit.*, 1982, p. 205.

34 M. Lader, Spectres of tolerance and dependence, *MIMS Magazine*, 15 August, 1979, pp. 31–5; P. Tyrer, D. Rutherford, and T. Huggett, Benzodiazepine withdrawal symptoms and propranolol, *The Lancet*, vol. 1, 1981, pp. 520–2.

35 Hooked on the happy pill, *Daily Mirror* (London), 18 March 1980; Why the happy pills have had their day, *Standard* (London), 16 October 1981.

36 T.V. Eye, Thames Television, 21 February 1980; Taking the Strain, BBC2, 7 July 1981.

37 J. Murray, *op. cit.*, pp. 855–6 noted that over half the sample of current and past users of psychotropic drugs also felt that these drugs had had undesired side-effects. Similar complaints were made by a fifth of the sample interviewed by C. Helman, *op. cit.*, p. 525.

38 W. Sharrock, Portraying the professional relationship, in D.C. Anderson (ed.), *Health Education in Practice*, Croom Helm, London, 1979.

39 G. Stimson and B. Webb, *Going to See the Doctor*, Routledge & Kegan Paul, London, 1975, p. 90; B. Webb and G. Stimson, People's accounts of medical encounters, in M. Wadsworth and D. Robinson (eds), *Studies in Everyday Medical Life*, Martin Robertson, London, 1976.

40 Although not mentioned earlier, the women we interviewed told us atrocity stories too. However, those stories were rarely about their current GP.

41 The notion of the deferential dialectic is borrowed from Bell and Newby who used it in a different context: namely, to describe the relationship between husbands and wives. See C. Bell and H. Newby, Husbands and wives: dynamics of deferential dialectic, in D. Barker and S. Allen (eds), *Dependence and Exploitation in Work and Marriage*, Longman, London, 1976.

42 E. Freidson, *Professional Dominance, the Social Structure of Medical Care*, Atherton Press, New York, 1970; M. Bloor and G. Horobin, Conflict and conflict resolution in doctor/patient interactions, in C. Cox and A. Mead, *A Sociology of Medical Practice*, Collier Macmillan, London, 1975; M. Bloor, Professional autonomy and client exclusion: a study in ENT clinics, in M. Wadsworth and D. Robinson (eds), *op. cit.*; P. West, The physician and the management of childhood epilepsy, in M. Wadsworth and D. Robinson (eds), *op. cit.*

43 T. Parsons, *op. cit.*, p. 464; R. Wilson, Patient-practitioner relationships, in H. Freeman *et al.* (eds), *Handbook of Medical Sociology*, Prentice Hall, Englewood Cliffs, N.J., 1963.

44 Our willingness to resurrect the notion of reciprocity indicates that we agree with Frankenberg that Parson's concepts should not be dismissed as useless simply because he 'failed to see the classes for the roles'. See R. Frankenberg, Functionalism and after? Theory and developments in social science applied to the health field, *International Journal of Health Services*, vol. 4, no. 3, 1974, pp. 411–27.

45 M. Jefferys, Social science and medical education in Britain: a sociologic analysis of their relationship, *International Journal of Health Services*, vol. 4, no. 3, 1974, pp. 549–63.

46 M. Stacey, with H. Homans, The sociology of health and illness: its present state, future prospects and potential for health research, *Sociology*, vol. 12, no. 2, 1978, pp. 281–307. At the same time they note the paradox that increasing faith in medicine has been paralleled by growing scepticism about its capacity as costs for professional services, pharmaceuticals, and apparatus soar.

47 P.M. Strong, Materialism and medical interaction: a critique of medicine, superstructure and micropolitics, *Social Science and Medicine*, vol. 13A, no. 6, 1979, pp. 613–19.

48 P.M. Strong, Sociological imperialism and the profession of medicine, *Social Science and Medicine*, vol. 13A, no. 2, 1979, pp. 199–215.

49 For a useful discussion of variations in ideological consistency see C.A. Rootes, The dominant ideology and its critics, *Sociology*, vol. 15, no. 3, 1981, pp. 436–44.

50 D. Wrong, The oversocialized concept of man, *American Sociological Review*, vol. 26, no. 2, 1961, pp. 183–93.

51 M. Balint, *op. cit.*

52 E. Goffman, The interaction order, *American Sociological Review*, vol. 48, no. 1, 1983, pp. 1–17.

53 That radicals using the concept of social control should be linked with functionalists might seem surprising to some. We are not the first to make such a link, however. See, for example, a discussion of the parallels between certain Marxist arguments and functionalist methods of explanation in N. Abercrombie, *Class, Structure and Knowledge*, Basil Blackwell, Oxford, 1980,

pp. 28–32. See also A. Giddens, *Central Problems in Social Theory*, Macmillan, London, 1979, pp. 111–12.

54 P. Cohen, *Modern Social Theory*, Heinemann, London, 1968, pp. 47–51; A. Giddens, *Studies in Social and Political Theory*, Hutchinson, London, 1977, pp. 109–12; A. Giddens, *op. cit.*, 1979, pp. 113–15; W. Skidmore, *Theoretical Thinking in Sociology*, Second Edition, Cambridge University Press, Cambridge, 1979, pp. 174–5.

## PART 6

Future trends in research on tranquilliser use

20

A personal view

Jonathan Gabe and Paul Williams

The papers in this collection demonstrate how research into tranquilliser use has developed in recent years, and illustrate how our understanding of the phenomenon has advanced. While much of this work has been important and instrumental in developing a social view of tranquilliser use, it is clear that the usual cliché 'more research is needed' applies here.

In this chapter, we shall make specific proposals for future work, and in so doing we draw on the comprehensive review by Cooperstock and Parnell (1982) and the survey of expert opinion on this topic conducted by Pole, Albrecht, and Williams (1984). Our proposals follow the structure of this book, namely long-term use, factors influencing use, alternatives to use, and the meaning of tranquilliser use. We shall discuss these four aspects in turn, after having drawn attention to the need for further work on problems of definition and nomenclature. It should be noted that no specific recommendations will be made for pharmacological research.

Definition and nomenclature

As Edwards, Arif, and Hodgson (1981) observe in their introduction to the WHO memorandum on the nomenclature and classification of drug- and alcohol-related problems, advances in definition and nomenclature 'facilitate not only epidemiological research and analysis, but also a greater understanding of disease aetiology, and improved management and decision-making in the health care system'. Definitions and nomenclature are especially problematic in the field of psychotropic drug use, where differing concepts may render comparison between studies difficult or of doubtful validity.

Pole, Albrecht, and Williams (1984) presented a set of twenty-four clinical terms/concepts relevant to research on benzodiazepine use, together with suggested definitions, to a panel of professionals selected because of their detailed knowledge of this area. While there was, in general, more concordance than might have been expected, disagreement was especially noted with regard to the definition of terms and concepts related to long-term use.

The classification of drugs also presents a problem, as is apparent from the papers presented in this book, as well as from a wider reading of the literature (Cooperstock and Parnell 1982). In general, taxonomic systems are developed by groups of researchers for their own purposes and to suit their own needs. Thus, laboratory scientists and clinicians have each generated their respective sets of definitions and classifications, but social scientists have yet to do so. We suggest that consideration be given to this issue. If such a 'social classification' is found to be necessary, it should be developed in consultation with workers from other disciplines so that the pharmacological, clinical, and social dimensions can be brought together in an attempt to devise a 'common language'.

Long-term use

A necessary prerequisite for research into long-term tranquilliser use is the development of a consensus about the interpretation of 'long term'. One approach is merely to seek a common view as to how long is 'long'; an alternative, more realistic approach is to regard the duration of use as a process rather than as a static criterion (Williams, this volume). Whichever of these two approaches to the duration of use is adopted, the material presented in this book makes it clear that an exclusively medical framework is inappropriate, and that a social framework is also required.

A start has already been made, in that sex and age differences in long-term use have been acknowledged for many years. However, as recognized by Cooperstock and Parnell (1982), this social mapping needs to be extended. Systematic studies are required to investigate the relationship between long-term use and social characteristics such as class, race, and marital status. These investigations can provide a background for a fuller social understanding of long-term tranquilliser use. Categories of long-term user, identified by social mapping, could be used as a basis for studying the 'career' of long-term users. Following Goffman (1961), the term 'career' is used in a broad sense to mean 'any social strand of a person's course through life'. Thus, in the present context, we would be concerned with the process of taking on and relinquishing the status of long-term user, and how this is related to the distribution and experience of various material and socio-cultural resources (Gabe and Thorogood, this volume). Consideration might also be given to the influence of networks of tranquilliser users (for example, among families and friends) and illicit markets for these drugs.

The long-term consequences of tranquilliser (especially benzodiazepine) use are as yet insufficiently understood. As described earlier in this book, it is now generally agreed that physical dependence on benzodiazepine tranquillisers can occur, but the precise characteristics of the syndrome, and the extent to which it occurs, require further study. To investigate the *characteristics* of the phenomenon, adequately controlled studies are essential, and greater attention should be paid to pre-treatment measurement of symptoms.

With regard to the *extent* of dependence on tranquillisers, further studies on representative samples are required. To date, most research has been conducted on samples which have been self-selected or referred to specialist psychiatric facilities. While this strategy is important for clinical description, data collected in this way cannot be used for statements about the extent or the broader social consequences of tranquilliser dependence.

These remarks so far apply primarily to physical dependence since, perhaps understandably, the literature on long-term adverse consequences of tranquillisers has been focused largely on this phenomenon, primarily as seen from a medical point of view. In our view, it is necesary to broaden the approach.

In particular, there is a pressing need for an enquiry into the long-term consequences of tranquilliser use that is broad-ranging, and which gives primacy to the point of view of the user. Banks *et al.* (1975), in the context of minor psychiatric illness, have drawn attention to the distinction, and indeed the contrast, between 'morbidity as diagnosed' (i.e. as seen through the eyes of doctors) and 'morbidity as experienced' (i.e. as seen through the eyes of the patient). Such a distinction is also important here.

Focusing on the experience of the long-term user directs attention towards considering the extent to which users regard themselves as being 'ill', 'morally culpable', or personally weak. Such self-definitions need to be seen within the context of the users' immediate and broader social networks.

In addition, the effects of long-term tranquilliser use on personal relationships need to be studied. To our knowledge, this is a very definite gap in the literature and, in particular, research effort could usefully be directed to exploring the extent to which long-term use affects social interaction within the family.

The broader social consequences of long-term tranquilliser use also need to be considered. For example, although much research has been done to investigate the effects of tranquillisers on concentration and skilled performance in laboratory and other artificial settings, relatively little is yet known about their contribution to events such as road accidents, and accidents at home and in industrial environments. Attention might be given, too, to the way in which tranquillisers may also be used as a form of social control in various institutional settings.

In the investigation of the consequences of long-term tranquilliser use, it may be valuable to adopt an economic approach – that is, an approach in which outcomes (consequences of long-term use) are first *listed* and then *valued* so that costs and benefits can be compared (see Drummond 1980 for a basic introduction to the cost–benefit approach). Values can be derived from different groups – patients, doctors, and others (see Holland 1985 for an account of quantitative methods of valuing outcomes). However, it should be borne in mind that values, which are closely related to attitudes, may be ambiguous and context-dependent (Gabe and Lipshitz-Phillips, this volume). Furthermore, the relationship between values/attitudes on the one hand, and behaviour on the other, is not always clear.

None the less, Pole, Albrecht, and Williams (1984) found that the attitudes of doctor and patient to tranquillisers were regarded as being among the most important issues for further research into long-term use. It may well be that a comparison of the value systems held by these various groups will throw light on why drugs continue to be prescribed and consumed in the absence of 'objective' indications for their use.

The prevention of unnecessary long-term tranquilliser use also requires further research effort. Apart from clarifying how 'necessary' and 'unnecessary' use is to be conceptualized, it is to be hoped that much of the work proposed above will help this process. Foremost among the questions that need to be considered is that of how to influence doctors' prescribing behaviour. Two proposals may be made. First, the effects of the limited list legislation on tranquilliser prescribing in general, and on the evolution of long-term use in particular, should be carefully studied. Second, further work on the effects of prescribing audit and feedback is required. There is now much evidence to show that the prescribing – and hence long-term use – of tranquillisers and other drugs is reduced as a response to providing doctors with information about their own level and pattern of prescribing (Harris *et al.* 1984). There is also evidence that the effect of such feedback is short lived (Harris *et al.* 1985); that is, when feedback is discontinued, prescribing returns to the pre-feedback level and pattern. As these authors observed:

'it seems as though doctors' prescribing habits are in a state of dynamic equilibrium, which is disturbed only when some strong new force is introduced ... the rapidity of the reversal (of the effects of feedback of information) is an indication of the power of whatever forces are counteracting them. To support more lasting changes in the way doctors prescribe it looks as though a more sustained intervention is required.'

We recommend that effort be directed towards identifying, characterizing, and testing such interventions.

Factors influencing tranquilliser use

Here we are primarily concerned with factors influencing the *initiation* of tranquilliser use. Although the most appropriate methodology for studying this issue is a longitudinal strategy, most of the studies to date have been cross-sectional surveys. We would argue that more of these studies, unless designed to test specific hypotheses, are unlikely to further our knowledge and understanding. Longitudinal studies are, in theory, to be recommended but, with the recent changes in prescribing patterns and the limited list legislation, samples of new users are proving difficult to obtain. In terms of epidemiological method, the situation is now similar to that of the investigator who wishes to study the aetiology of an uncommon disorder. Thus it may well be worth exploring whether case-control methodology (Schlesselman 1982) can be used to throw further light on factors influencing tranquilliser use.

In addition, there is a need for small-scale naturalistic studies of the consultation process, building on the work of Raynes (1978, 1979, 1980, and this volume). Such studies would focus on decision-making styles and the way in which these differ according to the social category of patient. Behaviour during the consultation, analysed in this way, could usefully be compared with interview data from doctors and patients concerning their attitudes towards prescribing and emotional problems. The relevance of the study of attitudes in this context is underlined by the findings of Pole, Albrecht, and Williams' (1984) survey of informed opinion, in which the 'attitude of prescribing physician towards tranquillisers' was regarded as the single most important influence on the extent of therapeutic use of tranquillisers. Patients' attitudes were also rated as an important topic for study.

These proposed studies are primarily concerned with the micro level. At the macro level, two influences on tranquilliser use need further consideration. First, the effects of medical education require study. Three aspects of the recent changes in medical education are relevant to the prescription of tranquillisers and other drugs. These are the increasing extent and clinical orientation of undergraduate pharmacology teaching, the development of social science courses within the undergraduate medical curriculum, and the expansion of postgraduate general practice vocational training. Second, further work on advertising should be undertaken in order to monitor shifts in content and style, and their effects on prescribing habits.

Alternatives to tranquilliser use

In recent years there has been a marked expansion in specialist attachment to general practice. In our Introduction to Part 4, we give a brief account of the involvement in primary care of social workers, clinical psychologists, counsellors, and others. This trend in the development of primary medical care, while having broader applications and implications, is of relevance to tranquilliser use. While there are as yet relatively few evaluative studies of these new approaches to the organization of services, such work as there is suggests that the attachment of such workers is usually associated with a reduction in tranquilliser prescribing. However, these studies have not always been adequately controlled and the follow-up period has sometimes been too short.

We suggest that further and larger scale evaluative studies could usefully focus on the extent to which the attachment of social workers, clinical psychologists, psychiatrists, counsellors, and others can provide patients with alternatives to tranquillisers. Such studies should be adequately controlled and the inclusion of a cost–benefit dimension is highly desirable.

As indicated earlier, it is not only professionals who can provide alternatives to tranquilliser use: consumers and ex-consumers of these drugs, organized in the form of self-help groups, are increasingly playing an important role. In her paper in this volume, Ettorre makes suggestions for future research in this area, including the proposal that the consequences of self-help groups' management of tranquilliser withdrawal be compared with that of general practitioner management.

However, it should be borne in mind that self-help groups, like many other forms of health care, are likely to appeal to and be utilized more by members of certain social categories than by members of others. For example, women are more likely than men to attend such groups, as are middle-class than working-class users. Attempts should therefore be made to develop self-help approaches which are acceptable to as broad a cross-section of users as possible.

The meaning of tranquilliser use

The study of meaning provides a new perspective on the use of tranquillisers: the work presented in Part 5 of this volume illustrates the initial development of this area. To our knowledge, Ruth Cooperstock was the first social scientist to recognize the importance of studying the ways in which tranquilliser users explain their own experiences and actions. Her recent untimely death has deprived the research community of a greatly valued member.

Building on her work as well as that of others, we would propose the following provisional research agenda. The processes by which people come to define themselves as 'anxious', and their explanations for it, need further exploration. Related to this, attention could usefully be given to examining people's ideas about the role of tranquillisers in treating 'anxiety' and how these compare with notions of drugs and illness in general.

The process of becoming a tranquilliser user –whether short-term or long-term – is an issue of considerable importance. Besides focusing on the role of doctors (in hospitals as well as in general practice), research effort could be directed to exploring the influence exerted by significant others in the home, the workplace, and elsewhere.

Finally, the study of the symbolic meaning of tranquillisers should be taken further by developing the work of Helman (this volume). Such work could pay particular attention to the way in which meanings vary according to social group.

Conclusion

The majority of the studies included in this book or referred to in the editorial material were conducted in North America or western Europe. We would hope that, in the future, more effective communication could be developed between workers in these countries and those in other areas, such as the Third World and eastern Europe. Such communication could encourage the study and understanding of tranquilliser use within a broader political and economic context.

References

Banks, M.H., Beresford, S.A., Morrell, D.C., Waller, J.J., and Watkins, C.J. (1975) Factors influencing demand for primary medical care in women aged 20–44 years: a preliminary report. *International Journal of Epidemiology* **4**(3):189–95.

Cooperstock, R. and Parnell, P. (1982) Research on psychotropic drugs: a review of findings and methods. *Social Science and Medicine* **16** (12):1179–196.

Drummond, M. (1980) *Principles of Economic Appraisal in Health Care.* Oxford: Oxford University Press.

Edwards, G., Arif, A., and Hodgson, R. (1981) Nomenclature and classification of drug- and alcohol-related problems: a WHO memorandum. *Bulletin of the World Health Organisation* **59**:225–42.

Goffman, E. (1961)*Asylums: Essays on the Social Situation of Mental Patients and Other Inmates.* Garden City, New York: Doubleday.

Harris, C., Fry, J., Jarman, B., and Woodman, E. (1985) Prescribing – a case for prolonged treatment. *Journal of the Royal College of General Practitioners* **35**(275):284–87.

Harris, C., Jarman, B., Woodman, E., White, P., and Fry, J. (1984) Prescribing – a suitable case for treatment. *Journal of the Royal College of General Practitioners* Occasional paper no. 24.

Holland, G. (1985) *Techniques of Health Status Measurement Using a Health Index*. London: Office of Health Economics.

Pole, D., Albrecht, H., and Williams, P. (1984) *Benzodiazepine Use: Opinions to Guide Further Research*. Basle: HealthEcon.

Raynes, N. (1978) General practice consultation study: some preliminary observations. *Social Science and Medicine* **12**(4):311–15.

Raynes, N. (1979) Factors affecting the prescribing of psychotropic drugs in general practice consultations. *Psychological Medicine* **9**(4):671–79.

Raynes, N. (1980) What can I do for you? In R. Mapes (ed.) *Prescribing Practice and Drug Usage*. London: Croom Helm.

Schlesselman, J.J. (1982) *Casecontrol Studies: Design, Conduct, Analysis*. New York: Oxford University Press.

© *1986 Jonathan Gabe and Paul Williams*

Name index

Subject index

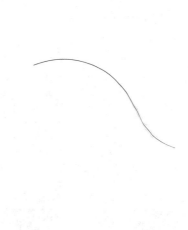